The Science
of SKINNY
Cookbook

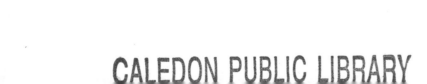

Also by Dee McCaffrey

The Science of Skinny

The Science
of SKINNY
Cookbook

**175 Healthy Recipes to Help You Stop Dieting—
and Eat for Life!**

DEE McCAFFREY, CDC

Da Capo
LIFE
LONG

DA CAPO LIFELONG
A Member of the Perseus Books Group

Designed by Linda Mark
Set in 12 point Adobe Jenson Pro by the Perseus Books
Group

Library of Congress Cataloging-in-Publication Data

McCaffrey, Dee.
  The science of skinny cookbook : 175 healthy recipes to
help you stop dieting—and eat for life! / Dee McCaffrey,
CDC.—First Da Capo Press edition.
     p. cm.
  Includes bibliographical references and index.
  ISBN 978-0-7382-1720-8 (paperback)—ISBN 978-
0-7382-1721-5 (e-book) 1. Reducing diets—Recipes.
2. Weight loss. I. Title.

  RM222.2.M4326 2014
  641.5'63—dc23
                         2014031656

First Da Capo Press edition 2014
Published by Da Capo Press
A Member of the Perseus Books Group
www.dacapopress.com

Da Capo Press books are available at special discounts for
bulk purchases in the U.S. by corporations, institutions,
and other organizations. For more information, please
contact the Special Markets Department at the Perseus
Books Group, 2300 Chestnut Street, Suite 200,
Philadelphia, PA, 19103, or call (800) 810-4145, ext.
5000, or e-mail special.markets@perseusbooks.com.

10 9 8 7 6 5 4 3 2 1

For my mother and truest friend, Carol,
who taught me how to turn a simple meal into a pleasurable feast

Contents

CHAPTER 14

Sweet Indulgences   251

Introduction

To be healthy, we need to prepare our own food, for ourselves and our families. This doesn't mean you have to spend hours in the kitchen, but you do need to spend some time there, preparing food with wisdom and love.

—SALLY FALLON, author of *Nourishing Traditions*

First of all: I love good food and I love to cook. When I sat down to write this cookbook, I knew that I wanted it to be something special—something more than just a collection of healthy recipes. I wanted it to be just as enlightening and educational as my previous book, *The Science of Skinny,* but with a fresh emphasis on the foods and cooking techniques that helped me lose 100 pounds and keep the weight off for over twenty years. My hope is that the information and recipes in this cookbook will inspire you into the kitchen to create something more than just today's breakfast or tomorrow's dinner. I want it to be your foundation for a natural *way of eating for life* that nourishes you in many ways.

While "skinny" figures prominently in the title and throughout (I'll explain more about that in the next chapter), this book is not only for those who want to shed pounds. Its message and the accompanying recipes are meant for anyone seeking to eat good food and improve their health. From my unique perspective as a chemist, nutritionist, and former obese person, I am on a personal mission to transform the way our nation approaches food, eating, and weight loss. One life at a time, one bite at a time, I teach people the importance of eating foods in their closest-to-natural form and how to shop for and prepare these foods for themselves and their families. My task, as I see it, is to help people understand and ultimately come to respect the important and powerful relationship between what we eat and how we feel, and to help them reclaim the innate connection we all inherently have with whole natural foods. This connection is what we ultimately need to feel in order to be inspired to make the nourishing food choices that bring about balanced health. Learning to value the quality of your food essentially means learning to value yourself—a more important factor in weight loss and improving your health than anything else.

I was once obese, so it should be no surprise that health has not always been my priority when it comes to food. However, spending time in the kitchen preparing meals for myself and others has always been important to me.

I am a home cook—the kind of cook who can look into the refrigerator or freezer, pull out an assortment of whatever is in there, and whip up a fairly tasty dish. No recipe required. Some may say that's a talent, but I prefer to think of it as a learned survival skill.

Money and food were not abundant when I was growing up, and we often had to make meals from just a few simple ingredients. Some of my recipes reflect that, while others show a more mature culinary purpose gleaned from my training as a nutrition educator, combining ingredients with both taste and optimal health in mind.

In addition to preparing processed-free meals for myself and my family, today I teach healthy cooking to large audiences and small groups around the country. For several years I've been the key presenter for the Culinary World at the annual American Diabetes Association Expo. For a time I offered my services as a private cook for individuals and families, and my husband and I ran our own organic meal delivery business called Dee's Healthy Gourmet, for which I was in charge of recipe creation, menu planning, and running the kitchen. All of this experience has afforded me the opportunity to create recipes with many different needs and preferences in mind. As many current eating styles fall under the umbrella of the "processed-free" philosophy introduced in my previous book, *The Science of Skinny*, you will find an eclectic variety of information, cooking techniques, and recipes that appeal to many different palates, from gluten-free, grain-free, and dairy-free to clean eating, diabetic-friendly, vegetarian, Paleo, and others.

You will also notice a general theme among the recipes: If you have the time and inclination, make your own. Staple items such as nut milks, broths, breads, condiments, sauces, salad dressings, snacks, and desserts are the types of foods and ingredients that may be hard to find in a processed-free form, even in natural food markets. If you are ready to try your hand at making your staples, the recipes await you.

For the most part, preparing processed-free food is not complicated nor does it take any more time than any other home cooking. After all, mixing and bake time are pretty much the same whether you're making peanut butter cookies with white flour, sugar, and vegetable shortenig, or you're making my recipe for Grain-Free Nutty Peanut Butter Cookies (page 252) using just peanut butter, egg, vanilla extract, and baking soda.

Whether you are a seasoned follower of *The Science of Skinny* or a newcomer to its tenets, *The Science of Skinny Cookbook* will provide you with a wealth of scrumptious recipes and new ideas for an eclectic repertoire of nourishing meals and snacks. The next chapter gives you a basic *Science of Skinny* overview. In following chapters, I'll introduce some of the scientifically proven skinny superfoods and ingredients and the basic cooking techniques, followed by the recipes themselves. At the end of the book, I've included a comprehensive Resources section (page 273) to help you find trusted brands of food products and cooking tools, as well as a list of helpful websites to support you in your transition to processed-free living.

Thank you for inviting me into your kitchen. I hope you enjoy preparing these recipes as much as I've enjoyed creating them!

Best of Health,
Dee McCaffrey

The Science:
Foods That Steal,
Foods That Heal

The food you eat can either be the safest and most powerful form
of medicine or the slowest form of poison.

—Ann Wigmore, author of *Why Suffer?*
How I Overcame Illness & Pain Naturally

ncient societies and our not-so-distant ancestors
(our great-grandparents) were intimately connected with their
food. They knew how to grow it, how to prepare it in order
to retain its valuable nutrients, and how to harness its health re-
storative properties. Many of our common foods, herbs, and spices
have long been considered sacred because they provide immediate
therapeutic benefits. Foods such as cacao (from which all chocolate
derives), quinoa, vanilla beans, purple potatoes, and even sugarcane
have recognized value that goes far beyond their taste. Modern science has now accumulated an abundant harvest of research proving
what the ancients knew all along—*food* is our best medicine. Nearly

every common plant food, and many animal foods, offer one or more therapeutic benefits—from alleviating everyday aches and pains to providing powerful protection against cancer, heart disease, diabetes, obesity, and many other chronic diseases.

But since the introduction of processed convenience foods, much of the traditional food wisdom has been lost along with the reverence for the very thing that sustains us. Within the last hundred years, we have gone from growing, harvesting, and preparing our own food with our own hands to consuming large quantities of mass-produced concoctions that are made in food laboratories. As a result, the Standard American Diet—appropriately acronymed SAD—is the worst diet humans have ever eaten. The consumption of nutrient-deficient, chemical-laden "foodstuffs" has created a rapid health crisis unlike anything seen in the annals of history.

Although the trend toward home and community gardening is resurging, far too many of us have no idea where our food comes from. We don't grow our own produce, and we don't know or care how our meat and dairy animals are raised (or tortured, depending on their source). Because of this disconnect, we have unwittingly allowed processed foods to become a dominant force in our culture and many of us have lost an important life skill—the ability to select, prepare, and cook real whole foods.

My ongoing passion, both personally and professionally, has been to cast new light on that age-old wisdom: Eating foods in their closest-to-natural form is the true path to sustained weight loss, and in fact the remedy for almost any health problem. I know this because I am living proof and because I have witnessed the remarkable health transformations many others have experienced simply by changing the types of foods they eat.

An Eye-Opening Box of Cake Mix

From the age of nine, and over the next twenty years, I was a compulsive eater who repeatedly failed at diets, yo-yoing my way into seemingly permanent obesity. By age thirty, I was carrying 210 pounds on my 4'10" petite body frame—that's nearly twice the normal weight for someone my height.

During that time, I was working my way through college at an environmental testing laboratory. (I was a late bloomer for college, not seriously starting on my chemistry degree until I was twenty-six.) Like most people, I had nary an inkling that the chemicals I used in my laboratory had any connection to the food on my plate. One evening that all changed when I was at home whipping up one of my favorite (and very frequent) indulgences at the time: deluxe angel food cake mix. You know the one—the highly processed convenient kind that lets baking novices turn out a perfect cake by just adding water to the mix.

Back then, reading food ingredient lists was not a common practice for me, or anyone for that matter, but for whatever reason, my eyes were drawn to the side of the box that evening. As I read through the list, skimming past the sugar and flour, my eyes fell upon three words I never expected to see in my food: *sodium lauryl sulfate*. I did a double take. *Sodium lauryl sulfate? Isn't that the detergent-like chemical I use to test for water pollutants?* Yes, it is. It is also used in cosmetics, shampoos, laundry detergents, and cleaning products. In high concentrations it's used in garage floor cleaners. And it's used as a whipping aid for powdered egg whites, so it's in every bite of many cakes made from boxed mixes.

That revelation did not sit well with me. As someone who had continually struggled with my weight, I was forced to question what effect sodium lauryl sulfate was having on my body. Could it, and perhaps other chemical food additives, be a contributing factor to my seemingly endless hunger and obesity? Twenty years ago, the answers to those questions were not easy to find. All I had to go on was my chemist instinct, and that instinct told me it couldn't be good.

The combination of the discovery of chemicals in my food and a strong desire to break free from the lifelong struggle with emotional eating and obesity was a perfect storm that shifted something inside me. From that point forward, I steadfastly removed processed foods from my life and replaced them with the real foods our bodies are designed to eat. Within thirteen months, I lost 100 pounds and gained a ton of health.

In the years that followed, I channeled my passions for food and health into a second career, returning to the classroom in 2000 to formally study nutrition at Bauman College. My chemistry background became extremely valuable in helping me to understand not only the inherent chemical nature of food itself, but also the many aspects of how foods and food additives interact with the body to create health or disease.

My experience and studies taught me a very important truth—in order to lose weight and gain health, we need do nothing more than approach eating as intelligently as the foods themselves have been designed by nature. Understanding how to properly care for and feed ourselves is one of our most important human responsibilities.

"Skinny" Is Not about a Diet

Webster's dictionary defines *skinny* as "lean or thin." Our current culture has adopted a more shallow definition, equating a "skinny" body with a "perfect" or "healthy" body. But this could not be farther from the truth—a large percentage of "lean or thin" people do not have bodies that are in perfect health. According to a 2012 report by the United Nations, up to 40 percent of normal weight (a.k.a. lean or thin) people have serious life-threatening health conditions brought on by a poor diet, such as diabetes, high cholesterol, hypertension, heart disease, cancer, fatty liver disease, and many others.[1] Many other lean or thin people, especially women, endanger their bodies in other ways in pursuit of a "perfect" body.

The attainment of your natural body weight should be part of a plan for overall wellness, so I've elevated the status of the word *skinny* and given it a more appropriate meaning—optimal health. To get and stay "skinny" by my definition means that you mindfully choose and eat the whole natural foods that will nourish your body to function at its best. And when you are optimally healthy, that health will be reflected in a body size that is optimal for you.

Foods That Steal, Foods That Heal

Healthful eating is not just about adding more fruits and vegetables to your plate. It's about respecting how your body is designed. At our core, we're all designed to eat real food. By that, I mean foods that haven't been highly processed, that aren't foreign to our DNA. But what actually constitutes a real food? Is the coconut milk that comes in a carton a real food? What about organic fat-free chicken broth with "No Added MSG" splashed across the packaging? Is organic milk that has been ultra-high temperature pasteurized to give it a long shelf life that doesn't require refrigeration a real food?

The answer is, it's complicated. In today's profit-driven food culture, there are many food "land mines" that we need to be aware of, whether we're shopping in a mainstream grocery store or in a natural food market.

The discovery of sodium lauryl sulfate in my angel food cake mix back in 1989 set me on a path to find out what else is in the foods most Americans eat each day and the effect they have on our health. What I learned blew me away. It changed the course of my life and eventually became the basis for *The Science of Skinny*. In 2007, my husband Michael and I founded Processed-Free America (see Resources, page 283)—a nonprofit organization dedicated to bringing a national awareness of the effect processed foods have on our health and the healing properties of natural whole foods. Our organization provides nutrition education and training to people of all ages and empowers them to take responsibility for their own health.

Our work is very important because the U.S. Food and Drug Administration (FDA) maintains a list of over 3,000 ingredients in its database titled "Everything Added to Food in the United States (EAFUS)." Some of these items are recognizable ingredients such as vinegar, salt, baking soda, and spices, but the majority of them are synthetic chemical concoctions that don't exist in nature. In addition to the thousands of chemicals on the EAFUS list, there are an unbelievable number of pesticides, herbicides, antibiotics, and hormone residues found in our produce, poultry, dairy, meat, and seafood. Many of these chemicals are what we call "anti-nutrients," so named because they inhibit the absorption of nutrients from foods, or they leach stored nutrients from our body, resulting in nutrient deficiencies. Some food additives have been linked to unforeseen and powerful chemical reactions in the body and the brain, leading to food addiction, chronic inflammation, weight gain, diabetes, heart disease, Parkinson's, Alzheimer's, cancer, and many other serious diseases.

To help you become a more confident and in-the-know food shopper, here's the lowdown on some of the most egregious foods that "steal":

REFINED SUGAR—You already know that white sugar is the bane of good health and weight loss. There's just no place for it in a processed-free lifestyle. The problem is that it's in practically every pre-prepared food. Sugar is added in one form or another to everything from bread, cereals, soups, ketchup, beverages, salad dressings, frozen foods, and more—and this also applies to many foods found in natural food markets. Many natural food manufacturers are just as guilty of adding way too much sugar to their products—in their case in the form of "natural" sugars such as agave and evaporated cane sugar. Both of these forms of sugar are very processed and not healthy or natural at all.

Refined forms of sugar are some of the most damaging anti-nutrients in our foods. First, they create an acidic body chemistry that forces the body to pull stored calcium from the bones to neutralize the acid (more on that a little later). This can lead to calcium deficiencies that have been linked to loss of bone density. But that seems to be the least of sugar's ill effects.

According to a group of prominent doctors, nutritionists, and biologists, sugar is a toxin that harms our organs and disrupts the body's usual hormonal cycles. The scientific evidence linking sugar to heart disease, cancer, diabetes, obesity, and fatty liver disease has been accumulating over the past few years. We now also have strong scientific proof that sugar is more addictive than heroin.

I recommend avoiding refined forms of sugar and opting for more natural sweeteners instead—those that provide your body with vitamins, minerals, and phytonutrients.

I've provided a detailed description of some of the best natural sweeteners on the market in chapter 3. However, these don't give license to replacing the same amount of refined sugars with natural forms. You should be seriously cutting down on the amount of all sugar, but when you do occasionally splurge, use a sweetener that provides your body with nutrients, rather than one that steals nutrients from you.

Check ingredient lists and avoid these forms of sugar:

Agave • Barley malt • Beet sugar • Brown sugar • Cane sugar • Cornstarch • Corn syrup • Corn syrup solids • Crystalline fructose • Dextrose • Evaporated cane juice • Evaporated cane sugar • Fructose • Fruit juice concentrates • Glucose • Honey • High-fructose corn syrup • Invert sugar • Maltodextrin • Maltose • Modified food starch • Molasses • Organic cane sugar • Refiner's syrup • Rice syrup • Rice syrup solids • Sorghum syrup • Sucrose • Sugar • Turbinado sugar

REFINED GRAINS (FLOURS AND STARCHES)—Like refined forms of sugar, refined grains like white flour and white rice lack the nutrients our bodies need to digest them. They break down quickly into simple sugars with many of the same ensuing health problems. They stimulate our hunger sensation but don't satisfy us. As a result, even though we fill up our bellies with white bread, rice, and pastas, the rest of our body isn't getting nourished, and even worse, we're being depleted of important nutrients our bodies need.

In addition to vitamins and minerals and other important nutrients, whole grains contain two important fibers—bran and germ—

necessary for their digestion. These health-giving fibers and nutrients are stripped away from grains during their refinement, leading to a substance that is so nutritionally depleted that manufacturers are required by federal law to add certain vitamins back in. That's why we see the word *enriched* on our food labels.

But enrichment does not replace all that is taken away. For example, a whole wheat kernel contains over 100 vitamins, minerals, and phytonutrients, in addition to essential oils, fibers, and enzymes, all of which act together, synergistically, to assist our body in digesting the wheat. Because those 100 vitamins, along with the fibers, are missing from white flour products, the body turns to its own bones and tissues in an effort to access the stored nutrients required to digest it.

The most common refined carbohydrates in the Standard American Diet (SAD) are wheat flour (i.e., enriched wheat flour), white rice, white rice flour, and degermed cornmeal. With the rise in the incidence of gluten intolerance (an adverse reaction to the protein portion of wheat, rye, and barley, called gluten), many people have simply switched from eating refined wheat flour products to products made from white rice flour, which doesn't contain gluten but is also refined and lacking nutrients. Eating gluten-free products does not necessarily spare you from the ravages of refined carbohydrates.

CANOLA OIL, PROCESSED COOKING OILS, AND PARTIALLY HYDROGENATED OIL (TRANS FATS)—Fats can be categorized in one of three ways: good, bad,

and ugly. Good fats are naturally occurring plant or animal fats that are unprocessed and vital for our health. Examples of good fats (which may surprise you) are avocados, virgin coconut oil, raw dairy and butter, raw nuts and seeds, olives and olive oil, eggs, fish, and grass-fed beef.

Bad fats are any oils that have been pressed from their sources and refined using heat, or those that have been heated to high temperatures for cooking. Heat changes the molecular structure of oils and renders them very unhealthy—so much so that they damage our cells and our DNA, leading to degenerative disease and cancer. Examples of bad fats (which may also surprise you) are canola oil, soybean oil, sunflower oil, safflower oil, corn oil, cottonseed oil, "vegetable oil," and the fats from animals that have been fed grains and sugars instead of their natural diet of green grass.

Ugly fats are trans fats, otherwise known as partially hydrogenated or fully hydrogenated oils. Trans fats are made through a process called hydrogenation. Hydrogenation turns a liquid oil (usually one of the bad oils) into a fat that is more solid and stable at room temperature. The result is a man-made fat that looks, tastes, and behaves like butter and coconut oil—two fats that have always been healthy but just got a bad rap because of some bad science back in the 1950s. Today, trans fat is out, and healthy forms of saturated fat are taking their rightful place back in the diets of clean eaters everywhere. But read ingredient lists carefully, because hydrogenated oils are still being used in some foods.

GENETICALLY MODIFIED FOODS—If you've ever wondered why so many people suffer from food sensitivities and allergies, it's because our food supply has undergone a recent radical change. In the mid-1990s, new food proteins were engineered and introduced into our food supply, unannounced and untested on humans and animals. These genetically modified organisms (GMOs) have had their genetic code (DNA) altered to give them characteristics they don't have naturally. In an effort to increase production and profits for food manufacturers, scientists artificially insert bacteria, viruses, and other genes into the DNA of common food crops such as corn, soybeans, canola (rapeseed), cottonseed, and sugar beets, which are then used to make over 80 percent of the foods most Americans eat. The genetically engineered growth hormone rBGH (recombinant bovine growth hormone) is used on dairy cows.

Corn, for instance, has been genetically modified to make its own pesticide within the plant itself, so that when an insect eats the corn, it explodes their stomachs and kills them from the inside out. Is that happening to people too? Some experts believe it is. The scary thing is that GMOs have never been tested for human safety, and food manufacturers are not required to inform consumers whether their food products contain GMOs.

These unlabeled genetically modified foods carry a high risk of triggering life-threatening allergic reactions, and evidence collected over the past decade now suggests that they are contributing to higher allergy rates. Milk is the number one food allergen in the United States. Soy and corn allergies rank right be-

hind it. GMOs have been linked to the alarming increases in allergies, attention deficit hyperactivity disorder (ADHD), cancer, asthma, and obesity.

It is estimated that genetically modified ingredients are found in 80 percent of processed foods. That's just one more reason to stop eating processed foods and begin following a "processed-free" lifestyle.

How else can you avoid GMOs? The USDA National Organic Program strictly prohibits the use of GMOs in any food carrying the USDA Organic seal. So if your food carries the organic seal, you know it's not made with GMOs. Also, organic growers and many other food companies are voluntarily labeling their products with a Non-GMO Project seal verifying that their foods do not contain genetically modified ingredients.

The best way to avoid GMOs is to avoid any food that contains ingredients made from the five major GMO crops (also called "at risk" ingredients): soybeans, canola (rapeseed), corn, cottonseed, and sugar made from sugar beets, all of which are typically used in processed foods. Unless these foods are grown organically, a large percentage of them are GMO.

ARTIFICIAL SWEETENERS—Although the FDA has deemed them safe, consumer advocacy groups and many nutrition and health experts beg to differ, claiming research on the safety of artificial sweeteners is flawed and doesn't account for how long-term use of these additives affects our health.

One hard fact that no one can dispute is that the sweet white powders that come packaged in pink, blue, and yellow packets don't exist anywhere in nature. Some of them are made from chemicals that are known to be not only harmful but truly toxic. All of them are wrought with documented negative health effects.

Here's a list of the most dangerous artificial sweeteners:

Saccharin (Sweet'N Low): Since being brought to market, saccharin has faced two bans and for a time it carried a cancer warning on its packaging due to evidence that it caused bladder cancer in laboratory animals. In 2000 saccharin was removed from the list of cancer-causing chemicals, no longer requiring a warning on its label because the evidence for bladder cancer was only seen in rats and not humans. However, in other rodent studies, saccharin has caused cancer of the uterus, ovaries, skin, blood vessels, and other organs. Also, it has been demonstrated that saccharin increases the potency of other cancer-causing chemicals. Despite the removal of the cancer warning, the carcinogenic nature of this man-made sweetener is still highly controversial.

Aspartame (Equal, NutraSweet): Early testing of aspartame was fraught with results showing that it was not safe, particularly that it induced brain tumors in mice. Even though the evidence mounted against the safety of aspartame, its use was approved in 1981.

By 1992, over 10,000 complaints had been filed with the FDA about food reactions pertaining to aspartame. Reported effects of what is now known to be aspartame poisoning include headaches, fibromyalgia, anxiety, memory loss, arthritis, abdominal pain, nausea, depression, heart palpitations, irritable bowel syndrome, seizures, neurological disorders, vision problems, brain tumors, and weight gain.

The Center for Science in the Public Interest (CSPI) places aspartame on its list of food additives to avoid, citing three independent studies conducted by researchers at the Ramazzini Foundation in Bologna, Italy, in 2005, 2007, and 2010 showing that rats and mice exposed to aspartame throughout their lifetime developed lymphomas, leukemias, kidney tumors, and breast, liver, and lung cancers.

Today, derivatives of aspartame are found in products like Neotame, AminoSweet, and the newest kid on the block, Advantame, which gained FDA approval in May 2014.

There are way too many question marks surrounding the safety of aspartame and its spinoff products. I steer clear of all of them, and I'm hoping you will too.

Acesulfame K (Sweet One, Sunette): Acesulfame K is made by combining a compound called acetoacetic acid with potassium (the letter K is the chemical symbol for the element potassium), using methylene chloride, a known carcinogen, as a solvent during the initial manufacturing step. There is concern among health advocates that methylene chloride residues may be present in the final product. Acesulfame K is also on the CSPI's avoid list, citing early studies that showed a potential link between the sweetener and development of multiple cancers in laboratory animals. It may also cause blood sugar attacks and has been shown to elevate cholesterol in laboratory animals. In addition, large doses of acetoacetamide, a breakdown product, have been shown to affect the thyroid in rats, rabbits, and dogs.

Sucralose (Splenda): The manufacturer of Splenda markets its sucralose product as being "natural" because it comes from sugar. The manufacturer is telling only a partial truth. Sucralose is a synthetic compound created by changing the molecular structure of sugar by adding chlorine atoms to it. The final product is a chlorinated compound with a molecular structure more resembling a pesticide than a sugar. In fact, the chemical structure of the chlorine in sucralose is almost the same as that in the now-banned pesticide DDT.

There have been no long-term studies of sucralose's effects on humans, whereas there have been over a hundred studies on animals, many of which revealed the same disturbing problems that are caused by pesticides. Studies on animals have shown that sucralose can cause shrinking of the thymus gland, the gland that is the very foundation of the immune system, and liver and kidney dysfunction.

A 2013 study out of Washington School of Medicine in St. Louis, Missouri, found that Splenda raises blood sugar levels, leading to insulin spikes, weight gain, and increased risk for diabetes—the exact opposite of what it is marketed to prevent.

Obesogens—One of the most recent dangers we are facing is the growing number of chemicals we are exposed to not only in our foods, but also in our food packaging, our cookware, our personal care products, and the environment. Many of these chemicals resemble our own hormones, including the hormones that help to control how many of our calories to burn right away and how many to store as fat for the body's energy needs. Certain compounds have been coined "obesogens" because they interfere with the regulatory system that controls our weight. They do this by several pathways:

- They encourage the body to store fat and reprogram cells to become fat cells.
- They prompt the liver to become insulin resistant, which makes the pancreas pump out more insulin that turns energy into fat all over the body.
- They alter the way your body manages hunger by preventing leptin (a hormone that reduces appetite) from being released from your fat cells to tell your body you are full.

Here are some common obesogens:

High-Fructose Corn Syrup (HFCS): High-fructose corn syrup shows up in many different types of foods, from soup and bread to soda, yogurt, ketchup, and snack foods. HFCS makes your liver insulin resistant and tampers with leptin to increase your hunger, setting up a vicious cycle where you crave more food that is then more easily turned into fat.

Monosodium Glutamate (MSG): This commonly used flavor enhancer triples the amount of insulin the body produces, creating the same problem as high-fructose corn syrup. The obesity effect of MSG is so well established and reproducible that scientists routinely use MSG to purposefully induce obesity in animals to study the effects of obesity and its complications. The weight gain from eating MSG has nothing to do with excess calories and everything to do with the alteration of fat-storing mechanisms. Yet it is legal and "approved" as a safe food additive! MSG is also a known excitotoxin (a chemical substance added to foods that overexcites neurons to the point of brain cell damage, and eventually, brain cell death!). In its various forms, MSG shows up everywhere in our food supply, even though you may never see it listed on an ingredient list. The tricky thing about MSG is that food manufacturers have a loophole that allows them to hide MSG in other food additives with different names, as long as the additive contains less than 79 percent MSG. For example, if a food additive called "seasonings" contains 78 percent MSG by weight, a food manufacturer does not have to list MSG in the ingredients, they only have to list "seasonings." Here are some of the myriad names of other food additives MSG may be hiding in:

• Anything "hydrolyzed" • Autolyzed yeast • Bouillon, stocks, and broths • Calcium caseinate • Gelatin • Hydrolyzed soy protein • Hydrolyzed yeast • Isolated soy protein • Maltodextrin • Natural flavorings • Seasonings • Sodium caseinate • Textured soy protein • Yeast extract

Other Known Obesogens: Bis-phenol A (a.k.a. BPA) is found in certain types of plastics and in the lining of cans used for canned foods, while perfluorooctanoates are found in nonstick cookware and greaseproof coatings, among other places, and in certain pesticides.

The bottom line is, man-made manipulated foods and ingredients don't honor how our body is designed; they are catalysts for poor health because not only do they not offer any health value, but they steal the health we already have. Replacing the foods that steal with the foods that heal, and putting those foods together into beautiful, tasty meals is what *The Science of Skinny Cookbook* is all about. It may sound complicated, but it's really just about staying away from processed foods. When we approach eating as intelligently as the foods themselves have been designed by nature, weight loss and good health become effortless and sustainable.

One of the main tenets of *The Science of Skinny* is this: The amount of vegetables you eat is directly proportional to the amount of weight you will lose and the amount of health you will gain. In the next chapter, I'll cover the foods that "heal"—skinny superfoods and all the great basics and ingredients you'll want to keep on hand to create the recipes, including fruits, nuts and seeds, legumes, beneficial fats and oils, organic animal foods, and herbs and spices. But before that, we need to talk a bit more about the science and how balancing your foods is the key to long-term health.

Alkalize and Liver-ize— Your Key to Optimal Health

The Science of Skinny focuses on two important body systems that lead to weight loss and optimal health—your body chemistry (pH) and the health of your main fat-burning and detoxifying organ (your liver). The foods you eat, the beverages you drink, and other things you ingest or come in contact with all affect your body's pH balance in either a positive (alkaline) way or a negative (acidic) way. Also, if your liver is overwhelmed with food additives, pesticides, medications, and other toxins, it becomes sluggish in its ability to detoxify, and it can't burn fat efficiently, leading to weight gain and other health issues. Eating foods in their closest-to-natural form provides the body with the nutrients needed to balance the body's pH, cleanse the liver of toxins, and easily restore the body to its natural state of health.

The term *pH* refers to the amount of acidity in a water-based medium. Human blood and body fluids are all water-based. Alkalinity basically means the absence of hydrogen, or the opposite of acidity.

The acid/alkaline scale (pH scale) ranges from 0 to 14, with 7 being neutral. A pH less than 7 is acidic; a pH greater than 7 is alkaline. Our bodies are designed to be slightly alkaline, at a pH of 7.4. Like the Richter scale that measures earthquakes, the pH scale is logarithmic, which means that a pH of 6.4 is ten times more acidic than a pH of 7.4, and a pH of 8.4 is ten times more alkaline than a pH of 7.4. Even small changes in pH can cause great damage or great health.

The normal functions of our body create small amounts of acid. For instance, when we exercise, our muscles create lactic acid. Breathing, cell building, and burning calories to fuel the metabolism are also normal functions of the body that create acid.

It is critical that the pH of the blood stays between 7.35 and 7.45, and even slight deviations can result in disease or death. To keep your blood in the ideal range, your body has a number of systems that are adept at neutralizing and eliminating excess acid from your blood. But sometimes that comes at a great cost to your health in other ways.

A healthy body stores adequate amounts of minerals in our bones, muscles, tissues, and teeth that can be drawn upon to neutralize the acidity created by normal body functions. These minerals, called the "alkaline reserve," include calcium, iron, magnesium, manganese, potassium, and sodium. But the minerals in our alkaline reserve are not infinite, and there is a limit to how much acid even a healthy body can cope with effectively. We need to replace these minerals regularly by eating the foods that contain them. To maintain our proper body pH, the majority of our foods should be alkaline forming, and the acid-forming foods should be minimized. Most fruits and vegetables are alkaline forming, whereas meats, grains, most fats, pasteurized dairy products, and all the junk foods—a typical diet for many people—are acid forming. The most acid-forming foods are refined carbohydrates—white sugar and white flour—in addition to sodas (especially diet sodas), artificial sweeteners, alcohol, coffee, and prescription drugs. Eating too many of the acid-forming foods and not enough of the alkaline-forming ones results in excess acidity, which overwhelms the body's alkaline reserve. It's like continuing to draw money out of a dwindling savings account without replacing it.

The alkaline reserve consists mainly of calcium, which is drawn from the bones, tissues, and teeth. When calcium is continually removed from the bones without adequate replacement, you end up with a calcium deficiency. Additionally, when your alkaline reserve becomes chronically low, your body is less able to neutralize additional acid coming in. As a result, other defense mechanisms are employed to protect your blood and organs from getting overly acidic. This may sound like a good thing—that your body is working hard to keep you alive despite your poor diet—but this is how many health problems begin.

To keep excess acid from entering your vital organs, your body inflates your fat cells, or creates new ones, and then quarantines the acid inside them. Storing acid in fat cells leads to weight gain and obesity. Your body then holds on to this fat as a way to continue protecting the organs. Hence, when your body is acidic, you gain weight that is very difficult to lose. Another place your body stores acid is in your muscles. Acidic muscles lead to low energy, muscle cramps, and chronic fatigue syndrome. Your body may also try to expel acid through the skin, causing hot flashes, strong perspiration, psoriasis, and rashes. Acidic body pH is responsible for arthritis, chronic fatigue, heart disease, strokes, gout, high cholesterol, diabetes, cancer, acid reflux, high blood pressure, obesity, and many, many more serious health problems.

To maintain the proper pH, your diet should consist mainly of alkaline-forming foods, which consist of most fruits, all vegetables (especially the dark green leafy types), and a few other foods including almonds, quinoa, virgin coconut oil, stevia, raw sugar cane, and sprouted grains. You also need to eat some healthy acid-forming foods to maintain the right balance of acid to alkaline. Acid-forming foods that are healthy include raw milk and dairy products, unsprouted whole grains, fruits such as blueberries and cranberries, hormone-free and antibiotic-free eggs, meat, poultry, and wild-caught fish. If you need to lose weight and restore your health, the goal for your daily food intake is to eat 80 percent alkaline-forming foods and 20 percent healthy acid-forming foods. Once you've achieved your pH balance, your diet should consist of 60 percent alkaline-forming foods and 40 percent acid-forming foods. The recipes in this cookbook highlight many of the alkaline-forming foods and healthy acid-forming foods, making it easy for you to maintain the right pH balance in your meals.

One important thing to note is this: A food's acid- or alkaline-forming tendency in the body has nothing to do with the actual pH of the food itself. For example, lemons are very acidic outside the body; however, the end products after digestion and assimilation are very alkaline, so lemons are alkaline forming in the body. The same goes for raw apple cider vinegar, which is acidic outside the body but very alkaline forming after digestion. Meat will test alkaline outside the body, before digestion, but it leaves an acidic residue in the body, so, like nearly all animal products, meat is acid forming.

The other body system we need to be mindful of is our liver and its role in keeping us clean and lean. If your liver is healthy, your weight loss will be effortless. The practice of keeping your liver clean is what I call "liver-izing." It simply involves choosing the right foods, beverages, spices, and herbs that specifically scrub, flush, and support the liver. These foods contain strong antioxidants that our liver needs to break down toxins so they can be safely flushed from the body. Liver-izing foods include dark green leafy vegetables, cruciferous vegetables (broccoli, Brussels sprouts, cabbage, and cauliflower), lemons, garlic, onions, eggs, red peppers, asparagus, avocados, walnuts, apples, oats, beets, carrots, brown rice, turmeric, milk thistle, and dandelion root. Many of these foods are also alkaline forming, so as you can see, when you build your meals around these important foods, you get skinny! You'll see all of these foods playing a starring role in a tasty way throughout many of the recipes I've included in this cookbook.

If all this talk about pH and liver-izing makes you think you're going to have to embark upon a strict diet plan without ever enjoying a dessert or treat again, stick with me—that's where "The Skinny" comes in! All you have to do is eat more liver-izing and alkaline-forming foods than you do acid-forming foods, and you are on your way to long-term health. It really is that simple.

Healthy Ingredients for Life

The next chapter helps you embark on a balanced and cleansing way of eating, one that's not based on restriction but is sustainable, satiating, and delicious. As you begin to eat foods in their more natural form, you'll be trying new foods and familiarizing yourself with new ingredients and products. You'll notice a reduction in cravings, those foods that steal will be a thing of the past, and you'll feel more energized and healthier overall.

The Skinny: Processed-Free Superfoods and Ingredients

Now that we've explored the science, it's time to turn to the grocery store and the kitchen to discuss the basic ingredients and tips to help you put the science into practice and reclaim your health.

Skinny Superfoods and Special Ingredients

Most of the vegetables, fruits, common whole grains, legumes, nuts, seeds, and other staple items used in these recipes can be found at your local farmers' market or supermarket, while other items, such as natural sweeteners, uncommon whole grains, sprouted flours and breads, and hormone-free meats and poultry may require a trip to the natural food market. If your natural food market does not carry a particular item that you want to try, ask if they can special order it for you.

If you live in an area where some of these ingredients are hard to find, consider ordering them online. (The Resources section on pages 273–283 lists several online natural food retailers.)

Key Vegetables

Asparagus: Known for its use in the treatment of arthritis and rheumatism, as well as for its cancer-fighting abilities, asparagus also contains high concentrations of the liver-cleansing compound glutathione and an amino acid called asparagine. These compounds quickly alkalize and cleanse the body, which excretes high amounts of toxins and asparagine's distinct odorous residue in the urine. For this reason, it was once thought that asparagus itself was toxic, but we now know that when the urine smells funny, it means the vegetable is doing its job well!

Beets and Beet Greens: Beets belong to the same family as chard and spinach. However, unlike those greens, both the root and the leaves of beets can be eaten. The beetroot, commonly just called the beet, has long been known for its healing effects on the liver. Beets protect the liver by breaking down fat deposits in the liver that are often associated with diabetes, high blood pressure, and alcohol consumption. The phytonutrients and high fiber in beets also are powerful cancer-fighting agents (especially against colon cancer) and can help protect against heart disease and birth defects.

Parsley: This vegetable is one of the highest alkalizing foods (whether raw or dried) and has many valuable health protective properties that are often ignored in its popular role as a plate garnish.

Sweet Potatoes: The sweet potato is not a member of the potato family and has quite different nutritional qualities than both the yam and the common spud. There is often much confusion between sweet potatoes and yams; the larger, moist-fleshed, orange-colored variety that is often called a yam is actually a sweet potato. Sweet potatoes contain a high content of vitamin C and beta-carotene, along with unique proteins that work synergistically to increase antioxidants in the body.

Cruciferous Vegetables: Eating cruciferous vegetables not only helps you alkalize and liver-ize, but these are some of the most powerful cancer-fighting foods. This special family of vegetables consists of bok choy, broccoli, Brussels sprouts, cabbages, cauliflower, collards, kale, mustard greens, radishes, rutabagas, and turnips. These vegetables contain multiple nutrients and phytonutrients that are essential in helping you burn fat—especially the dreaded belly fat associated with a sluggish liver.

Carrots and Pumpkin: Eating these two bright orange foods is an easy and natural way to cleanse the liver. Their most important component, beta-carotene, which the body converts to vitamin A, is a powerful healing antioxidant that improves the overall tissue health within the liver, as well as detoxifies it. Both vegetables have also been shown to protect against heart disease and cancer.

Garlic and Onions: Although they are strong on the breath, these veggies are packed with a unique combination of cancer-fighting antioxidants and sulfur compounds that give them their distinct odors—namely allicin, alliin, and others. These, along with vitamin C, vitamin B6, and the antioxidant mineral selenium in garlic, have the ability to activate liver enzymes that flush toxins from the body; hence, these are powerful liver-supportive vegetables. Related vegetables include leeks, shallots, scallions/green onions, and chives, which all have some measure of the same health benefits of garlic and onions.

Red Bell Peppers: Red bell peppers are much sweeter and contain significantly higher levels of vitamin C, beta-carotene, vitamin K, and B vitamins than their green counterpart. Red bell peppers also contain lycopene, which offers protection against cancer and heart disease. As with the other vegetables high in beta-carotene, red bell peppers are strong liver cleansers.

Avocados: Although technically a fruit, many people eat avocados as a vegetable. Avocados contain the vitamins and minerals of green vegetables and the protein of meat, and they provide one of the healthiest forms of beneficial fat. They also have nearly twenty vitamins, minerals, and phytonutrients, including vitamin A (the potent antioxidant) B vitamins including folate, lutein (a phytonutrient important for the eyes), magne-

sium; and 60 percent more potassium than a banana. One medium-size avocado contains a whopping 15 grams of fiber, making it one of the most fiber-rich fruits on the planet.

Key Fruits

Apples: The phytonutrients called polyphenols, found in both the skin and flesh of apples, have powerful antioxidant properties that protect against clogging of the arteries and other cardiovascular problems. Apples' strong antioxidant benefits are also related to their ability to lower the risk of asthma and lung cancer. In addition, in study after study, apple consumption is consistently associated with a reduced risk of heart disease, lung cancer, asthma, and type 2 diabetes, compared with other fruits and vegetables.

Dates: Dates contain more than fifteen minerals, with high amounts of alkaline-forming calcium, magnesium, potassium, copper, manganese, and iron; thus, they are among the most alkalizing foods. Dates also have a high amount of the antioxidant mineral selenium, which is known to help fight cancer and build the immune system. Dates are also surprisingly rich in carotenoids, which convert to vitamin A in the body and act as antioxidants.

Watermelon: High in potassium, watermelon is *the* most alkaline-forming fruit, which means you should frequently partake of it when it is in season. It is highly concentrated with some of the most powerful antioxidants in nature, including vitamin C, beta-carotene, and lycopene.

The debate has ended. Organic foods really do contain more nutrients. A comprehensive study of the nutrient content in organic foods published in the July 2014 issue of the *British Journal of Nutrition* found that overall, organic fruits, vegetables, and whole grains contained 17 percent more antioxidants than their conventionally grown counterparts, and for some antioxidants the difference was even larger. A class of compounds known as flavanones, for example, were 69 percent higher in the organic produce. However, the main reason to choose organic produce over conventional is to avoid the residues of toxic pesticides and herbicides that are sprayed on conventionally grown crops. The study also showed that pesticide residues were several times higher on conventionally grown produce.

Many pesticides are known obesogens, and even small doses can cause other serious damage to human health, such as cancers of the reproductive, endocrine, and immune systems. Pesticides pose particular risks to pregnant women and young children, with evidence linking ingestion of pesticide residues on produce to pediatric cancers, decreased cognitive function, and behavioral problems. Antioxidants, on the other hand, have been shown to prevent the development of cancer, heart disease, diabetes, and many other serious diseases.

The challenge many of us are faced with is the high cost of organic produce. That's where the Environmental Working Group's (EWG) Shopper's Guide to Pesticides in Produce comes in handy. The EWG, a non-profit advocacy group, publishes a list of forty-eight common conventionally grown produce items that have been tested for residues of pesticides and herbicides. In order to get the most realistic residue values, tests are performed after the produce has been washed, peeled, and otherwise cleaned in the same manner as you would at home. After testing, the produce is ranked from highest to lowest concentrations of residues. The top 12 items on list—the ones that have the highest levels of pesticide residues—are dubbed "The Dirty Dozen." The EWG's studies show that we can lower our pesticide exposure by 90 percent if we avoid eating the conventionally grown Dirty Dozen and opt for their organic counterparts instead. They also include a "Plus" category that highlights two produce items—leafy greens (kale and collard greens) and hot peppers—that are frequently contaminated with trace levels of highly hazardous pesticides that are toxic to the human nervous system. If you eat these items frequently, EWG recommends opting for organic.

The bottom 15 items on the list—the ones that have low to no pesticide residues are dubbed "The Clean 15." The EWG deems these produce items safe to consume conventionally grown.

The EWG's 2014 Guide to Pesticides in Produce is on page 19. Note that the most contaminated item on the Dirty Dozen list is apples and the least contaminated item on the Clean 15 list is avocado. These are two of my super skinny foods, so when prioritizing where to spend your dollars, go organic on the apples and conventional on the avocados!

THE DIRTY DOZEN
(ranked from most to least residues):
1. Apples
2. Strawberries
3. Grapes
4. Celery
5. Peaches
6. Spinach
7. Sweet bell peppers
8. Nectarines (imported)
9. Cucumbers
10. Cherry tomatoes
11. Snap peas (imported)
12. Potatoes
Plus: Kale/collard greens and hot peppers

THE CLEAN 15
(ranked from least to most residues):
1. Avocados
2. Sweet corn
3. Pineapples
4. Cabbage
5. Sweet peas (frozen)
6. Onions
7. Asparagus
8. Mangoes
9. Papayas
10. Kiwi
11. Eggplant
12. Grapefruit
13. Cantaloupe
14. Cauliflower
15. Sweet potatoes

The EWG typically publishes their annual updated list in the month of June. For the most current list, go to www.foodnews.org, or download the free Dirty Dozen mobile app.

SOURCE: Environmental Working Group, www.foodnews.org.

. . . .

Legumes

Legumes contain both soluble and insoluble fiber, and a 1-cup serving of legumes contains anywhere from 11 to 15 grams of total fiber (nearly one-third of your recommended daily fiber intake). When combined with whole grains, legumes form a complete protein, providing between 14 and 17 grams of protein (equivalent to the amount in 2 ounces of chicken or fish). The almost magical protein-fiber combination in legumes, coupled with their high antioxidant content, has been shown to be a very powerful food weapon against many of today's common diseases.

Fats and Oils

Virgin Coconut Oil (and All Things Coconut): Coconut oil provides health benefits that surpass even those of other highly regarded oils. While it's true that coconut oil is a saturated fat, it's a plant source of saturated fat with a unique molecular structure that is very different from the type of saturated fats that come from animal foods. This unique structure, called medium-chain triglycerides (MCTs), is what provides many of coconut oil's health benefits. Coconut oil has been shown to protect against heart disease, cancer, diabetes, osteoporosis, and a host of other degenerative diseases. It does *not* raise the evil LDL cholesterol, but in fact increases the good HDL. Additionally, MCTs do not store easily as fat in your body; instead they get burned for energy immediately. This gives coconut oil a unique ability to promote weight loss by improving metabolism and help you burn more of your stored fat.

About half of the MCTs in coconut oil are a special type of fat called lauric acid, which converts in the body into a powerful compound called monolaurin. Monolaurin strengthens the immune system, wards off colds and flu, and destroys viruses and bacteria. As if these virtues weren't enough, the MCTs in coconut oil also act as antioxidants, which protect your body from free radical damage and a host of degenerative diseases, including cancer.

Molecularly, saturated fats are the most stable of all the different types of fats and can withstand the highest cooking temperatures of any fat or oil. Most of my recipes call for virgin coconut oil for sautéing, stir-frying, and baking because of its remarkable stability and resistance to oxidation. Most other oils, especially the polyunsaturated oils, become rancid and produce harmful free radicals when heated to cooking temperatures. Coconut oil is the amazing exception. It has a very high temperature threshold and is able to take heat up to about 350°F on the stovetop and 400°F in the oven without breaking down the way other oils do.

There are several types of coconut oil on the market, and you may be wondering which type is best. If you want the maximum health benefits from coconut oil (high antioxidant content, quick energy, increased metabolism, weight loss support, thyroid support, and strengthened immune system), then go with virgin coconut oil. There is no industry standard and no official classification or difference between "virgin coconut oil" and "extra-virgin coconut oil" like there is in the olive oil industry. So when you see "extra-virgin coconut oil" on a label, that's just a marketing term that is used to appeal to consumers, but the oil itself is no better or different from those labeled "virgin coconut oil."

Virgin coconut oil is unrefined; it is produced by pressing fresh coconut meat, called non-copra, without the use of chemicals. It contains the highest amount of lauric acid and offers the most health benefits. Because it is unrefined, virgin coconut oil will have the slight scent and taste of coconut. In my recipes and throughout this book, I will use the term "virgin coconut oil" since this is the term used on most labels, and it is the common term used in all the peer-reviewed studies on coconut oil.

Refined coconut oil is a more processed type of coconut oil that is produced from what is called copra, or dried coconut meat. After the oil is pressed from the copra, high heat and chemical solvents are used to remove impurities and prolong the shelf life. The components responsible for the scent and taste of coconut are also removed during this process, along with much of the lauric acid. This type of coconut oil is referred to as RBD, which stands for refined, bleached, and deodorized. Due to the fact that some of the less stable components have been removed from the oil, RBD coconut oil has a higher smoke point than virgin coconut oil. However, this type of chemical processing disrupts the balance of the MCTs, so RBD coconut oil does not have the same health benefits as virgin coconut oil.

I do not recommend using refined coconut oil, with one exception. An online company (see Resources, page 277) produces a refined coconut oil using a traditional pressing method that does not use chemicals. The oil is steam deodorized, rather than chemically extracted with solvents, to remove the scent and taste components, and the process leaves the lauric acid and many of the other MCTs intact. The end result is a high-quality refined coconut oil without the scent and taste of coconut, which many people prefer. This type of refined coconut oil is perfect for use in recipes where you want a tasteless oil.

You may have seen a product called Liquid Coconut Oil or Medium Chain Triglyceride (MCT) Oil sitting next to the jars of virgin coconut oil on the store shelf. Another name for this type of coconut oil is fractionated coconut oil. Liquid coconut oil is not real coconut oil—it is a manufactured product that has had the lauric acid removed. Depending on the company producing it, the removal is done either through chemical means or steaming. Lauric acid makes up 50 percent of the composition of coconut oil, and it is also the most stable saturated fat component, which is why coconut oil is typically solid at room temperature. When the lauric acid is removed from coconut oil, what remains are the types of fats that stay liquid at room temperature but are not really unique to coconut oil. Two of the fats are

MCTs called caprylic acid and capric acid, which together have a lower melting point. These MCTs can be found more abundantly in goat milk than in coconut oil. The other fats that remain in liquid coconut oil are not saturated fats—they are monounsaturated fats similar to the type found in olive oil, and polyunsaturated fats similar to the type found in corn and soybean oil. Neither of these types of oil is suitable for cooking, due to their less stable molecular structures, which are damaged by heat and become very damaging to our bodies when consumed. The bottom line is that liquid coconut oil is a refined oil that is lacking the most valuable component of real coconut oil. It does not have the health benefits of real coconut oil, and therefore I don't recommend it.

Omega-3 Fats (Fish Oil, Flaxseed Oil, and Flaxseeds): Taking fish oil supplements and adding flaxseed oil and flaxseeds or chia seeds to your meals will ensure that you are getting the proper amount of omega-3 fats every day.

Extra-Virgin Olive Oil: Aside from coconut oil, olive oil is one of the most digestible of all the fats. It contributes to the prevention of heart disease and cancer and has been used as a remedy for a wide variety of ailments.

Organic Butter: You may be surprised to see butter on this list. But there are many healthful properties of this maligned fat. Butter contains vitamin A, which is needed for the health of the thyroid and adrenal glands, both of which play a role in the proper functioning of the heart. Butter also contains vitamin E and the mineral selenium, which are strong antioxidants that protect us against free radical damage. Additionally, butter is a good source of iodine. Butter has many other health benefits, from improving the immune system and preventing cancer to assisting the body in the absorption of calcium and in building strong bones.

Grains and Grain Products

Quinoa: While it is often referred to and eaten as a grain, quinoa is technically the seed of a plant. Quinoa is one of only a few alkaline-forming grains, owing to its high content of magnesium. Since low levels of magnesium are associated with increased rates of high blood pressure and heart disease, this tiny grain can offer yet another way to protect against strokes and heart attacks. Other nutrients contained in quinoa are folate, manganese, iron, copper, and phosphorous. It is a good source of fiber and a protein powerhouse, containing all of the essential amino acids needed to make a complete protein. Bonus: As quinoa is technically a seed, it does not contain gluten.

Oat Bran: The most virtuous and versatile component of the oat resides in its outer layer—the bran. Since 1963, study after study has proven that oat bran significantly lowers cholesterol and leads to weight loss.

Other Key Foods

Almonds: Almonds help lower cholesterol and reduce the risk of heart disease, stabilize blood sugar levels, protect against diabetes, promote weight loss, and prevent gallstones. Almonds are one of only a few alkaline-forming nuts, owing to their high content of calcium, magnesium, and potassium. They are also high in fiber and protein. It is very important to eat almonds and any other nuts *in their raw form.*

Raw, Unfiltered Apple Cider Vinegar: Raw apple cider vinegar is made from pressing fresh apples; therefore, it is not surprising that this vinegar contains as many health benefits as the apple itself. For this reason, it has been used for generations as a natural remedy for a number of ailments. In particular, raw apple cider vinegar has been known to reduce sinus infections, lower cholesterol, fight allergies, alleviate symptoms of arthritis and gout, prevent and dissolve kidney stones, clear urinary tract infections, and strengthen the immune system.

Wild-Caught Salmon: Salmon is an incredibly healthful fish full of essential omega-3 fatty acids, but you need to make sure that you are eating wild-caught salmon instead of farm-raised salmon. Wild salmon roam freely in the ocean and fresh waters and eat algae and tiny crustaceans called krill, which provide the salmon with astaxanthin, a powerful phytonutrient that gives them their orange-pinkish color. Astaxanthin is known as a super-antioxidant with a long list of health benefits, including reducing inflammation and joint pain, protecting the brain from dementia and Alzheimer's, preventing cancer, improving blood sugar levels in diabetics, and improving athletic endurance, to name just a few.

Buyer beware: Farm-raised salmon do not have a natural dietary source of astaxanthin, so they are fed pellets of grain-based "fish food" with a dose of synthetic astaxanthin to artificially add color to their flesh. That's why you'll notice a statement on the packaging of farmed fish that says "Farm Raised, Color Added." Synthetic forms of astaxanthin are made from petrochemicals or GMO yeast. That doesn't sound very appetizing, does it?

Organic Eggs: Banish the boring egg-white-only omelets, and start eating whole eggs! Organic eggs contain nearly all known nutrients except for vitamin C and are a nearly perfect form of protein. They are good sources of the fat-soluble vitamins A and D, plus they contain essential fatty acids. While many people have been afraid to eat eggs due to their high cholesterol levels, studies suggest that eggs contain several nutrients that promote heart health and actually lower the risk of heart disease.

Plain Organic Whole Milk Yogurt: Yogurt is a fermented dairy product made by adding bacterial cultures to milk. These "live and active" cultures carry on the conversion of the milk's lactose sugar into lactic acid. The lactic acid bacteria that are traditionally used to make yogurt—*Lactobacillus bulgaricus, Lactobacillus acidophilus, Bifidobacterium lactis,* and *Streptococcus thermophilus*—are also responsible for many of yogurt's health benefits.

Here's a list of some ingredients that may be new to you:

AGAR-AGAR: This clear, flavorless gelling agent is a vegetarian alternative to animal-based gelatin. Also called *kanten* or Japanese gelatin, it is made from a combination of various sea vegetables with strong thickening properties. Agar-agar comes in powdered, flake, or stick form. You can find it in the Asian section of your natural food market, Asian grocery stores, and online.

ALMOND MEAL: Almond meal is made by coarsely grinding whole raw almonds to the consistency of cornmeal. It can also be made from the pulp leftover from making almond milk. Almond meal can be used to make raw cookies, cakes, crackers, and pâté, or it can be sprinkled on foods or blended into smoothies. It works well as a flour alternative for grain-free/gluten-free baked goods such as cookies, brownies, pancakes, and more.

Almond meal is available in natural food markets; however, making it yourself can give you the nutritional advantage of using soaked and dried almonds. Bonus: It's easy and more economical! For instructions, see page 71.

Note: Although often used interchangeably with the term *almond flour*, almond meal and almond flour are not the same thing. Almond meal is more coarsely ground and typically (but not necessarily) retains the brown almond skins. Almond flour, on the other hand, is made from blanched almonds (nuts that have had their skins removed) and is finely ground to produce a nut flour that is commonly used to make baked goods that have the appearance of those made with their refined white flour counterparts.

Arrowroot: A dried and powdered root of a tropical American plant, this natural thickening agent is a healthy unrefined alternative to cornstarch. Its high calcium content and trace minerals make it an alkaline-forming food that is the most easily digested of all starches. It can be used to thicken sauces, gravies, pie fillings, and puddings. It can also be used to replace part of the flour in recipes for cookies and other baked goods and is especially useful as a binder in gluten-free baking mixes. It has a neutral taste and makes shiny, transparent sauces. You can find arrowroot in the spice or baking section of your grocery store, natural food market, and online.

Blackstrap Molasses (Unsulphured): Blackstrap molasses is the dark, viscous syrup that lends the signature robust flavor to gingerbread and baked beans. It is packed with significant amounts of the antioxidants and alkalizing minerals found in natural sugarcane—namely, calcium, iron, magnesium, manganese, and potassium. It also contains good amounts of B vitamins, copper, chromium, and selenium.

Blackstrap molasses is best known for its high iron content: just 1 tablespoon provides 20 percent of the recommended daily value for iron—more than a serving of red meat.

Perhaps one of the most valuable properties of blackstrap molasses is its high concentration of polyphenols—plant compounds with powerful antioxidant properties and numerous potential health benefits, including the prevention of cancer, especially prostate and breast cancer.[1]

When used as a supplemental form of nutrients, the recommended dosage is 1 tablespoon per day (this also provides 18 percent of the recommended daily value of calcium).

Cacao Nibs: Cacao (pronounced "ka-KOW") is the scientific name of the fruit that bears the seeds from which all chocolate is derived. After the seeds (a.k.a. cocoa beans) are fermented, dried, and roasted, they are crushed and shelled. These "nibs" are the whole food form of chocolate before undergoing further processes to make cocoa powder and chocolate confections.

Cacao nibs contain 47 percent solids and 53 percent fat (cocoa butter). The solid part of the nib contains the famous dark chocolate antioxidants and other health protective compounds, while the fat is the healthy type that protects against heart disease and strokes, and also contains vitamin E and other antioxidants.

You can use cacao nibs in recipes in place of chocolate chips; sprinkle them into granola, trail mix, yogurt, and homemade ice cream; and blend them into smoothies and shakes. They're also great in savory sauces like mole and chili and can even be sprinkled on salads. Cacao nibs can be purchased in packages or from the bulk bins at natural food markets and are also available online.

Cocoa (Cacao) Powder: Cocoa powder is produced by intensely grinding cacao nibs into a thick cocoa paste, then separating out most of the cocoa butter using a hydraulic press. This process leaves a dry, pressed mass, which is then pulverized and sifted into a powder. Cocoa powder has very high amounts of antioxidants.

Note: All cocoa powders are not created equal. Some cocoa powder is treated with a chemical called alkali to remove the cocoa's natural bitterness and give it a milder flavor. Unfortunately, this chemical process, called Dutch process, also significantly reduces the antioxidant content and health value of cocoa powder; therefore, Dutch cocoa is not recommended for your processed-free recipes. Read ingredient lists carefully.

One more thing to note about cocoa (and dark chocolate) is that casein, a protein found in cow's milk, interferes with the absorption of the antioxidants in cocoa powder. Therefore, if you want to reap the benefits of cocoa's antioxidants, use a non-dairy milk such as almond milk, coconut milk, or hemp milk for making milkshakes, smoothies, hot cocoa, and other recipes. The whey protein in milk does not interfere with the absorption of cocoa's antioxidants, so a high-quality whey protein concentrate can still be beneficial with cocoa powder.

Raw cacao powder can be found at natural food markets and is also available online. High-quality natural unsweetened cocoa powder can be found in most grocery stores.

CAROB: Commonly known as a caffeine-free alternative to cocoa, carob can replace cocoa powder in recipes, but its flavor is more caramel and honey-like. Carob shares some of the same health benefits as cocoa, with similar anticancer properties as some of the compounds in cocoa.[2] These compounds also offer significant protection against heart dis-

ease by stopping the formation of LDL (bad) cholesterol and lowering blood pressure. But when it comes to calcium and fiber, carob beats cocoa—it has three times as much calcium and four times as much fiber ounce for ounce. The main appeal of carob over cocoa is that it does not contain the central nervous system stimulant caffeine or the muscle stimulant theobromine. All in all, carob makes a wonderful substitute for cocoa, and it can be used interchangeably in most recipes calling for cocoa. It can be found in most natural food markets and in some mainstream grocery stores, as well as online.

COCONUT CREAM CONCENTRATE: Sometimes referred to as "coconut butter" or "coconut manna," coconut cream concentrate is a thick, smooth, creamy paste that is made from ground dried coconut meat. Coconut cream concentrate is a versatile culinary ingredient. It can be mixed into recipes for soups, breads, cookies, muffins, frosting, smoothies, ice cream, and candies, and it also makes a great spread on toast, muffins, and crackers. It can also be blended with water to make instant coconut milk. There are about as many ways to use coconut cream concentrate as there are people thinking up ways to use it! You can find coconut cream concentrate in natural food markets and online.

Note: Coconut cream concentrate is not to be confused with coconut cream, which is a thick creamy liquid that comes in a can and typically contains added sugar.

GELATIN (UNFLAVORED): Gelatin is made of collagen, the protein that occurs naturally in bones and connective tissue, as well as in skin. It is a good source of protein and contains twenty of the twenty-two amino acids, including arginine and glycine. Unflavored gelatin gives body and texture to puddings, mousses, broths, and gelée-style dishes like molds. Recommended uses include thickening soups, sauces, and stews or adding to smoothies.

The best gelatin is produced from the highest quality grass-fed cows tested to be free of mad cow disease. This gelatin is produced in a way that virtually eliminates the formation of glutamic acid/MSG by-products.

HERBAMARE: Herbamare is my favorite staple seasoning salt. It is prepared by combining fresh, organically grown herbs with natural sea salt. Herbamare makes life easy when you want to season food without chopping fresh herbs or rummaging through your pantry for dried ones. It can be used in place of salt to season everything from broths, vegetables, salad dressings, meats, fish, poultry, grains, and more.

MASA HARINA: This is the traditional corn flour used to make tortillas, tamales, and other Mexican staples. To make masa harina, field corn (or maize) is dried and then treated in a solution of lime and water to loosen the hulls from the kernels and soften the corn. In addition, the lime reacts with the corn so that the nutrient niacin can be assimilated by the digestive tract.

The soaked maize is then washed, and the wet corn is ground into a dough, called masa. When dried and powdered, fresh masa becomes masa harina.

NUTRITIONAL YEAST: This deactivated yeast enhances many foods with its unique cheesy flavor and powerhouse of nutrients, including B-complex vitamins, protein, and fiber. It's especially popular with vegans and vegetarians as a stand-in for the cheese flavor in foods (its flaky texture and tangy taste are remarkably similar to Parmesan cheese), but it can be enjoyed by everyone. Sprinkle it into dishes such as soup, quinoa, stir-fry, dressings, sauces, pastas, scrambled eggs, popcorn, and more!

OATS: You probably already know that oats help lower cholesterol, lower blood pressure, stabilize blood sugar, and assist in weight loss. They are also lower in carbohydrates and higher in protein and healthy fats than most other whole grains.

Oats contain more than twenty unique polyphenols called avenanthramides, which have strong antioxidant, anti-inflammatory, and anti-itching properties.

Here's the lowdown on all the different types of oats and a list of their health benefits.

Whole Oat Groats: Oat groats are the most whole form of the oat grain and the starting material for all of the different types of "cut" oats. They take longer to cook than any of the "cut" varieties of oats.

Steel Cut Oats (Irish Oatmeal): When groats are cut into two or three pieces with a sharp metal blade, steel cut oats are formed.

Their cooking time is shorter than oat groats because water can more easily penetrate the smaller pieces, but they still take about 30 minutes to cook. Steel cut oats, interchangeably called Irish oatmeal, make a porridge with a chewy, nutty texture.

Scottish Oatmeal: Rather than cutting groats with a steel blade, the Scottish tradition is to stone-grind them, creating broken bits of varying sizes, which results in a porridge with a creamier texture than steel cut oats.

Rolled Oats (Old Fashioned): Rolled oats (also known as old-fashioned oats) are created when oat groats are softened by steaming, then run through metal rollers to flatten them into flakes. This process stabilizes the healthy oils in the oats, allowing them to stay fresh longer. Due to the steaming and the greater surface area, rolled oats cook in about fifteen minutes.

Rolled Oats (Quick or Instant): Rolling the oat flakes even thinner creates quick oats, which cook in under five minutes. Instant oats are also rolled thinner than old-fashioned oats, but they are then "cooked and dried" requiring no further cooking—just add hot water and stir. The Whole Grain Council says the nutrient content stays the same (all cuts of oats are all whole grains), but the time it takes for the body to digest and break down the starches in these types of oats is significantly less and could be problematic for those who are diabetic or carbohydrate

sensitive. Also, many brands of instant oatmeal contain added sugar.

Oat Bran: The outer layer of the whole oat groat contains the bran. Unique to oats, and in particular to oat bran, are special antioxidant compounds that help prevent free radicals from damaging cholesterol, providing another powerful mechanism for oat bran to reduce the risk of heart disease. Oat bran is high in fiber.

Young Thai Coconut: Also known as green or immature coconuts, the young Thai coconuts you'll typically find in stores have a white "husk" that is cone-shaped at the top. They are different from mature coconuts, which are the more familiar-looking brown, hairy variety. Young coconuts have more water inside of them than mature coconuts, and their meat is very soft, moist, and creamy. Due to its firmness, mature coconut meat can be grated, shredded, or cut into chunks for snacking or using in recipes, while young coconut meat is better suited for making creamy concoctions such as puddings, custards, smoothies, and yogurt. Both types can be blended with the coconut's water to make coconut milk.

Natural coconut water from young coconuts is the highest known source of five key electrolytes: sodium, potassium, calcium, magnesium, and phosphorus. It is packed with more potassium than a banana or fifteen sport drinks. It is also a good source of vitamin C, riboflavin, thiamin, and vitamin B6, and it even contains some protein.

The meat of a young coconut is high in antioxidants and lauric acid, a medium-chain fat that is known for its antiviral, antibacterial immune-boosting properties.

You can find young Thai coconuts at natural food markets, but the best place to shop for them is in Asian markets, where they are typically more affordable. When selecting a young coconut, choose one that feels heavy and full of liquid and has a bright, off-white husk without dark spots or pink discoloration. The husk should appear well hydrated, without any sunken or dry spots. Chill young coconuts in the refrigerator once you get them home until you are ready to use them. For instructions on opening a young coconut, see page 65; you'll find tips for opening a mature coconut on page 66.

Skinny for Life Pantry List

To make it easy for you, here is a full list of Skinny ingredients that are used in the recipes and/or that you'll want to have around to create your own healthy, inspired dishes.

All vegetables and most of the fruits listed are alkaline forming.

SKINNY FOR LIFE PANTRY LIST

Dark Green Leafy Vegetables

Arugula
Beet greens
Bok choy
Butterhead lettuce
Cabbage, green and red
Chard, all types
Chinese cabbage (napa cabbage)
Collard greens
Dandelion greens
Endive
Escarole
Frisée
Green loose-leaf lettuce
Kale
Mustard greens
Radicchio
Red loose-leaf lettuce
Romaine lettuce
Spinach
Spring mix
Turnip greens
Watercress
Kelp and seaweeds

Rainbow Vegetables

Alfalfa sprouts
Artichokes
Asparagus

Bamboo shoots
Bean sprouts
Beets
Bell peppers (all colors)
Broccoli
Brussels sprouts
Carrots
Cauliflower
Celery
Chives
Cucumbers
Daikon
Eggplant
Jicama
Kohlrabi
Leeks
Mexican gray squash
Mushrooms
Okra
Onions, all types
Parsley
Radishes
Rhubarb
Rutabagas
Sauerkraut
Scallions/green onions
Shallots
Snap peas

Snow peas
Sorrel
Sprouts, all types
String beans, green and yellow
Tomatoes
Turnips
Water chestnuts
Yellow summer squash
Zucchini

Starchy Vegetables

Parsnips
Pumpkin
Spaghetti squash
Sweet potato or yam
Winter squash

Legumes

Beans, all types
Lentils, all types
Split peas

Whole Grains

Amaranth
Barley
Brown rice
Buckwheat
Bulgur
Corn kernels
Corn on the cob
Cornmeal, whole grain with germ
Kamut
Millet
Oats
Polenta
Quinoa
Red rice
Rye
Spelt
Wild rice
Whole wheat

Fruits

Apples
Apricots
Bananas
Berries
- Blackberries
- Blueberries
- Cranberries
- Raspberries
- Strawberries
Cherries
Dates
Figs, fresh or dried
Grapefruit
Grapes, all types
Kiwifruit
Lemons
Limes
Mangos
Melons
- Cantaloupe
- Honeydew
- Watermelon
Nectarines
Oranges
Papayas
Peaches
Pears
Persimmons
Pineapples
Plums
Prunes
Raisins
Tangelos
Tangerines

High-Quality Protein

Fish (wild caught is best)

Cod
Grouper
Haddock
Halibut
Herring
Mackerel
Mahimahi
Orange roughy
Sardines, canned in water or olive oil only
Salmon, fresh
Salmon, canned in water
Sea bass
Snapper
Sole
Tilapia
Trout
Whitefish
Tuna, fresh
Tuna, canned in water only

(continues)

Poultry

Chicken
Chicken, canned (no additives)
Chicken or turkey bacon (no nitrates or nitrites)
Chicken or turkey sausage (no pork casings, nitrates, or nitrites)
Chicken or turkey deli meats and hot dogs (no synthetic additives, nitrates, or nitrites)
Cornish game hen
Duck
Turkey

Meat (all lean types)

Beef
Beef deli meats and hot dogs (no synthetic additives, pork casings, nitrates, or nitrites)
Buffalo
Lamb
Liver (must be organic)
Veal
Venison

Other Protein Foods

Eggs

Dairy

Plain organic whole milk yogurt
Plain organic whole milk yogurt, Greek-style
Whole-milk goat yogurt

Fermented soy foods

Miso
Tamari sauce
Tempeh

Protein Powders

Brown rice protein powder (unsweetened or naturally sweetened brands only)
Goat whey protein powder concentrate (unsweetened or naturally sweetened brands only)
Hemp protein powder (unsweetened or naturally sweetened brands only)
Whey protein powder concentrate (NOT isolate; unsweetened or naturally sweetened brands only)

Health-Promoting Fats and Oils

Virgin Coconut Oil and Coconut Products

Omega-3

Hemp seed oil
High-lignan flaxseed oil

Other Health-Promoting Fats and Oils

Avocado
Butter, organic
Extra-virgin olive oil
Organic butter
Peanut oil, expeller pressed, unrefined
Sesame oil, expeller pressed, unrefined

Nuts and Seeds

Almonds
Brazil nuts
Cashews
Chia seeds
Flaxseeds
Hazelnuts
Hemp seeds
Macadamias
Nut and seed butters, includes sesame tahini
Peanuts, dry roasted, unsalted
Pecans
Pine nuts
Pistachios
Pumpkin seeds (pepitas)
Sesame seeds (includes tahini)
Sunflower seeds
Walnuts

Alkalizing and Liver-izing Herbs and Spices

These herbs and spices are thermogenic, meaning they create heat in the body, raise metabolism, and burn fat.

Allspice
Anise
Bay leaves
Cardamom
Cayenne
Cilantro/Coriander
Cinnamon
Cloves
Curry powder
Dill
Fennel
Garlic
Ginger
Mustard, dried
Turmeric

3

Processed-Free Kitchen Essentials

N ow that you know how to stock your pantry, here are some tips for prepping the rest of your kitchen. Below you'll find suggestions for equipment, as well as basic cooking techniques and strategies for making your own favorite recipes optimally nutritious. I have listed websites and more information about my recommended brands of appliances and gadgets in Resources (page 273).

Cookware, Gadgets, and Equipment

First things first: I suggest you replace aluminum and/or Teflon-coated cookware with stainless steel, cast iron, or Pyrex instead. Teflon contains a synthetic polymer called polytetrafluoroethylene (PTFE), a known obesogen. It releases toxic substances into the environment, and quite likely into food. Aluminum easily leaches into the food you are cooking, which is bad news as aluminum is known to inhibit the body's use of calcium and magnesium—the very minerals that are needed to build bones and neutralize acidity in the body. I recommend non-coated stainless-steel and cast-iron cookware for stovetop cooking, and glass, CorningWare, or Pyrex for the oven.

Time-Saving Appliances

These kitchen appliances aren't essential to have, but they certainly can help make things easier!

BLENDER: The ultimate kitchen appliance is a Vitamix, a high-powered blender that can do everything from grind flaxseeds, coffee beans, and grains to make ice cream and soups in a matter of minutes. It is the best blender for making smoothies, as it can blend whole fruits and vegetables, including stems and peels, into creamy drinks, retaining all of the valuable nutrients. The Vitamix is definitely a major purchase, but it is well worth the investment. If you're not ready to commit to a high-powered blender, a regular blender or an immersion blender will work for most smoothies and soups.

BLUAPPLE: This produce saver has been a saving grace for me. The Bluapple is an absorbent pouch housed in a small blue apple-shaped plastic container that can be placed in your crisper drawers, on the shelves in your refrigerator, or anywhere you keep fruits and veg-

etables. The Bluapple absorbs ethylene gas and extends the useful storage life of your produce up to three times longer than normal. This really works! I've had lettuce and other greens last up to two weeks, and carrots, celery, and other hardy vegetables stay fresh for up to a month.

FOOD PROCESSOR: These handy machines with S-shaped blades and grating attachments make chopping vegetables a snap, and they can also blend and purée foods easily. Any food processor on the market will do the trick.

JUICER: Most of my juicing recipes do require a juicer. Like a high-powered blender, a juicer may be an appliance you're not sure about, but it is a solid investment in your long-term health since juicing will help increase your daily veggie intake exponentially. There's a wide range of juicers on the market; you don't need to break the bank!

RICE COOKER: There are many rice cookers on the market, but not all are created equal. Most have aluminum and nonstick inner cooking pots. There are a few companies, such as Lotus Foods, that manufacture rice cookers and vegetable steamers with inner cooking pots made of stainless steel.

SLOW COOKER: These timesaving appliances are fairly inexpensive and quite versatile. They're great in winter months for cooking soups, beans, stews, casseroles, and even oatmeal, but they are just as helpful during the hot summer months when you don't want to turn on the oven. Slow cookers are also great for cooking in bulk, then freezing the extra for future meals.

Food Preparation Tips and Techniques

Cooking with Oils

Of all the components of healthy foods, oils are the most fragile. When subjected to high heat, the oil molecules react with the oxygen in the air, turning them into harmful, damaging molecules called free radicals. When consumed, free radicals cause inflammation in the body and damage our DNA. This sets the stage for obesity, diabetes, heart disease, cancer, Alzheimer's, and other very serious degenerative diseases.

There are three types of oils—saturated, monounsaturated, and polyunsaturated. The polyunsaturated oils are the most fragile and susceptible to damage by heat.

Most of the cooking oils sitting in bottles on your supermarket shelf, or those that are used in packaged or bottled foods, contain polyunsaturated oils. They have been heated to very high temperatures and treated with chemicals during processing. They already contain hundreds if not thousands of free radicals. When further heated for cooking, they are damaged even more. Some of these oils include corn oil, canola oil, safflower oil, sunflower oil, soybean oil, vegetable oil, and any type of hydrogenated oil (otherwise known as trans fat). For this reason, I don't recommend using these types of oils for cooking.

Monounsaturated oils, like extra-virgin olive oil, sesame oil, peanut oil, and avocado oil are healthy only when they are not heated too high; therefore, I only recommend using these oils if they are unrefined and expeller pressed or cold pressed. This means that no heat or chemicals were used during pressing, and therefore they are less likely to contain free radicals. Monounsaturated fats are more stable than polyunsaturated fats, but they are still susceptible to becoming damaged if too much heat is applied.

Saturated fats are the only type of oil that can withstand the high temperatures of cooking and baking. These include coconut oil, palm fruit oil, butter, and ghee (clarified butter). Saturated fats are the most stable oils of all. Their molecular structure is strong and sturdy, and they do not react with the air even when heated. However, even these fats have a temperature threshold and should not be heated above 400°F.

Many cooking oils are marketed as being good for cooking because they have a high smoke point (assuming they can be used at high temperatures without becoming rancid and producing free radicals). Such oils may be important to modern chefs, but what they fail to understand is that the smoke point of an oil or fat has nothing to do with its health benefits or its safety for cooking at higher temperatures.

Rather than using smoke point as the determining factor for high-heat cooking, be aware of the composition of the oil. As a general rule, if an oil is polyunsaturated, then it is not good for cooking, regardless of the smoke point listed on the bottle. Many oils contain compounds in them that can raise the smoke point, but free radicals can form in the oil at lower temperatures.

However, there are some ways to protect monounsaturated oils from getting too hot, so you can use some olive oil or sesame oil to cook with when you want a different flavor. To help you in the kitchen, here are some of my rules for cooking with oils:

- Never allow the oil to touch a hot pan. Preheat your empty pan over medium heat.
- Have your vegetables and/or meat ready (as if for stir-frying), so the pan doesn't heat excessively while you are busy with prep.
- Put some water or broth into the pan first, enough to cover the bottom, to cool the pan down to 212°F. The liquid creates a barrier between the hot pan and the oil; that way, the oil never gets as hot as the pan.
- Toss in your vegetables and/or meat.
- Drizzle in a bit of your favorite oil after you've added the other ingredients, and stir it around so it's always moving and doesn't have a chance to burn. This minimizes the damage to the oil and preserves the flavor.

As a rule of thumb, you should never see smoke coming off your oil. If you do, that means you are burning it and creating free radicals. You can smell the difference between smoking oil and steam coming off your food.

And finally, you should never see any black or brown residue in your pan after you've cooked with oil. If you do, that means you burned your oil and created free radicals.

Soaking and Sprouting Whole Grains, Legumes, Nuts, and Seeds

Have you ever heard someone say, "I like nuts, but they don't like me"? What about the phrase, "Beans beans, the magical fruit, the more you eat, the more you toot"? Well, say goodbye to Beano! You won't be needing it or any other gas-reducing medication when you soak beans before cooking! The reason these foods create gastrointestinal discomfort is because they contain compounds that are difficult for us to digest. All seeds (nuts, grains, and legumes are seeds of plants too) are most nutritious and digestible if soaked prior to eating and cooking.

As a way of preserving and protecting themselves in the wild until conditions are right to start the growth cycle, seeds are equipped with an arsenal of self-defense mechanisms known as anti-nutrients, which are contained in the outer seed coating (or bran, in the case of grains). When placed in water or planted in the ground, a seed will begin to germinate. Once the germination process starts, natural enzyme activity eliminates the anti-nutrients from the outer seed coating and transforms the long-term storage properties of the seed into simpler molecules that are easily digested. Soaking mimics the natural germination process that occurs in nature, unlocking important enzymes and nutrients.

Before I go into how to soak these foods, I want to explain what the anti-nutrients are, why they can be harmful to your health, and why soaking is an important practice. The main anti-nutrients are enzyme inhibitors, phytates, and lectins.

Enzyme Inhibitors: Plant seeds, especially nuts and seeds, contain enzyme inhibitors that ward off predators. These inhibitors block enzyme function, particularly the enzymes required to digest proteins, which can put a real strain on the digestive system if consumed in excess. The inability to digest proteins can lead to chronic inflammation, insulin resistance, impaired digestion, immune suppression, increased allergies, severe intestinal issues, and declined mental function.

Phytates (Phytic Acid): The best known anti-nutrient found in nuts, seeds, and grains is phytic acid (phytates), a compound that protects the plant seed from premature germination. When you eat foods containing phytates, they combine with calcium, magnesium, copper, iron, and especially zinc in the intestinal tract and block their absorption. Phytates also have the potential to block protein absorption.

Over time, regularly consuming foods that contain phytates can lead to serious mineral deficiencies and cause a wide array of health problems including bone loss, digestive issues, autoimmune diseases, allergies, skin irritations, decaying teeth, and hormone disruption.

However, seeds, nuts, legumes, and grains also contain a dormant enzyme called phytase, which is activated by soaking. Once activated, phytase breaks down phytates so that they no longer inhibit the absorption of nutrients.

Lectins: Lectins are basically carbohydrate-binding proteins that are present in nearly all foods, both plant and animal. In plants, they act as built-in pesticides that nature intended for warding off predators. These types of lectins are highly concentrated in grains (especially wheat), beans (especially soybeans), and nuts. When consumed in large quantities, they are very harmful to the small intestine. They stick to the lining of the small intestine and damage the sensitive villi that are responsible for transporting nutrients into the bloodstream.

Over time, lectins lead to a condition called "leaky gut syndrome," which means that the delicate lining of the small intestine has become so damaged and perforated that undigested food particles, proteins, toxins, and other pathogens are able to "leak" into the bloodstream and bind to tissues and organs throughout the body. This triggers inflammation in the body as a way to protect the affected tissue. Because of this, lectins are also linked with autoimmune disorders like irritable bowel syndrome, Crohn's disease, ulcerative colitis, thyroid disorders, fibromyalgia, arthritis, lupus, and many others.

When soaked, the vital proteins, vitamins (especially B vitamins), enzymes, and minerals are unlocked, making them ten times more nutritious than in their raw unsoaked form. Soaking also releases their dormant energy and greatly increases their digestibility.

It is not imperative that you soak grains or nuts and seeds, but to receive the highest amount of nutrition and experience optimal digestion, I highly recommend it.

General Soaking Guidelines

You'll notice that when you soak your beans, grains, nuts, and seeds for many hours, a foamy scum forms on top of the soak water. What is that scum? Anti-nutrients, that's what! That's why it's important to drain and rinse off the soak water before cooking.

Grains: Soaking grains is most optimal by starting with hot water and an acid medium, such as lemon juice, raw organic unfiltered apple cider vinegar, coconut vinegar, brown rice vinegar, or fresh whey left over from making yogurt. The water only needs to be hot initially; you don't have to keep it hot for the entire soak time. Drain off the soak water and rinse the grains before cooking.

Beans/Legumes: Beans and legumes require VERY HOT water initially for soaking, and most require a twenty-four-hour soaking time, rinsing and changing the treated soak water every eight hours if possible. Hot water only needs to be used initially for the first soak. For subsequent soakings, room temperature water can be used. If you can't rinse and change the water every eight hours, don't worry about it. The more important thing is the soaking itself.

The acidification of the soak water depends on the type of bean—lentils, chickpeas (a.k.a. garbanzo beans), black beans, and smaller beans such as adzuki, red beans, and navy beans should be treated with an acid medium, such as lemon juice, raw organic unfiltered apple cider vinegar, coconut vinegar, brown rice vinegar, or liquid whey left over from making yogurt. All other larger, kidney-shaped beans plus split peas require a pinch of baking soda. The baking soda should be added to the last soaking period, not at the beginning. Do not use baking soda for smaller beans because they will cook too fast and become mushy.

Raw Nuts and Seeds: Raw nuts and seeds are best soaked in a brine (salt solution) to reduce enzyme inhibitors and increase digestibility. The salt also lends a nice flavor to the nuts and seeds. It is important to only use a high-quality sea salt or Himalayan pink salt and not iodized table salt.

Soaking Guide

For water temperatures and approximate soaking times, refer to the chart on page 38.

Place grains, beans, nuts, or seeds in a large glass or ceramic bowl.

Fill the bowl with purified water to cover 1 inch above whatever you are soaking.

If the water should be heated (see General Soaking Guidelines, page 36), first heat the water on the stove in a pot to the estimated temperature. Please do not heat your water in the microwave. Pour the heated water over whatever you are soaking.

For grains, small beans, and lentils, add 1 tablespoon of acid (lemon juice, raw organic unfiltered apple cider vinegar, coconut vinegar, brown rice vinegar, or whey) to the water.

For large beans, add ½ to 1 teaspoon of baking soda to the water.

For nuts and seeds, add 1 to 2 teaspoons of salt.

Cover the bowl with a cheesecloth or other light towel and let soak on the kitchen counter for the recommended amount of time listed in the chart on page 38.

Add more water after a few hours if the grains, beans, nuts, or seeds have absorbed most of the water.

Beans: The soak water should be changed every 8 hours for beans. Make sure to thoroughly rinse the beans each time you change the soak water (to get rid of the scummy anti-nutrients). If using baking soda for larger beans, add it to the last soaking period.

Always rinse thoroughly before cooking or drying.

Drying Nuts and Seeds

Unlike grains and beans, you won't be cooking your nuts and seeds right after soaking, so it's important to dry them thoroughly and properly.

Drain off the water, rinse, and dry the soaked nuts or seeds by blotting them with a towel and then spreading them on a baking sheet. Put them in the oven with the oven light on. DO NOT TURN ON THE OVEN. You can leave them in the oven all day to dry while you are away or all night while you are asleep. The light will create a very low heat (no higher than 120°F) and will allow them to dry but won't harm the delicate oils contained within them. It is very important to eat nuts and seeds in their raw form, never roasting them at high heats.

Alternatively, if you have a food dehydrator, you can dry your nuts and seeds in it.

Soaked and dried nuts and seeds should be stored in the refrigerator. Make sure they are completely dry, otherwise they will get moldy very quickly.

Soaking Times and Temperatures

	WATER TEMPERATURE	SOAK TIME (HOURS)
NUTS		
Almonds	Warm	12–18
Brazil nuts	See Notes Below	
Cashews	See Notes Below	
Hazelnuts	See Notes Below	
Macadamia nuts	See Notes Below	
Peanuts	Room Temperature	12
Pecans	Warm	12–18
Pine Nuts	See Notes Below	
Pistachios	See Notes Below	
Walnuts	Warm	12–18
SEEDS		
Chia or Salba seeds	Room Temperature	1
Flaxseeds	Room Temperature	2–3
Hemp seeds	See Notes Below	
Pumpkin seeds (pepitas)	Room Temperature	6–8
Sesame seeds	Room Temperature	6–8
Sunflower seeds	Room Temperature	6–8
GRAINS		
Amaranth	Warm	18
Barley, hulled	Warm	18
Barley, pearled	Warm	18
Buckwheat	Warm	8
Cornmeal	Warm	18
Farro	Warm	24
Millet	Warm	18
Oats, groats	Warm	12–18
Oats, rolled or steel cut	Warm	8–12
Quinoa	Warm	4–6
Rice, brown	Warm	18–24
Rice, wild	Warm	24–36
Rye, berries	Warm	24
Spelt	Warm	24
Teff	Warm	18
Triticale	Warm	24
Wheat, whole berries	Warm	24

	WATER TEMPERATURE	SOAK TIME (HOURS)
Wheat, bulgur	Warm	24
Wheat, cracked	Warm	24
Wheat, couscous	Warm	24
BEANS		
Adzuki	Hot	24
Anasazi	Hot	24
Black beans	Hot	24
Black-eyed peas	Hot	24
Cannellini	Hot	24
Chickpeas	Hot	24
Green peas, whole	Hot	24
Green peas, split	Warm	12–18 See Note
Kidney	Hot	24
Lentils, brown	Warm	6-8 See Note
Lentils, green or red	Warm	2–6
Lima	Hot	24
Mung, whole	Warm	12 See Note
Mung, split	Warm	6
Navy	Hot	24
Northern	Hot	24
Pinto	Hot	24

Notes on Nuts and Seeds: There are also different schools of thought about the need to soak certain types of nuts and seeds. Most sources agree that Brazil nuts, cashews, hazelnuts, hemp seeds, macadamia nuts, pine nuts, and pistachios do not need to be soaked because they don't contain high amounts of phytates. Shelled Brazil nuts and cashews are not truly raw when you buy them because a tremendous amount of heat is used to extract them from their shells before packaging. In the process, the phytates are destroyed, making soaking unnecessary.

The only time you may want to soak these nuts would be when using them in a recipe in which you need the nuts to be softer so they can easily be blended, as in a nut milk, sauce, dressing, or creamy spread. In that case, the soak time should be no longer than 2 hours. I know from personal experience that soaking cashews too long makes them slimy and unappetizing.

Notes on Legumes: There are varying schools of thought about whether lentils, split peas, and mung beans require presoaking. Some sources say they don't require soaking because they contain less oligosaccharides (large carbohydrate molecules that are difficult for our bodies to break down). The larger the legume, the more oligosaccharides, and the longer soaking time helps to break them down prior to cooking. In my experience, lentils and split peas tend to turn mushy quickly if they are soaked too long. Presoaking is still beneficial to neutralize anti-nutrients, but the length of soaking time is much shorter for these smaller legumes.

Cooking Grains

Once your grains have been soaked, drained, and rinsed, place the grains in a pot with a fitted lid, add the designated amount of cooking liquid, bring to a boil, reduce the heat to a low simmer, cover, and cook for the designated amount of time. If any foam develops on top, skim it off and discard it because it can contain released anti-nutrients.

To 1 cup of this whole grain:	Add this much water or broth (cups), plus a dash of sea salt:	Bring to a boil, then reduce heat to simmer, cover, and cook for: (cooking times will be shorter with presoaking)	Yields this amount of cooked grain (cups):
Amaranth	2½–3	20–25 minutes	2½
Barley, hulled	3	60–75 minutes	2½
Buckwheat groats (kasha)	2	15 minutes	2½
Cornmeal, fine grind	4–4½	8–10 minutes	2½
Cornmeal, coarse grind (polenta)	4–4½	20–25 minutes	2½
Corn grits, white	4	15 minutes	3–4
Farro	4	Soak overnight, then cook 45–60 minutes	3
Kamut	4	Soak overnight, then cook 45–60 minutes	3
Millet, hulled	2½	25–35 minutes	4
Oat bran	2½	5 minutes	2
Oat groats (steel cut)	3	40–50 minutes	3½
Oats, steel cut (Irish)	4	30 minutes	4
Oats, Scottish	3	30 minutes	4
Oats, rolled	2	15	2
Quinoa	2	15–20 minutes	2¾
Rice, brown basmati	2½	35–45 minutes	3
Rice, brown long grain	2½	45–55 minutes	3
Rice, brown short grain	2–2½	45–55 minutes	3
Rice, wild	3	50–60 mintues	3½
Rye, berries	3–4	Soak overnight, then cook for 1 hour	3
Spelt berries	4	Soak overnight, then cook for 1 hour	3
Teff	3	15 minutes	3
Triticale, berries	3	1 hour, 45 minutes	2½

To 1 cup of this whole grain:	Add this much water or broth (cups), plus a dash of sea salt:	Bring to a boil, then reduce heat to simmer, cover, and cook for: (cooking times will be shorter with presoaking)	Yields this amount of cooked grain (cups):
Whole wheat, berries	4	Soak overnight, then cook 45–60 minutes	3
Whole wheat, bulgur	2	15 minutes	2½
Whole wheat couscous	1½	Bring water to a boil. Remove from heat, cover, and let sit 15 minutes.	3
Whole wheat, cracked	2	20–25 minutes	2¼

Soaking and Drying Oats to Use for Baking

If you like to make cookies, granola, oatmeal, breads, and muffins with rolled oats, this preparation step will ensure that you always have properly soaked oats on hand when you need them for a recipe.

Add the desired amount of oats to a large mixing bowl. Add 1 cup of water and stir to moisten the oats. You may need to add more water, but you don't need too much. The idea is to simply wet the oats until they are all slightly damp, rather than submerged. Add in small amounts of water a little at a time until you've reached the desired moistness.

Add in 1 tablespoon of an acidic medium, such as organic whole milk yogurt, lemon juice, or vinegar for every 1 cup of oats used and mix to combine. For example, if you are soaking 4 cups of oats, you would add 4 tablespoons of acid. Yogurt is my preferred acid medium for soaking oats because it adds a nice flavor, but if you are dairy intolerant you should use lemon juice or vinegar.

Cover the oats and allow them to soak at room temperature for at least 24 hours, but don't let them soak more than 30 hours, as they will begin to mold.

Spread the oats in a thin layer on baking sheets lined with parchment paper and place in the oven on the lowest setting possible until they are completely dry (about 8 to 12 hours depending on the temperature of your oven). The lowest temperature setting on my oven is 170°F; yours may be lower. If you have a food dehydrator, you can dry the oats at 110°F. Drying time will depend on your dehydrator.

Check the oats periodically while they are drying, and break up any small clumps that are sticking together with your hands or the back of a spoon to ensure they dry completely.

Once the oats are completely dry, remove them from the oven or dehydrator, allow to cool completely, and then store them in an airtight container in your pantry as you normally would any other grains. Use within 1 month or store in the freezer to extend their shelf life up to 6 months.

Cooking Beans and Legumes

Soaking beans not only breaks down anti-nutrients, it also reduces the cooking time a bit. Even more importantly, presoaking helps the beans cook more evenly and become completely tender all the way through.

To cook, place soaked, rinsed, and drained beans or legumes in a stockpot and add the designated amount of water. Bring the beans to a boil, then reduce the heat to a very gentle simmer for the rest of the cooking time. You should barely see movement in the water. Along with presoaking, simmering the beans gently helps them cook evenly until tender, retain their shape without getting too mushy, and keep their skins intact.

Don't add salt until the beans or legumes are almost finished cooking. The best time to add the salt is when the beans or legumes are tender enough to eat but still too firm to really be enjoyable, around the last half hour of cooking.

If you use a pressure cooker, you still need to soak your beans, legumes, or grains. While the pressure cooker will take less time to cook them, it does not remove anti-nutrients. Put the beans in the pressure cooker with three times as much water as beans. Cook at 15 pounds of pressure for 30 minutes for small beans. For large beans, such as lima or fava beans, pressure cook for about 40 minutes.

To 1 cup of these soaked beans/legumes:	Add this much water (cups):	Bring to a boil, then reduce heat to a gentle boil and cook for:	Yields this amount of cooked beans/legumes (cups):
Adzuki (Aduki)	4	45–55 minutes	3
Anasazi	2½–3	45–55 minutes	2¼
Black beans	4	1–1½ hours	2¼
Black-eyed peas	3	1 hour	2
Cannellini (white kidney beans)	3	45 minutes	2½
Fava beans, skins removed	3	40–50 minutes	1⅔
Chickpeas	4	1–3 hours	2
Great Northern beans	3½	1½ hours	2⅔
Green peas, whole	6	1–2 hours	2
Kidney beans	3	1 hour	2¼
Lentils, brown	2¼	20–25 minutes	2¼
Lentils, green	2	20–25 minutes	2
Lentils, red or yellow	3	15–20 minutes	2–2½
Lima beans, large	4	45–60 minutes	2

To 1 cup of these soaked beans/legumes:	Add this much water (cups):	Bring to a boil, then reduce heat to a gentle boil and cook for:	Yields this amount of cooked beans/legumes (cups):
Lima beans, small	4	50–60 minutes	3
Lima beans	4	1 hour	2
Mung beans	2½	1 hour	2
Navy beans	3	45–60 minutes	2⅔
Pink beans	3	50–60 minutes	2¾
Pinto beans	3	1–1½ hour	2⅔

Converting Your Own Recipes into Processed-Free Fare

The most valuable thing I've learned from cooking processed-free food is that there is almost always a healthy ingredient that can replace a processed one. Often your modified recipes turn out better than the original. (Try my Grain-Free Almond Spice Cookies, page 253, and you'll know what I mean!) Take, for example, my processed-free version of the Almond Joy candy bar, Joyful Chocolate Almond Bars (page 264). Here are the ingredients in my recipe: unsweetened shredded coconut, virgin coconut oil, coconut nectar or raw honey, vanilla extract, sea salt, unsweetened cocoa powder, liquid stevia, and raw almonds.

Now here's the ingredient list of the popular commercial version of this treat: corn syrup, milk chocolate (sugar; cocoa butter; chocolate; milk; lactose; milk fat; nonfat milk; soy lecithin; PGPR, emulsifier); coconut; sugar; almonds (roasted in cocoa butter and/or sunflower oil); contains 2 percent or less of: partially hydrogenated vegetable oil (soybean and palm oil); whey (milk); cocoa; salt; natural and artificial flavor; chocolate; soy lecithin; hydrolyzed milk protein; sodium metabisulfite, to maintain freshness; sulfur dioxide, to maintain freshness; caramel color.

Which would you rather put into your body?

The following guidelines will help you make healthy changes to any recipe.

Instead of this:	You can use this:
Butter, melted	Virgin coconut oil, melted
	Flaxseed oil (not for cooking; to be added after cooking—i.e., drizzled on cooked cereals, vegetables, or baked potatoes)
Butter, solid	Virgin coconut oil, solid
	Non-hydrogenated palm oil shortening
Buttermilk	Add 1 tablespoon lemon juice or raw organic unfiltered apple cider vinegar to a measuring cup, then add enough organic milk, unsweetened almond milk, or coconut milk to bring the volume to 1 cup. Let sit for 10 minutes to curdle.
Canola oil or other vegetable cooking oils	Virgin coconut oil, palm oil, or organic butter
Chocolate chips	85 percent or higher cacao dark chocolate bar with less than 6 grams of sugar per serving, cut into small pieces
	Raw cacao nibs
Cocoa powder	Carob powder
	Carob tastes similar to cocoa or chocolate but not exactly the same. Therefore, you should be familiar with the difference in flavor before attempting to substitute one for the other in a recipe. When substituting carob for chocolate, use 3 tablespoons carob powder plus 2 tablespoons water or milk for every ounce of unsweetened chocolate called for in the recipe.
Coffee	Dandy Blend herbal coffee alternative
	Teeccino herbal coffee alternative
Cornstarch	Arrowroot
	Arrowroot must be dissolved in a small amount of cold water before adding to recipes, otherwise it will clump and not thicken properly. Dissolve 1 tablespoon arrowroot with 1 or 2 tablespoons water and stir until it makes a slurry. Whisk into your simmering liquid until it thickens. You may need to add more, depending on the volume of your recipe.
Cake flour	Most cake flours are made from a combination of refined white flour and cornstarch. To replace this, you can use a combination of white whole wheat flour and arrowroot.
	For every cup of flour called for in a cake recipe, substitute ¾ cup white whole wheat flour and 2 tablespoons arrowroot powder, sifted together. This substitution can also be used for muffin and scone recipes.

Instead of this:	You can use this:
Eggs, for baking	Chia seeds or ground flaxseeds For each egg needed, combine 1 tablespoon whole chia seeds or gound flaxseeds with 3 tablespoons water. Let sit for 10 minutes to form a gel, then add to recipe. Fruit purées such as applesauce, banana, and pumpkin.
Heavy whipping cream Whipped cream Nondairy whipped topping	Coconut milk (use the full-fat version, not the light version) When placed in the refrigerator, the creamy fat layer inside a can of full-fat coconut milk will rise to the top. This can be separated from the liquid part of the milk, then whipped with an electric mixer just like whipping cream to make an all-natural nondairy whipped topping. Please note: The full-fat version of coconut milk must be used to make whipping cream. The light versions do not have enough of a cream layer.
Mayonnaise (most commercially available mayonnaise contains canola oil or soybean oil)	Truly Healthy Organic Mayonnaise (page 159) Mashed avocado Plain yogurt
Milk	Unsweetened almond milk Coconut milk Unsweetened rice milk Unsweetened hemp milk
Milk, evaporated or condensed	Coconut milk
Nondairy coffee creamers	Coconut milk Unsweetened almond milk Coconut cream concentrate
Pasta made from white flour	Brown rice pasta Quinoa pasta Whole spelt pasta Corn pasta Whole wheat pasta Sprouted grain pasta There are many commercially available whole grain pastas that can easily replace regular pasta. Try different types to see which ones have the taste and texture desired for your dish. Brown rice pastas are the most like white flour pastas in texture and taste, while sprouted grain pastas are the most dense and chewy.

(continues)

(continued)

Instead of this:	You can use this:
Philadelphia cream cheese	Organic Neufchâtel
Pumpkin pie spice	1½ teaspoons ground cinnamon ¾ teaspoon ground ginger ¼ teaspoon ground nutmeg ¼ teaspoon ground cloves
Refined white sugar	See the natural sweeteners chart on page 47.
Sour cream	Yogurt
Unflavored gelatin	Agar-agar Agar-agar comes in powdered form or flakes. 1 tablespoon gelatin granules = 2 tablespoons agar-agar flakes = 1 teaspoon agar-agar powder To gel 2 cups of liquid, dissolve 1 tablespoon agar-agar flakes or 1 teaspoon agar-agar powder in 4 tablespoons hot water. Bring water to a boil. Simmer for 1 to 5 minutes for powder and 10 to 15 minutes for flakes. Add to recipe, mix well, then let it cool to set. It dissolves in hot liquid but does not require refrigeration to gel; it will thicken and set at room temperature.
White flour, including: All-purpose flour Enriched unbleached flour Bread flour Cake flour	Whole grain flours, sprouted or unsprouted, including: Whole wheat flour White whole wheat flour Sprouted wheat flour Sprouted white wheat flour Whole wheat pastry flour

Natural Sweeteners

Eating processed-free doesn't mean going without sweets. However, when we do indulge our sweet tooth, it is best to do it with sweeteners that will nourish us, rather than deplete us. These sweeteners, which can be used in a variety of ways to replace white sugar, are balanced by a wide range of nutrients that slow down the absorption of their naturally occurring sugars into the bloodstream and provide the body with nutrients. They can be found at natural food markets and online. See Resources (page 279) for recommended brands.

Sweetener	Why It's Healthy	How to Use It
Traditional barley malt syrup, organic	This dark brown syrup is made from sprouted barley. It is a whole grain sweetener made by an ancient technique that uses only water and the grain's own enzymes created during the sprouting process to produce a thick, nutrient-rich syrup that is about half as sweet as refined sugar and has a consistency and flavor similar to molasses. It's important to use only traditional 100 percent barley malt syrup made from sprouted barley—not barley/corn malt syrup, which is made using pharmaceutical, artificially produced enzymes and other chemicals to speed and increase production.	Barley malt syrup is a versatile sweetener. It's great in granola and on pancakes, in cookies, popcorn balls, and caramel corn. It can also be used to sweeten homemade chocolate. It makes moist spice cakes, gingerbread, whole grain breads, muffins, and dark breads like pumpernickel. It is also delicious in baked beans and barbecue sauces and with roasted or baked sweet potatoes and winter squash. It can also be used in home brewing. Substitute 1½ cups barley malt syrup for every 1 cup white sugar called for. Reduce liquid in recipe by ¼ cup and add ¼ teaspoon baking soda per cup barley malt syrup used. If a lighter, sweeter flavor is desired, barley malt syrup can be combined with another natural sweetener.
Blackstrap molasses, unsulphured	This viscous sweetener is produced as a by-product of the sugar-refining process. It contains most, if not all, of the redeeming value of the original sugarcane—such as B vitamins, calcium, iron, magnesium, potassium, chromium, and antioxidants. See page 24 for more of blackstrap molasses' health-promoting properties.	Blackstrap molasses is an excellent sweetener in baked beans, quick breads, cookies, cakes, and pies. It can also be added to shakes and smoothies. Given the bold taste that molasses will provide your recipe, it is advisable that only a portion of the required sugar in any recipe be replaced, as molasses can substantially change the taste of baked goods. Use 1 tablespoon molasses to replace ½ cup sugar.

(continues)

(continued)

Sweetener	Why It's Healthy	How to Use It
Brown rice syrup	Brown rice syrup is produced by fermenting brown rice that has been ground and cooked with special enzymes that disintegrate the natural starch of the grain to produce a lightly sweet, amber-colored syrup with a mild butterscotch flavor. It has only half the sweetness of sugar. Sweeteners made from malted grains retain at least some of the nutrients found in the whole grain as well as complex sugars, which take longer to digest, helping to keep blood sugar levels even. Two tablespoons of brown rice syrup provides 3 percent of the daily requirement of sodium and potassium. Brown rice syrup is a complex sugar that is absorbed and utilized more slowly than simple sugars and has a low glycemic index (25). Complex sugars are also more easily used by the body for energy, which means less is stored as fat for later use. However, diabetics still need to use it sparingly and with caution.	Brown rice syrup is nice drizzled over pancakes or waffles, or use it in recipes for cookies, granola, pies, puddings, and ice cream. Baked goods made with brown rice syrup tend to be hard or very crisp. It is not recommended for use in cakes or any type of bread, as it produces a gooey center. Substitute brown rice syrup in place of sugar, honey, corn syrup, maple syrup, or regular molasses (not blackstrap). To substitute sugar, use 1¼ cups brown rice syrup for 1 cup sugar. Reduce the liquid by ¼ cup.
Coconut nectar	This thick, syrupy liquid is a naturally sweet, nutrient-rich "sap" that is tapped from the blossoms that grow on coconut palm trees. As it comes from the flowers and not the coconut itself, it has no coconut flavor. Its mild taste is similar to butterscotch or caramel. Coconut nectar's glycemic index is low (35). It contains 17 amino acids, minerals, vitamin C, and B vitamins. Coconut nectar is considered a raw, enzymatically alive sweetener that has been minimally evaporated to remove moisture and thicken the nectar.	Coconut nectar can be drizzled over pancakes and waffles and added to beverages, and it works well in recipes for muffins, quick breads, and ice cream. It can be used in a 1:1 ratio to replace the liquid sweetener in any recipe. To replace white sugar, it is better to use the dehydrated version called coconut sugar (see below).
Coconut crystals, a.k.a. coconut sugar and palm sugar	When coconut nectar is evaporated down to its crystalline form, the end result is coconut crystals. They are brown or sandy-colored coarse crystals closely resembling organic whole cane sugar. They have a caramel taste similar to nectar, with the same low glycemic index and nutritional benefits.	Coconut crystals are the ideal sweetener to use in cookies, granola, muffins, brownies, quick breads, ice cream, and other desserts. They can be used in a 1:1 ratio to replace white or brown sugar in any recipe. (If your recipe calls for both white and brown sugar, you can replace both with coconut sugar.)

Sweetener	Why It's Healthy	How to Use It
Date sugar	The term sugar is really a misnomer here—this should actually be called ground dehydrated dates. It is simply the whole fruit that has been dried and ground into moist, coarse granules, and thus contains all of the nutrients and health benefits that dates bestow. It is high in fiber and contains a host of vitamins and minerals, including iron. (See page 17 for more on dates' nutritional benefits.) However, while dates are healthy, they should be consumed in small quantities, so small amounts of date sugar should also be the rule. The best date sugar is made from raw unsulphured dates.	Date sugar makes a great sprinkle or topping for fresh fruits, yogurt, hot cereals, and more. It does not work well for coating anything that will be baked, such as granola, as it can burn easily if exposed to high heat. It lends a unique flavor and sweetness that pairs well with whole grains, so it is a perfect sweetener to replace white or brown sugar in homemade bread recipes. It can be used in a 1:1 ratio to replace white or brown sugar, but some people have found that a 1:1 ratio is too sweet, so you may want to reduce it to ⅔ cup date sugar for every cup of white sugar called for in a recipe. Date sugar may also be used in combination with other sweeteners. Because it's not really a sugar, date sugar does not dissolve in liquids. As it naturally absorbs moisture, it tends to clump in storage, but it breaks up easily and can be re-ground in a blender or food processor, if necessary.
Organic whole cane sugar, unrefined and unbleached Organic Sucanat	Organic whole cane sugar is real raw sugar in its closest-to-natural form. It is produced by pressing the juice from raw sugarcane and evaporating off the water using low heat, not boiling. This method retains many of the vitamins, minerals, and antioxidants contained in sugarcane juice. The granules are coarse and amber colored with a mild molasses-like taste. Sucanat is a trade name that stands for SUgar CAne NATural. It is essentially the same sugar as organic whole cane sugar, but the two are packaged and sold by two different companies.	This is the sweetener I use most in my baking because of its rich flavor, relatively low cost, ease of substitution, and high nutrient value. Because it is real sugar, it can replace white sugar in virtually anything. It is especially great in cookies, muffins, quick breads, chocolate-based recipes, and barbecue sauces. It has the same sweetness as refined sugar and can be used in a 1:1 ratio to replace white or brown sugar in any recipe. If your recipe calls for both white and brown sugar, you can replace both with this unrefined sugar.

(continues)

(continued)

Sweetener	Why It's Healthy	How to Use It
Raw honey *Note: The best raw honey comes from local sources. Check your natural food market or farmers' market for locally produced raw honey.*	Raw honey refers to honey as it exists in the beehive and that has not been heat pasteurized or heated above 105°F during production or storage. Like coconut nectar, raw honey is an enzymatically alive raw food that is high in antioxidants, vitamins, and minerals. The taste of raw honey is more pure and delicious than pasteurized honey. It is 20 to 60 percent sweeter than white sugar, so less is needed for the same amount of sweetness. Some raw honey is solid and creamy and some is clear and pourable; it depends on the variety. Raw honey is not recommended for people with diabetes, as it can adversely affect blood sugar levels. Raw honey should not be given to children under one year of age because it can cause infant botulism, a rare and serious form of bacterial food poisoning that affects a baby's nervous system. Once a child reaches one year old, their digestive system is mature enough to kill any botulism germs.	Raw honey has many wonderful food uses. Its rich creaminess makes a nice spread on bread or muffins. It can be used to sweeten things like yogurt, smoothies, almond milk, and hot or iced beverages. It can also be used to make chocolate or other raw desserts. A little bit of honey goes a long way, so it's best not to overindulge. If using raw honey for baking, the heat will cause a loss of nutrients; however, it is still better to use raw honey for baking than pasteurized honey, as pasteurized honey is void of any nutrients whatsoever. (Putting raw honey in a cup of warm water or tea will not destroy its nutrients.) To replace white sugar with honey in baking, use half as much honey as white sugar in recipes. Reduce the liquid in the recipe by ¼ cup, but if there is no liquid to reduce, add 3 to 4 tablespoons additional whole grain flour or meal for each ½ cup honey used. Also add ⅛ teaspoon baking soda per ½ cup honey. Reduce the oven temperature by 25°F and adjust the baking time.
Pure maple syrup	Pure maple syrup is the product of the sap from sugar maple, red maple, or black maple trees. The syrup is made by collecting a quantity of sap and then carefully boiling it without chemicals or preservatives until the sap is reduced to a syrup. Pure maple syrup contains calcium, zinc, and manganese, as well as more than 20 antioxidant compounds reported to have anticancer, antibacterial, and antidiabetic properties.	Pure maple syrup can be used in all baked goods and is wonderful in cakes and pies. Substitute ⅔ to ¾ cup maple syrup for 1 cup white sugar. Reduce the liquid in the recipe by 3 tablespoons and add ¼ teaspoon baking soda per cup of maple syrup. It is great drizzled on whole grain pancakes and waffles.

Sweetener	Why It's Healthy	How to Use It

Stevia
 	
Note: A company called SweetLeaf produces the best-tasting and most unprocessed form of liquid stevia extract called Stevia Clear. They also offer a variety of naturally flavored liquid stevia extracts called Sweet Drops. These make a great addition to teas, herbal coffee, sparkling water, yogurt, and a variety of recipes. See Resources (page 279) for more info.
	Stevia is an herb that has been used for centuries in South America for its sweetening and medicinal properties. Its sweetness comes from compounds in the plant's leaves called glycosides, which are 200 to 300 times sweeter than sugar. As it is an herb, stevia has no calories and does not affect blood sugar levels. This is the best sweetener for diabetics.
	
	Stevia's leaves contain many nutrients, including chromium, calcium, magnesium, potassium, iron, beta-carotene, vitamin C, niacin, protein, and antioxidants.
	
	Stevia can be purchased in several forms: as a fresh live plant; as dried leaves in bulk or in tea bags; as a dark unfiltered liquid extract; as a clear filtered liquid extract; as a white powder in bulk form; as a white powder in individual packets; and as dissolvable tablets.
		The leaves of the stevia plant can be eaten fresh or put in teas and foods.
		
		Liquid and powder forms of stevia can be added to yogurt, hot cereal, sparkling water, cold or hot beverages, sauces, smoothies, and recipes for baked goods.
		
		Stevia can be used in cooking and baking. It is heat stable to 400°F.
		
		For use in baking, use the following approximate measurements for using stevia in place of sugar:
		
		1 cup sugar =
		  1 teaspoon stevia liquid extract
		  1½ to 2 tablespoons white stevia powder
		  18 to 24 individual stevia packets
		  2 teaspoons dark stevia concentrate (use to replace brown sugar)
		
		If you are using stevia to replace sugar in one of your favorite recipes, you will have to experiment and make some adjustments. The small amounts of stevia don't add the type of volume that a cup of sugar does, therefore the volume of sugar needs to be replaced. If your recipe calls for 1 cup sugar, you can use ⅓ cup mashed bananas, unsweetened applesauce, apple butter, plain yogurt, sour cream, cream cheese, oatmeal, or whatever else you think will work as the volume replacement.
		
		Also, stevia does not activate yeast, so it can't replace sugar in yeast bread recipes.

THESE RECIPES COVER A BROAD CULINARY spectrum—some are super quick and easy, some are more challenging and require more time and planning. Many are suitable for diabetics and those with gluten sensitivities. The main point is to use whole-food ingredients that have high nutrient value and to enjoy the fruits of your labor (pun intended).

When eggs are called for in a recipe, I recommend using large eggs (preferably organic and pastured). I also recommend using grass-fed organic beef; pasture-raised poultry; organic dairy products such as butter, cheese, and yogurt; and wild-caught fish whenever possible. I want you to know, however, that most of the recipes can be made using conventional ingredients if those are your only options.

For my own cooking, I try to buy the best food I can afford, but I do watch my pennies and sometimes even go for the least expensive options. However, I do prioritize. I make sure to always buy organic dairy products, grass-fed if I can get them, and when available I buy raw cheeses either from the grocery store or the farmers' market. If the type of cheese I want to use in a recipe is not available raw, then my next best choice is organic.

I don't use cow's milk in any of my recipes for muffins, pancakes, waffles, or other baked goods, but it can be used in place of the specified nondairy milks if you want to use it. Just substitute the same amount of cow's milk in any recipe calling for nondairy milk.

I always buy organic lettuce, celery, and carrots, as they are on the Environmental Working Group's (EWG) Dirty Dozen list. I also opt for organic apples, strawberries, and grapes. If I'm using citrus zest or peel in a recipe, I use an organic citrus. And since I recommend leaving the skins on potatoes, those are on the top of my organic list as well. I try to keep in mind the other produce items on the Dirty Dozen list, but buying everything organic is cost prohibitive and not always realistic or necessary.

In the previous chapters, I've introduced you to the concepts of soaking nuts, seeds, legumes, and grains to neutralize antinutrients and increase digestibility. In my recipes, I refer to nuts and seeds as "raw, preferably soaked and dried," which is the ideal and most nutritious way to consume them. However, I realize that soaking and drying may be new food preparation techniques for you, and you may not have the time or ability to do it. It is still better to use nuts and seeds in their raw unsoaked form than in their roasted form. Always purchase raw nuts and seeds to use in recipes. And if you can, please do soak and dry them first according to the instructions on page 37. Similarly, the whole grains and whole grain flours in the recipes should ideally be soaked and/or sprouted ahead of time before using in the recipes. Sprouted grain flours can be purchased in natural food markets, which can save you some time. Again, if these techniques are new to you, you can use regular unsprouted whole grains and whole grain flours in the recipes when indicated. For instance, if a recipe calls for sprouted wheat flour, you can use traditional or white whole wheat flour interchangeably in most cases. The idea of introducing you to the traditional food preparation techniques is to provide your body with the optimal nutritional benefits from your foods.

Having said that, there is one staple pantry item that I like to splurge on—organic canned beans from Eden Foods. These are the only canned beans I know of that are soaked overnight in purified water before cooking. They also come in BPA-free cans. For these reasons, Eden Foods is the brand of canned beans I use in my recipes when I don't have time to soak and cook beans myself. However, any brand of canned beans will work in the recipes.

Finally, I have included a number of dessert recipes that are definitely in the "splurge" category because I know those occasions will come up, and when they do I want you to feel good about treating yourself and those you invite to your table to a nutrient-dense, high-quality indulgence that will nourish your body rather than deplete it in the way most sweet treats do. While my cookies and other treats are definitely healthier than any you can buy in a store, please don't assume that you should make and eat them as everyday fare.

4

Foundational Do-It-Yourself Recipes

Here are recipes for some key staple ingredients, all of which are used in several recipes throughout this book. I specifically selected these because their grocery store counterparts are not as healthy as they are marketed to be; these homemade staples are much higher in nutrients and flavor when freshly prepared yourself. I am not suggesting that you should never buy a jar of nut butter or a can of coconut milk, but if you have the inclination, you'll find that many of these staple items are very quick and easy to make yourself. All it takes is a little preplanning, and soon you'll be stocking your fridge and freezer with homemade items you use frequently.

NUTRIENT-RICH BROTHS

Broths are an indispensable cooking staple, so much so that you'll find a large pot of broth simmering in the kitchen of most five-star restaurants. But there is much more to broth than just the taste. When prepared the traditional way, by simmering over low heat for many hours, broth is more like a superfood.

Almost every culture throughout history has used broth for its nutritional significance and culinary versatility, and today many societies around the world still consume broth regularly for those same reasons. Consuming broth is also one of the most economical ways to boost your intake of nutrients that are essential to good health.

Vegetable broth has many merits of its own, but broth made from the bones of animals has unique and unrivaled health benefits. Typically made from the bones of chicken or beef, it can also be made from lamb or fish bones. The cooking water is acidified with a small amount of raw organic unfiltered apple cider vinegar or lemon juice to draw the minerals and other nutrients out of the bones while they cook. The finished broth is rich in calcium, magnesium, and other trace minerals, and gelatin—a protein substance that has numerous regenerative healing effects on the body, including healing the lining of the intestinal tract, boosting the immune system, and breaking up cholesterol buildup in the arteries. Gelatin also contains glucosamine and chondroitin, two compounds that help alleviate the degenerative effects of arthritis and joint pain by helping to rebuild joint cartilage in our bodies. Push the supplements aside and opt for a warm cup of homemade broth instead!

While store-bought broths may be more convenient and easy to use, they don't provide the health-building properties that traditionally prepared broths have been revered for throughout history. Even the organic varieties contain added sugar, refined cooking oils, and questionable flavor-enhancing additives such as yeast extract and "natural flavorings" (two hidden sources of monosodium glutamate) to make up for the poor quality of the broth. For these reasons, I offer you the following simple recipes for making your own broth, both meat- and vegetable-based.

CHICKEN BROTH

Homemade, nutrient-dense bone broth is easy and inexpensive to make. For the price of one chicken, you get the meat plus several quarts of broth.

There are two ways to make chicken broth: (1) By using the remaining bones from a whole roasted chicken or from baked or grilled chicken parts, after you've removed all the meat. When

I roast a chicken, I remove all the usable meat to use for meals, and then I save the carcass with all the remaining little pieces of meat still clinging to the bones. The bones can be saved in the refrigerator if you are going to make broth the next day or frozen for up to a month to make broth later. (2) By using a whole uncooked chicken or uncooked chicken parts with bones. An optional nutritional boost can be had from adding two chicken feet, which will lend a much higher concentration of nutrient-rich gelatin. Chicken feet are difficult to find in regular stores, but you can ask your butcher if he has any. There are also online sources to buy high-quality chickens and chicken feet (see Resources, page 274).

Select high-quality organic chicken if possible, although the bones from a store-bought rotisserie chicken are fine. One chicken carcass will make anywhere from 1½ to 3 quarts of chicken broth. The general guideline is 2 pounds of bones (about 2 to 3 full chicken carcasses) per gallon of water.

The following procedures use a slow cooker, but you can also make these in a stockpot on the stove. The cooking time is just as long, but when you use a slow cooker you don't have to worry about leaving your stove on for six to twenty-four hours. If you don't have a slow cooker and are uncomfortable leaving your stove on for the length of time required to cook the broth, you can let it cook while you are at home, turn off the heat when you leave the house or while sleeping, and then turn the heat back on when you are home and awake. Do this as many times as you need to until you've reached the cumulative number of hours of cooking time. The only downside to doing it this way is that every time you turn the stove back on, you have to bring the broth up to a boil again and skim the scum off the top before turning the heat back down to the slow simmer. This technique is safe and has been practiced in homes around the world for generations.

CHICKEN BROTH MADE FROM LEFTOVER CHICKEN BONES

• Makes 4 quarts, using a 6-quart slow cooker •

1 chicken carcass from a roasted chicken	4 garlic cloves
1 medium yellow onion, cut in half	2 bay leaves
1 to 2 celery stalks, cut in half	¼ cup raw organic unfiltered apple cider vinegar
1 to 2 small carrots, cut in half	1 bunch fresh curly parsley

Place all ingredients except the parsley in a slow cooker. Cover with enough water to come within about 2 inches of the top of the slow cooker. Let everything soak for 30 minutes before turning on the slow cooker.

Set to low heat and cook for a minimum of 6 hours and up to 24 hours. (You can let it cook overnight and all the next day while you are at work.) This can also be cooked on the stovetop: Let the bones soak in the pot first for 30 minutes, the same as with the slow cooker method. Bring the pot to a boil, skim off any foam that forms, then reduce the heat to a low simmer and cook for 6 to 24 hours.

About 10 minutes before taking the broth off the heat, add the bunch of parsley.

Remove the carcass (or bones) from the slow cooker and discard.

Pass the broth through a fine-mesh strainer or a regular strainer lined with cheesecloth into a large bowl. Discard the vegetables—there are no more nutrients left in them, as they all went into the broth.

Place the broth in the refrigerator to chill until the fat congeals on top. Scrape the fat off with a spoon. Store the broth in quart-size jars or half-gallon containers. Refrigerate the broth up to 5 days or store in the freezer if not using it right away (see page 61 for tips on freezing broth).

Making turkey broth follows the same process, so don't throw out that Thanksgiving turkey carcass!

CHICKEN BROTH MADE FROM A WHOLE UNCOOKED CHICKEN

THE IDEA HERE IS THE SAME EXCEPT THAT YOU'RE USING AN UNCOOKED CHICKEN. YOU CAN USE chicken parts as well, as long as they have the bones.

• Makes 4 quarts, using a 6-quart slow cooker •

1 whole uncooked chicken	4 celery stalks, cut in half
¼ cup raw organic unfiltered apple cider vinegar	4 small carrots, cut in half
1 tablespoon sea salt	4 garlic cloves
2 teaspoons freshly ground black pepper	2 bay leaves
1 medium yellow onion, cut in half	1 bunch fresh curly parsley

Rinse and pat dry the chicken and place it in the slow cooker. If your chicken included the neck and giblets, you can add those as well. Top the chicken with the vinegar, salt, and pepper. Add the rest of the ingredients except the parsley and enough water to cover everything. Let soak for 30 minutes before turning on the slow cooker.

Set to low heat and cook for a minimum of 8 hours and up to 24 hours. (You can let it cook overnight and all the next day while you are at work.) This can also be cooked on the stovetop: Let the chicken soak in the pot first for 30 minutes, the same as with the slow cooker method. Bring the pot to a boil, skim off any foam that forms, then reduce the heat to a low simmer and cook for 6 to 24 hours.

About 10 minutes before taking the broth off the heat, add the bunch of parsley.

Take the chicken out of the broth, let it cool, and remove the meat from the bones to use for meals. The soft bones may be given to pets or discarded.

Strain, chill, scrape off the fat, and store as above.

BEEF BROTH

AKING BEEF BROTH FOLLOWS THE SAME PROCEDURE AS MAKING CHICKEN BROTH. YOU CAN USE meat with bones on it, bones leftover from pieces of meat that you've already eaten, or you can purchase "soup bones" from a butcher or local farm. The best bones are from grass-fed organic beef. You may also use lamb, buffalo, and venison bones to make different broths, but the method will be the same.

• Makes 4 quarts, using a 6-quart slow cooker •

1 yellow onion, chopped	3 to 4 pounds beef bones
4 small carrots, chopped	Pinch of sea salt
4 celery stalks, chopped	¼ cup raw organic unfiltered apple
6 garlic cloves, chopped	cider vinegar
2 bay leaves	1 bunch fresh curly parsley

Place the vegetables in the bottom of the slow cooker, then add the bay leaves and the bones. Sprinkle the salt over the bones, then pour the vinegar over them. Fill the slow cooker with enough water to cover the bones. Let soak for 30 minutes.

Set the slow cooker to low heat and cook for 8 to 10 hours.

About 10 minutes before taking the broth off the heat, add the parsley.

When done, strain the broth through a fine-mesh strainer into a large bowl. Let cool, then place the broth in the refrigerator to chill until the fat congeals on top. Scrape the fat off with a spoon. Store the broth in quart-size jars or half-gallon containers. Refrigerate the broth up to 5 days or store in the freezer if not using it right away (see page 61 for tips on freezing broth).

Stovetop method: Bring the pot to a boil, skim off any foam that forms, then reduce the heat to a low simmer and cook for a minimum of 12 hours and as long as 72 hours. See page 57 for notes on long cooking time.

VEGETABLE BROTH

WELL-PREPARED VEGETABLE BROTH PROVIDES YOU WITH MANY ALKALINE-FORMING AND LIVER-supporting nutrients that cleanse your body, speed up weight loss, and increase energy. Like bone broth, it can be enjoyed by the cup or used to make meals.

Vegetable broth is the easiest of the broths to make and is the most versatile in its uses. Its flavor lends itself well to both vegetarian and meat-based soups, stews, grain dishes, and sautés.

It is also the most economical because you can use almost any vegetable, especially the not-so-pretty pieces of vegetables left over from making salads or other recipes. As I do with saving the bones from my chickens and beef, I have a dedicated container in the freezer for saving the ends of celery, carrots, fennel, leeks, and onions, kale stems, and the sliced-off tops of garlic heads used to make roasted garlic. When I have enough scraps and enough time, I make a big pot of broth.

When you make your own vegetable broth, you can significantly limit the salt you add or skip it altogether. Using a small amount of dried sea vegetables, such as kelp, nori, or kombu, can lend a natural salty flavor while adding a rich source of natural iodine and alkaline-forming minerals such as calcium and magnesium. Onions, leeks, and herbs (fresh or dried) such as parsley, oregano, basil, and thyme also add flavor without adding salt.

Fresh garlic is a vegetable broth–flavoring essential—you can use an entire head of garlic, and you don't need to spend time peeling the tight skins off of each clove. Simply remove the outer papery husks and crack them open to expose the insides of the clove by smashing them with the side of a chef's knife, then toss them into the pot, skins and all.

The vegetables and amounts below are a guideline for making a nutrient-rich vegetable broth, but don't feel limited by what's listed. The beauty of vegetable broth is that you can use whatever you have on hand.

• Makes 2 quarts (recipe can be doubled, tripled, or
quadrupled to make a large quantity of broth) •

4 large carrots, sliced (about 2 cups)

2 to 3 large celery stalks, including leaves, chopped (about 1 cup)

1 large yellow onion, cut into chunks (about 2 cups)

2 medium red potatoes, quartered

2 leeks, cut into chunks (white and light-green parts only; about 2 cups)

2 cups chopped greens with stems: kale, beet greens, collard greens, chard, dandelion, or other greens

1 garlic head, cloves separated and smashed (remove excess paper, but skins can be left on)

2 bay leaves

4 to 6 sprigs fresh thyme, or 2 teaspoons dried thyme

Large handful of fresh curly parsley sprigs

½ to 1 teaspoon sea salt or Herbamare, or 1 handful of dried seaweed: nori, kelp, or kombu (optional)

½ teaspoon whole peppercorns

10 cups water

Place all the vegetables into the slow cooker. Add the bay leaves, herbs, salt, if using, and peppercorns. Pour in the water to cover everything, place the lid on the slow cooker, and cook on the low setting for 8 to 12 hours. Turn off the heat. Place a fine-mesh strainer over a large bowl or line a colander with cheesecloth and place over the bowl. Carefully strain the broth. Let the vegetables drain over the bowl for 5 minutes or more. Squeeze any remaining broth from the vegetables by pressing them with your hands or the back of a large spoon. Discard the vegetables. Transfer the broth to storage containers and let cool completely before putting the lid on. The broth can be stored in the refrigerator for up to 3 days or in the freezer for up to 3 months (see below for tips on freezing broth).

Stovetop Method: Combine all the ingredients in a large stockpot. Bring to a boil, reduce the heat to medium, and simmer uncovered for 1½ hours. Turn off the heat, strain, and store as described above.

VARIATIONS

- Instead of celery, use 1 large fennel bulb, including leaves, coarsely chopped.
- Instead of parsley, use 2 sprigs of fresh oregano (or 2 teaspoons dried) and 2 tablespoons of chopped fresh basil leaves (or 2 teaspoons dried).
- Instead of potatoes, use other root veggies such as turnips, parsnips, or rutabagas and/or 2 cups of cubed winter squash such as butternut, acorn, or pumpkin.

TIPS FOR FREEZING AND THAWING BROTH

- *The best containers for freezing broth are glass mason jars or freezer-safe Pyrex.*
- *Do not fill the containers all the way. As the broth freezes, it will expand, so it is important to leave plenty of air space above the broth for expansion during freezing. A general rule is to leave at least 1 inch of air space above the liquid.*
- *Leave the lids off the containers and let the broth completely cool to room temperature before freezing. Even slight warmth can cause the containers to break in the freezer.*
- *If you have time to plan ahead, the best way to thaw frozen broth stored in glass containers is to leave it in the refrigerator overnight.*
- *For quick thawing in a pinch, place the glass container in a big bowl of cool or room temperature water and let it sit for about 10 minutes. Do not place frozen containers of broth into warm or hot water initially, as the quick change in temperature will cause the glass to break. After 10 minutes, you can replace the cold water in the bowl with warm water and let it sit for a few minutes. After that, you can replace the water in the bowl with hot water to hasten the thawing process.*

BETTER-THAN-BOXED ALMOND/NUT MILK

Almond milk makes a tasty, nutritious alternative to dairy milk, and you'll see it used in a variety of recipes throughout this book. While the use of a commercially prepared almond milk is convenient, you should be aware that many of them contain synthetic vitamins and a stabilizing agent called carrageenan—a food additive that has recently been linked to a host of digestive diseases and colon cancer.

With this basic recipe, you can make other nut milks (Brazil, cashew, hazelnut, macadamia, pecan, pistachio) and experiment with different flavor varieties, such as vanilla, chocolate, strawberry, etc.

• Makes 3 to 4 cups •

1 cup raw almonds	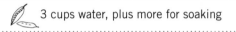 3 cups water, plus more for soaking

Place the almonds in a large bowl and add enough water to cover them well. Cover the bowl with a towel and leave the almonds in a cool place or in the refrigerator to soak for at least 8 hours and up to 24 hours (see the chart and notes on pages 38–39 for soaking times for other nuts). Soaking will plump the almonds and soften them in addition to increasing the nutritional value of the milk. If you don't want to strain the pulp from your almond milk, it is recommended to let them soak for the full 24 hours.

When ready to make the almond milk, drain the almonds in a colander and rinse them well with water. Shake as much water off the almonds as possible.

Place the 3 cups of fresh water in a blender and add the soaked almonds. Blend on high speed for a few minutes, or until the mixture is well blended and smooth. You will see the almond pulp suspended in the milk, and when you remove the cover of your blender, the top of the milk will be frothy.

Notes:

You may want to invest in a nut-milk strainer bag (about $7 to $12 online; see Resources, page 282)—a fine-mesh nylon bag that makes straining the almond pulp easy and is highly recommended. Once you have blended the almond milk and removed the cover from your blender, the nut-milk strainer bag slips over the top of the blender so you can just invert the contents into the bag and collect the almond milk in another large container. The nut-milk bag has a drawstring to keep it closed and makes squeezing all of the almond milk out of the bag clean and efficient. Nut-milk strainer bags are easy to clean and can be reused many times.

Strain the almond milk through a fine-mesh sieve, cheesecloth, or nut-milk bag strainer (see notes) into your original bowl or another large container, such as a pitcher. Press or squeeze as much of the milk from the almond pulp as possible. You can discard the almond pulp or save it for a variety of uses (see below).

Store it in a tightly sealed container in the refrigerator and use it within a week. You will need to stir or shake the almond milk every time you use it since it does settle.

FLAVOR VARIATIONS

- To flavor or sweeten the almond milk, pour it back into the clean blender and add 2 pitted dates (or desired amount of other sweetener) and 1 teaspoon vanilla or almond extract. Blend again until the sweetener and flavors are incorporated. Store as directed above.

- For chocolate almond milk: Add 2 pitted dates (or desired amount of other sweetener), 1 teaspoon pure vanilla extract, and 2 teaspoons unsweetened cocoa powder.

- For strawberry almond milk: Add 2 pitted dates (or desired amount of other sweetener), 1 teaspoon pure vanilla extract, and ½ cup fresh or frozen strawberries.

 ### USES FOR LEFTOVER ALMOND PULP

ALTHOUGH MANY OF THE NUTRIENTS AND flavor from the almonds goes into the milk, the leftover pulp still has valuable fiber and nutrients that can enhance other foods. You can simply store the almond pulp in an air-tight container in your refrigerator and use it within a few days, or it can be stored for up to one month in the freezer for use later. Here's a few ideas for using your leftover almond pulp:

- Add 1 to 2 tablespoons into your cup of yogurt.

- Experiment with adding small amounts (about ¼ cup) to muffin batters and quick breads for added moisture.
- Add ¼ cup to granola before baking.
- Add 1 to 2 tablespoons to pancake batter.
- Stir 1 to 2 tablespoons into hot cereals during the last minute of cooking.
- Use it in Lavender-Spiced Almond Pulp Crackers (page 141).
- Dehydrate it and turn it into almond meal (see page 72).

COCONUT MILK

AT FIRST GLANCE YOU MAY THINK THAT MAKING YOUR OWN COCONUT MILK IS A DIFFICULT TASK INVOLVING real whole coconuts and a big machete. That *is* one way to make coconut milk, but there are easier ways that are less dangerous! As with making your own almond milk, homemade coconut milk helps you avoid the myriad food additives that are often added to the commercial varieties (see the sidebar on page 67 for a list of coconut milk ingredients to avoid). Coconut milk provides your body with medium-chain triglycerides (MCTs), a healthy type of saturated fat with a long list of health benefits, including weight loss and improved thyroid function. You'll see coconut milk used in many of the recipes, so it's nice to be able to whip up a cup or two whenever you need it.

Here you'll find four ways to make homemade coconut milk, with the easiest and most convenient way first.

COCONUT MILK FROM
COCONUT CREAM CONCENTRATE

COCONUT CREAM CONCENTRATE IS ALSO KNOWN AS COCONUT BUTTER; YOU'LL FIND IT IN JARS at natural food markets and online. The flavor of this coconut milk depends on the brand of coconut cream concentrate you use (see the Resources section on page 281 for recommended brands). The nice thing about making coconut milk this way is that you can control how thick or thin you want it, and you can make as much or as little as you need.

• Makes 1 cup •

1 cup water	1 to 2 teaspoons coconut cream concentrate (listed in headnote)

Put the ingredients in a blender and blend until smooth and creamy. If the milk is not thick and creamy enough for you, add more coconut cream concentrate; if it's too thick, add more water. Store it in the refrigerator for up to 4 days. Since there are no fillers, gums, or stabilizers in homemade coconut milk, the cream may separate from the water when stored in the refrigerator, so you may need to shake, stir, or blend it again on your next use.

COCONUT MILK FROM
UNSWEETENED SHREDDED COCONUT

THE KEY IS TO USE THE NATURAL, UNSWEETENED VARIETY OF SHREDDED COCONUT. THIS RECIPE also yields coconut pulp. If you want to reuse the pulp, it can be dehydrated into coconut flour, which you can then use in baking. See the recipe on page 72 for how to dehydrate almond pulp to make flour. The method is the same for coconut pulp.

• Makes 2 cups •

2 cups unsweetened shredded coconut	2 cups hot (not boiling) water

Put the shredded coconut in a blender and add the hot water. Blend on high for 3 minutes, or until thick and creamy.

Place a colander in a bowl and line it with four thicknesses of cheesecloth. Pour the blended coconut milk mixture into the cheesecloth and let the milk collect in the bowl underneath. Take up the corners of the cheesecloth to make a sack holding the coconut pulp and then twist it to gently squeeze out the rest of the milk into the bowl. Alternatively, you can use a nut-milk strainer bag.

The coconut milk will be warm, but you can drink or use it immediately in a recipe. Store it in the refrigerator for up to 4 days. Since there are no fillers, gums, or stabilizers in homemade coconut milk, it may separate when stored in the refrigerator, so you may need to shake, stir, or blend the milk again on your next use.

COCONUT MILK FROM A YOUNG THAI COCONUT

THIS IS THE BEST AND MOST AUTHENTIC TYPE OF COCONUT MILK, AS IT IS THE WAY MOST commercially prepared coconut milk is made. It does involve cracking open the coconut, which requires a cleaver or a large chef's knife and a bit of courage (see note)! Young coconuts are distinguishable from mature coconuts because they have a white, fibrous coconut husk instead of a dark, hairy outer shell. The husk often has a cone-shaped point at the top of the coconut and is leveled on the bottom, allowing the coconut to be set on a flat surface.

• Makes about 1 quart •

2 young Thai coconuts

Crack open the coconuts (see note) and pour the coconut water into your blender. Take a large metal spoon and scrape out the soft coconut meat from the inside of the coconut and place it in the blender with the coconut water. Blend on high until the coconut milk is smooth and creamy. Drink immediately or use in a recipe. Store in the refrigerator for up to 4 days.

> **NOTE: HOW TO CRACK A YOUNG COCONUT**
>
> *Cracking open a young coconut requires practice, but once you learn, it's very easy. These are general guidelines; there are many online tutorials and YouTube videos that can help you master the technique. To crack open a young coconut, place the coconut on a hard flat surface with the point facing up. Hold the coconut at the bottom with one hand and hold your cleaver or chef's knife in the other hand. Being very careful, whack around the base of the cone-shaped top to make deep cuts all around the cone. If needed, use your knife to cut through any spots that you missed. You should then be able to stick the tip of your knife through the coconut husk and move it around to lift off the top of the cone.*

COCONUT MILK FROM A MATURE COCONUT

THIS METHOD ALSO INVOLVES CRACKING OPEN A COCONUT. IT IS THE MOST LABOR-INTENSIVE METHOD and is more suited for those who want to be adventuresome in the kitchen. It requires a sharp knife and an ice pick or a hammer. Strong arms are recommended! Mature coconuts are the round, brown hairy coconuts you are probably most familiar with. They are hard on the outside, and the inside flesh is also hard. When selecting a coconut for making coconut milk, hold it up to your ear and shake it. If you hear the sloshing of the coconut water inside, you've got one that's nice and fresh.

This recipe will yield coconut pulp, which can be dehydrated into dried shredded coconut for use in recipes. See the recipe on page 72 for how to dehydrate almond pulp. The method is the same for coconut pulp.

• Makes about 1 quart •

2 brown mature coconuts 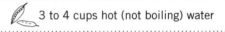 3 to 4 cups hot (not boiling) water

Puncture and crack the coconuts and remove the flesh (see note), then place the pieces of coconut meat and the coconut water in a blender. Add the hot water and blend until the coconut and water forms a smooth, creamy slurry.

Place a colander in a bowl and line it with four thicknesses of cheesecloth. Pour the blended coconut milk mixture into the cheesecloth and let the milk collect in the bowl underneath. Take up the corners of the cheesecloth to make a sack holding the coconut pulp and then twist it to gently squeeze out the rest of the milk into the bowl. Alternatively, you can use a nut-milk strainer bag.

The coconut milk will be warm, but you can drink or use it immediately in a recipe. Store in the refrigerator for up to 4 days.

> **NOTE: HOW TO CRACK A MATURE COCONUT**
>
> *To crack open a mature coconut, it is very helpful to first put it in the freezer for an hour; this helps separate the meat from the shell.*
>
> *Find the "eyes" on the top of the coconut (three small relatively soft spots that are positioned like the finger holes in a bowling ball). One of the eyes will be the softest. Puncture that one and one other with a sharp knife or ice pick. Drain the coconut water into a bowl or large glass. Taste the water; if it doesn't taste sweet, then the coconut is rancid and should not be used to make milk.*
>
> *Wrap the coconut in a towel and place it on a hard surface—a driveway or cement patio is ideal— then whack it near its center with a hammer or rolling pin until it cracks open. Pry the meat away from the shell with an oyster knife or any dull knife. (There's also a tool you can buy called a coconut meat removal knife; see Resources, page 282.) Use a vegetable peeler or sharp knife to peel off any remaining brown membrane that adheres to the coconut meat. Cut the coconut meat into small pieces for easier blending.*

BUYING COCONUT MILK?
READ INGREDIENT LISTS CAREFULLY!

WHEN IT COMES TO COCONUT MILK, nothing beats making your own, but if you have to purchase coconut milk, read ingredient lists carefully and look for brands with no additives (see Resources, page 281). Many popular commercial varieties contain one or more of the following fillers, stabilizers, or synthetic vitamins and minerals, making these types of coconut milk a food that steals rather than a food that heals:

calcium phosphate
magnesium phosphate
potassium metabisulfite
sodium metabisulfite
sulphur dioxide
carrageenan
guar gum
citric acid
ascorbic acid
synthetic vitamins and minerals

ORGANIC YOGURT

I'M EMBARRASSED TO ADMIT HOW LONG IT TOOK ME TO START MAKING MY OWN YOGURT AT HOME. I was hesitant to start because I thought it was too complicated, involving an electric blanket, special containers, or a yogurt maker. As it turns out, you don't need any of those things to make delicious yogurt, and the procedure is amazingly simple.

It makes economical and nutritional sense to make yogurt yourself.

Homemade yogurt is teeming with the probiotics that give yogurt its many touted health benefits, from improving digestive health and reducing the risk of colon cancer to lowering LDL (bad) cholesterol, boosting the immune system, and aiding in weight loss. A good percentage of commercially available yogurts found in grocery stores have very little probiotics in them, especially those that are sweetened and flavored.

Homemade yogurt will be creamy but not thick, and a little on the tart side. The flavor truly depends on the milk that you use; raw, grass-fed organic milk from a local dairy is great for making yogurt, but if you don't have access to this type of high-quality milk, a store-bought pasteurized organic milk will be fine. The procedure is only slightly different for raw milk versus pasteurized milk, and I have outlined the steps for making both types of yogurt in the following recipes.

The only equipment you need is a stockpot, a basic instant-read food thermometer with a temperature range of 0°F to 220°F, some clean glass jars with tight-fitting lids (such as mason jars), an oven or slow cooker, and a starter culture (I use store-bought plain organic whole milk yogurt). You can also purchase powdered thermophilic (heat-loving) starter cultures from an online company.

PLAIN YOGURT FROM
PASTEURIZED ORGANIC WHOLE MILK

• Makes 2 quarts •

2 quarts (½ gallon) pasteurized organic whole milk

½ cup store-bought organic plain, unsweetened whole milk yogurt with live active cultures (no additives, thickeners, or gums), or 4 tablespoons Greek or Bulgarian powdered thermophilic yogurt starter

Prep your storage containers. Make sure your jars and lids are clean and sterile; fresh out of the dishwasher is ideal.

Pour the 2 quarts of milk into a large stockpot. Slowly bring the temperature up to 160°F, stirring occasionally, and hold the milk at this temperature for a few minutes to sterilize it. It is absolutely crucial that you get the temp to 160°F to kill off any bad bacteria that may have formed. Do not let the milk burn.

Remove the milk from the heat and let it cool to 110°F, stirring occasionally to release steam. The cooling period may take up to 1 hour.

Once the milk reaches 110°F, whisk in the starter culture. Whisk the entire mixture briskly to fully incorporate the starter mixture into the warm milk. Make sure the temperature is 110°F; if it's any higher, it may kill the starter bacteria, and if it's too cool, the starter bacteria will not thrive.

Pour the entire mixture into one large glass jar or several smaller glass jars with tight-fitting lids.

If you're using a yogurt maker, simply pour the mixture into the yogurt maker's containers and culture it according to the manufacturer's instructions for about 8 to 12 hours.

To use your oven, turn it on to the lowest setting (mine goes down to 170°F). When it reaches temperature, turn the oven off and turn on the oven light. The light will generate just enough heat in the oven to maintain an oven temperature of about 110°F, which is needed for the yogurt to culture and stay active. Place the jar(s) in the oven, close the door, and leave undisturbed for 10 to 12 hours, at which point the yogurt is done.

To use a slow cooker, place the jar(s) in the center of the slow cooker and pour warm water (about 110°F) into the ceramic insert until it reaches just below the lid of your jar(s). (Do not turn the slow cooker on.) Place a towel over the jar(s) and slow cooker, to act as a lid and to provide extra insulation. Leave in a warm spot in your kitchen to culture for 8 to 12 hours.

The longer the yogurt cultures, the more firm and tart it becomes as the probiotics consume more of the milk sugar (lactose). Therefore, if you want yogurt with less lactose, more firmness, and a stronger flavor, allow it to culture longer. You may want to experiment with the culturing time, somewhere between 8 and 12 hours, to produce yogurt that suits your taste and texture preferences.

Once the culturing period is complete, transfer the jar(s) of warm yogurt to the refrigerator and allow them to completely chill, about 2 to 3 hours. The yogurt will thicken as it chills but will not be as thick as store-bought yogurts that contain pectin, gelatin, milk solids, and other thickeners. There may also be a layer of liquid whey on top of the yogurt, which you can stir into the yogurt or strain off and save.

If you prefer a thicker yogurt, such as Greek-style yogurt, simply drain the finished yogurt in a few layers of cheesecloth after it has been chilled. Save the liquid whey to use in smoothies. Whey is a nutritious source of easily absorbable protein, vitamins, minerals, enzymes, and probiotics.

Flavor and sweeten as desired. The yogurt will keep in the refrigerator for about 10 days, but you'll probably eat it all before then!

PLAIN YOGURT FROM ORGANIC RAW WHOLE MILK

• Makes 2 quarts •

2 quarts (½ gallon) organic raw whole milk

½ cup store-bought organic plain, unsweetened whole milk yogurt with live active cultures (no additives, thickeners, or gums), or 4 tablespoons Greek or Bulgarian powdered thermophilic yogurt starter

Prep your storage containers. Make sure your jars and lids are clean and sterile; fresh out of the dishwasher is ideal.

Prepare the yogurt as above by pouring the raw milk into a large stockpot. To maintain the native probiotics in the milk, gently heat the milk only to 110°F; do not allow the temperature to go any higher.

Turn off the heat, add in the starter culture, and whisk to thoroughly combine the mixture. Transfer the yogurt mixture to clean jar(s) and incubate in the same manner as above for the same amount of time. Once the culturing period is complete, transfer the jar(s) to the refrigerator to chill for several hours. Drain, if desired, to make thicker yogurt. Sweeten or flavor to taste.

FLAVOR VARIATIONS

The possibilities for flavoring yogurt are endless. You can stir in a teaspoon of 100 percent fruit jam or simply add in your own bite-size fresh fruits. Yogurt can be sweetened with stevia, maple syrup, coconut nectar, raw honey, or other natural sweeteners of your choice, and natural extracts such as coconut, vanilla, almond, lemon, orange, and peppermint add some exciting flavors. You can also use flavored liquid stevia extracts to make your own sugar-free yogurt flavors, such as toffee, watermelon, chocolate, and vanilla crème. Here are just a few of my favorites:

- Sugar-Free Vanilla: To 1 cup yogurt, add 1 teaspoon pure vanilla extract plus a few drops of liquid stevia extract to taste. Or use a vanilla-flavored liquid stevia extract and omit the vanilla extract.

- Honey Lemon: To 1 cup yogurt, add 1 teaspoon pure vanilla extract, 1 teaspoon raw honey, 1 teaspoon freshly grated lemon zest, and 1 teaspoon freshly squeezed lemon juice.

- Maple Cinnamon: To 1 cup yogurt, add 1 teaspoon ground cinnamon and 1 teaspoon pure maple syrup.

- Coconut Cacao: To 1 cup yogurt, add 1 teaspoon pure vanilla extract, a few drops liquid stevia extract or 1 teaspoon coconut nectar, 1 tablespoon unsweetened shredded coconut, and 1 heaping teaspoon raw cacao nibs.

- Vanilla Rose with Peaches and Walnuts: To 1 cup yogurt, add 1 teaspoon pure vanilla extract, 1 teaspoon raw honey, and 1 teaspoon rose water. Serve with fresh peach slices and a sprinkle of raw walnuts.

FRESH PUMPKIN PURÉE

IF YOU'VE NEVER MADE YOUR OWN PUMPKIN PURÉE TO USE IN YOUR PIES, BREADS, SOUPS, AND other pumpkin recipes, you're in for a treat. While canned pumpkin purée is convenient and works great in a pinch, the nutrients and flavor of fresh pumpkin purée are far superior. Cooking and puréeing pumpkins is as easy as pie, so when they're in season, be sure to stock up.

There are several ways to cook the pumpkin: steam on the stovetop, bake in the oven, or use a pressure cooker. I've listed all three methods below.

• Makes 2 to 3 cups •

1 pie pumpkin (also known as sugar pie
  pumpkin) (about 2½ pounds)

TO PREPARE THE PUMPKIN FOR COOKING:

Cut the pumpkin in half and scrape out the seeds, discarding the stem section and stringy pulp. An ice cream scoop or a melon baller works great for this. Save the seeds to dry and toast.

TO COOK THE PUMPKIN, CHOOSE ONE OF THESE METHODS:

STEAMING

Put a couple of inches of water in a large pot, place the pumpkin halves flesh-side up in the pot, cover, and bring up the heat to boil the water. You may need to cut the pumpkin into more pieces to make it fit into the pot. Steam for 15 to 20 minutes, or until firm but tender enough to easily pierce through the peel with a fork. Remove the pumpkin to a large bowl to cool to room temperature.

BAKING

Preheat the oven to 350°F. Place the pumpkin halves flesh-side up in a shallow baking dish and fill with ½ inch of water to help prevent it from drying out. Bake for 45 minutes to an hour, until tender enough to easily pierce through the peel with a fork. Remove the pumpkin to a large bowl to cool to room temperature.

PRESSURE COOKING

Follow the manufacturer's instructions for cooking squash and allow to cool to room temperature.

Regardless of how you've cooked the pumpkin, once it's cooled, scoop the cooked pumpkin away from the peel.

Discard or compost the peels.

If your scooped pumpkin is watery (there should not be any free water), you may want to let it sit for 30 minutes in a colander and then pour off any free water.

Using a food processor, blender, or immersion blender, purée the pumpkin until smooth and creamy. The pumpkin purée is now ready to be used as you would canned pumpkin in any recipe that calls for it. You can refrigerate fresh pumpkin purée for up to 3 days or store it in the freezer up to 6 months. If using frozen pumpkin purée, you may need to drain it again in a colander after it has been thawed to remove any excess water that has accumulated.

HOMEMADE ALMOND MEAL

THE FRESHNESS OF HOMEMADE ALMOND MEAL CAN'T BE BEAT, AND THERE ARE TWO EASY WAYS TO make it yourself. One way is to grind whole raw almonds, and the other is to dry and grind the almond pulp left over from making your own almond milk.

ALMOND MEAL FROM WHOLE ALMONDS

IT TAKES ONLY ABOUT FIVE MINUTES TO GRIND ALMONDS IN A FOOD PROCESSOR OR HIGH-POWERED blender. This recipe is easy to customize—1 cup whole almonds yields 1 cup almond meal—so you can add more or less as needed. Grinding nuts creates a higher surface-area exposure of their oils to oxygen and light, and they can easily become rancid if not stored properly. Be sure to store any unused portion of almond meal in an airtight container in the refrigerator or freezer. Refrigerated, it will keep for up to two months, and up to six months in the freezer.

• Makes 1 cup •

1 cup whole raw almonds (preferably soaked and dried)

Place the almonds in a food processor or high-powered blender. Pulse the almonds until they are ground into the consistency of cornmeal. The meal should be fluffy and just barely hold together. Be careful not to overblend, otherwise you'll make almond butter!

ALMOND MEAL USING LEFTOVER PULP FROM HOMEMADE ALMOND MILK

YOU CAN MAKE YOUR OWN ALMOND MEAL BY DEHYDRATING THE LEFTOVER PULP FROM MAKING almond milk. This can be done right after making your almond milk, or you can save the wet pulp in an airtight container in your refrigerator or freezer until you have time to dehydrate it. The wet pulp will last about two days in the refrigerator and up to three months in the freezer. I typically wait until I have saved three or four batches of pulp in the freezer and then dehydrate all of them at once using this method.

• Makes about ½ cup •

½ cup packed moist almond pulp (yield from
    making almond milk from 1 cup
    whole almonds)

Set your oven to the lowest heat setting (mine goes down to 170°F; yours may go lower).

First, spread the almond pulp out on a dry baking sheet into as thin a layer as possible. Let the pulp dehydrate in the oven for about 2 hours, depending on your oven temperature. After 2 hours, check the almond pulp by rubbing it between your fingers. If it is still moist, put it back in the oven for another 30 to 60 minutes, or until it has dried completely (in my oven it takes about 3 hours total).

If using a dehydrator, dry at 115°F for 4 to 8 hours, or until completely dry.

Once the almond pulp is completely dry, place the chunks into a food processor, high-powered blender, or coffee grinder. Grind the chunks until they form a fine-textured flour. Store in an airtight container in the refrigerator for up to 2 months and in the freezer for up to 6 months.

HOMEMADE NUT AND SEED BUTTERS

IT TAKES LESS THAN FIFTEEN MINUTES TO MAKE YOUR OWN NUT OR SEED BUTTER, IT'S LESS COSTLY than store-bought (especially if it's organic), and when it comes to taste, jarred varieties just cannot compare. The only special equipment you need is a basic food processor with an

S-shaped blade. The procedure is super simple, but nuts and seeds go through a few different texture stages before they become the smooth spreadable goodness you know and love—you'll see detailed notes in the instructions.

You can apply this basic technique to make any of your favorite nut or seed butters—almonds, peanuts, cashews, macadamias, pistachios, hazelnuts, pumpkin seeds, sunflower seeds, and others. You can also make mixtures containing more than one type of nut or seed. Ideally, the nuts should be soaked and dried before being made into nut butter, but unsoaked raw nuts may still be used. With the exception of peanuts, do not use commercially roasted nuts.

Processing times may vary, depending on the power of your food processor.

• Makes 1¼ cups •

2 cups raw nuts or seeds

½ teaspoon sea salt or Himalayan pink salt
   (optional)

1 tablespoon raw honey or coconut nectar
   (optional)

Stage 1: Place the nuts or seeds in the bowl of a food processor. Pulse a few times to chop them into small pieces. If you prefer a chunky nut/seed butter, you can remove ½ cup of the chopped nuts/seeds and set them aside to add back in later.

Stage 2: Run the food processor continuously for 2 minutes. Stop and scrape down the sides and bottom of the bowl. At this stage, the butter will look like a crumbly meal.

Stage 3: Run the food processor continuously for another 2 minutes, then stop and scrape down the sides again. At this stage, the butter will start to clump together. You'll be able to see the beginnings of actual nut butter.

Stage 4: Run the food processor continuously for another 2 minutes, then stop and scrape down the sides again. At this stage, the butter will be very thick and glossy. There will still be some loose crumbs in the bowl, but most of it should be sticking together, almost forming a dough at this point.

Stage 5: Run the food processor continuously for another 2 minutes. At this stage, the butter should begin to form a ball.

Stage 6: Continue processing for another 2 minutes. At this stage, the butter "ball" should begin to spread out and redistribute in the bowl of the food processor as the nuts'/seeds' oils are being released. The mixture will take on a thick, grainy texture.

Stage 7: Continue processing for another 2 minutes. By this time, the nuts/seeds have released their oil and the butter should be smooth, creamy, and ready to consume.

Stage 8: If using, sprinkle the salt and/or honey over the top of the butter and process again until the salt and/or honey are completely mixed in. Stop and adjust to taste if needed. If you reserved chopped nuts for a chunky butter, add them in and pulse a few times to incorporate them into the butter.

Stage 9: Transfer the butter to a container with a tight-fitting lid and keep refrigerated. Most butters will keep for up to 2 to 3 weeks in the refrigerator (see storage note on page 74).

Using the technique on the previous page, try these delicious combinations.

Pecan, Pistachio, and Pumpkin Seed Butter

Makes about 1¼ cups

½ cup raw pecans

1 cup raw pistachios

½ cup raw pumpkin seeds

½ teaspoon sea salt (optional)

Process as above.

Triple Seed Spread

This is a recipe for a delicious protein- and omega-packed seed butter; you can swap out whatever seeds you like, but the method is the same.

Makes about 1¼ cups

½ cup raw sunflower seeds

1 cup raw pumpkin seeds

¼ cup freshly ground golden flaxseeds

3 to 4 tablespoons virgin coconut oil

Sea salt or Himalayan pink salt (optional)

If desired, toast the sunflower seeds and pumpkin seeds before making the butter. Place all three types of seeds in the bowl of a food processor.

Turn on the food processor and process for 1 minute. Stop and scrape down the sides and bottom of the bowl. Continue processing, and with the food processor still running, slowly add in the oil, a little bit at a time, until the seed butter is creamy and smooth (you may need more or less oil), stopping to scrape down the sides of the bowl as needed. This seed butter will take less time than nut butter, about 6 or 7 minutes total.

Taste, add salt if desired, and process again quickly to incorporate the salt.

> **NOTES:**
> - *If you are using raw nuts that have been previously soaked and dried, you may need to add a small amount of virgin coconut oil (about 1 tablespoon) in stage 7.*
> - *Store nut and seed butters in containers with tight-fitting lids and keep them in the refrigerator. Almond butter and peanut butter have longer storage times than butters made from other nuts; they will keep in the refrigerator for 3 weeks. Other nut and all seed butters ideally should be stored in a dark container; they will keep in the refrigerator for about 2 weeks.*

ROASTED BELL PEPPERS AND CHILE PEPPERS

ROASTING PEPPERS IS VERY EASY TO DO AT HOME. THE METHOD IS THE SAME WHETHER YOU ARE roasting bell peppers or any type of chile pepper, such as Anaheim chiles, Hatch green chiles, or jalapeños. Roasted peppers add great flavor to hummus, salsas, salads, chili, eggs, tacos, wraps, or anything else you can think of. Once they're roasted and peeled, they can be frozen for later use, so you'll always have some on hand when you need them.

• Makes 4 roasted peppers •

4 peppers, washed and dried

Preheat the oven to 375°F and line a baking sheet with parchment paper. Lay the peppers on their sides on the parchment, stems pointing sideways. Bake the peppers for 20 minutes, turn them over, and bake for 20 minutes more. The skins should be charred and soft, and the peppers should look slightly collapsed. Remove from the oven.

The next step is to trap the heat from the peppers in a contained system so that the steam will loosen the charred skins and make them easy to peel off. You can steam the peppers in one of several ways:

Inverted-Bowl Method: While the peppers are still hot from the oven, lift the parchment paper from the baking sheet with the peppers still on it and place it on a large cutting board or heat-proof counter top. Push all the peppers as close together as possible (you can even stack some on top of each other), then invert a large sturdy glass or stainless-steel mixing bowl over top of them, like a dome, to trap the steam inside.

Bag or Pouch Method: Alternatively, you can just wrap the peppers in the parchment paper and then place the whole thing in a paper bag and seal the top by rolling it closed. You can also wrap the pepper-parchment package with aluminum foil or plastic wrap, or place it in a resealable plastic bag, to make a sealed steaming "envelope" for the peppers.

Whichever method you use, allow the peppers to steam for 15 to 20 minutes.

Gently peel off the charred skins with your fingers, then slice one side of the pepper vertically from top to bottom so that it opens up and you can lay the whole pepper flat. Pull the stem from the top of the pepper (the stem and a clump of seeds should loosen easily). Scoop out any remaining seeds with a spoon or knife.

Use the peppers right away or store them in the refrigerator for up to 3 days. Freeze for up to 6 months.

ROASTED GARLIC

ROASTING TRANSFORMS THE SHARP PUNGENT FLAVOR OF RAW GARLIC INTO A SMOKY SWEET TASTE akin to caramelized onions. Roasted garlic can be eaten on its own, or it can lend its distinguishable flavor to a variety of recipes. The soft cloves can be spread directly onto bread or crackers, or they can be mixed with butter, olive oil, or coconut oil to make a flavorful infusion. Like roasted peppers, roasted garlic is perfect for salsas, hummus, chili, and soups. It can also be mixed into soft cheeses or used to flavor mayonnaise, potatoes, and salad dressings.

To be efficient and ensure that you always have plenty of roasted garlic on hand for your recipes, you can roast a large quantity of garlic heads and freeze them, rather than roasting just a few cloves for the recipe at hand.

• Makes 2 servings •

1 garlic head   1 to 2 teaspoons virgin coconut oil, melted

Garlic can be roasted in the oven or in a slow cooker.

To roast garlic in the oven, preheat the oven to 375°F.

Cut a small amount, about ¼ inch, off the top of the head of garlic to expose the ends of each clove (save and freeze those little tops to use for making vegetable broth).

Place the head of garlic, cut-side up, on a baking dish. Drizzle the exposed cloves with the melted coconut oil. Cover the baking dish with foil and bake for 35 minutes.

To roast in a slow cooker, wrap the garlic head in a piece of parchment paper, then wrap with aluminum foil (the parchment paper serves as a barrier between the foil and the garlic). Place the wrapped garlic into the slow cooker and cook on the low setting for 4 to 5 hours.

Remove the foil and parchment and let the garlic cool long enough to be handled, about 10 minutes. Grab the bottom of the garlic head and gently squeeze the cloves out from their casings.

To store roasted garlic in the refrigerator, place the cloves into a small glass jar with a tight-fitting lid and pour in enough extra-virgin olive oil to cover all the cloves. Secure the lid and refrigerate for up to 2 weeks.

To freeze a whole head of garlic, do not squeeze the cloves out of their casings. Place the whole head in a freezer-safe container.

To freeze individual cloves, squeeze them out of their casings, place on a plate or baking sheet, and place in the freezer until frozen. Then transfer them to a jar or other freezer-safe container. Freezing individually beforehand keeps them from sticking together during storage. Roasted garlic can be frozen for up to 3 months.

5

Beneficial Beverages and Brews

Whether your beverages are for hydration, refreshment, or mere enjoyment, they should still be just as healthful as your food. As you will discover in this chapter, there are many creative ways to make delicious nutrient-rich beverages at home to replace the processed stuff that comes from bottles, baristas, and soda fountains. From a variety of antioxidant-packed brews like Hibiscus Ginger Tea (page 79) to your own homemade Processed-Free Peppermint Mocha (page 85), you will find something here to please your palate and quench your desire for something more than just plain water. And finally, if you need a change of pace from plain water, you can drink Naturally Flavored Vitamin Water (page 81) to help meet your daily quota.

VITALITY VINEGAR TONIC
WITH VARIATIONS

OWING TO ITS ALKALIZING PROPERTIES, RAW ORGANIC UNFILTERED APPLE CIDER VINEGAR ADDED to water is a powerful and effective food weapon for lowering cholesterol, stabilizing blood sugar levels, and alleviating arthritis. (In fact, a recent study found that an apple cider vinegar drink is more effective at lowering fasting blood glucose levels, more economical, and less toxic than some of the leading diabetes drugs!) I recommend consuming it daily for its natural cleansing, healing, and energizing qualities. On its own, the plain tonic is quite tart, so you may want to add other flavorful alkalizing ingredients.

• Makes 1 (8-ounce) serving•

2 teaspoons raw organic unfiltered apple cider vinegar

8 ounces water, chilled or at room temperature

½ teaspoon raw honey or coconut nectar, or a few drops of liquid stevia extract (optional, to tame the tartness)

Combine, stir, and drink.

FLAVOR VARIATIONS

- Apple Cinnamon: Reduce water by ¼ cup, then add ¼ cup organic unfiltered apple juice and ½ teaspoon ground cinnamon.
- Concord Grape: Reduce water by ¼ cup, then add ¼ cup organic Concord grape juice.
- Honey Lemon Ginger: Add 1 tablespoon freshly squeezed lemon juice, 1 teaspoon raw honey, and ½ teaspoon freshly grated ginger.
- Blackstrap Molasses: Add 1 teaspoon unsulphured blackstrap molasses.

FRESH MINT TEA

WHENEVER I BUY A BUNCH OF MINT LEAVES TO USE IN A RECIPE, I INEVITABLY HAVE SOME LEFT over. That's when I make fresh mint tea! The flavor and health benefits of fresh mint leaves are far superior to the dried form of this refreshing herb. Fresh mint tea can be served hot or iced and can be made as a single serving or a whole pot, depending on how much fresh mint you have on hand. Try different varieties of the herb, such as peppermint, apple mint, chocolate mint, and orange mint.

• Makes 4 cups •

4 to 5 fresh mint stalks (stems and leaves)   4 cups boiling water

To release the mint oil in the leaves, roll the mint stalks between your palms a few times before placing them, stems and all, into your teapot, saucepan, or heat-proof bowl (or tea cup if you're making a single serving). Pour the boiling water over the mint stalks until your pot or cup is full. Cover the teapot (or pan, bowl, or cup), let the leaves steep for 5 minutes, then serve immediately or chill and serve over ice.

HIBISCUS GINGER TEA

THE DRIED FLOWERS OF HIBISCUS ARE HIGH IN VITAMIN C, POTASSIUM, AND CALCIUM. THEY GET THEIR deep crimson color and tangy tart flavor from a group of natural pigments called anthocyanins—strong antioxidants that have been clinically studied for their role in lowering cholesterol and blood pressure, stabilizing blood sugar level in diabetics, and aiding in weight loss. Hibiscus is naturally caffeine-free and can be enjoyed hot or chilled.

• Makes 3 quarts •

- 2 quarts (8 cups) water
- 1 (½-inch) piece fresh ginger, peeled and finely grated
- 1 cup dried hibiscus flowers (also known as hibiscus tea)
- 1 teaspoon liquid stevia extract (optional)
- Juice of 1 lime (about 2 tablespoons)

Bring the water and ginger to a boil in a large pot over high heat. Remove from the heat and stir in the hibiscus flowers. Let steep for 10 minutes.

Strain the tea through a fine-mesh strainer into a large pitcher or bowl. Stir in the stevia and lime juice and set aside to cool. Refrigerate until ready to drink. Serve over ice.

SUGAR-FREE BLACKBERRY LEMONADE

CE-COLD LEMONADE IS A THIRST QUENCHER FOR THOSE HOT SUMMER DAYS. THIS VARIATION MAKES it even more enticing with the heart-protective power of blackberry juice. Compounds in blackberry juice called anthocyanins increase the juice's antioxidant activity and protect your cardiovascular system from the damage caused by free radicals. Sweet!

• Makes 4 (16-ounce) servings •

- 2 quarts (8 cups) water
- 8 lemons
- ¾ cup blackberries
- 1 teaspoon liquid stevia extract, or more to taste

Fill a 2-quart pitcher with the water. Squeeze the juice from the lemons into the water. Add the stevia.

Set aside 8 blackberries for garnish. Mash or purée the remaining blackberries, add them to the pitcher, and stir to mix thoroughly. Serve over ice. Garnish each glass with a couple fresh blackberries.

NATURALLY FLAVORED VITAMIN WATER

WE ALL KNOW HOW IMPORTANT DRINKING WATER EVERY DAY IS FOR OUR HEALTH, BUT SOMETIMES plain water gets a bit boring. Naturally flavored vitamin water to the rescue! Naturally flavored vitamin water is better for your health in many ways (it's hydrating, alkalizing, and full of REAL vitamins, not synthetic versions) and is surprisingly easy to make yourself. It is especially helpful for transitioning away from sodas, sugary juices, and flavored powdered drink mixes.

With just a few fresh or frozen ingredients and some water, you can make your own exciting infusions in an endless variety of flavors. Here's a basic recipe that you can easily customize. You'll want to have a 2-quart sun tea jar or other large glass jar with a lid (mason jars work great) for the water, as well as a wooden spoon or kitchen mallet for gently mashing fruit and herbs. The tamper from a Vitamix works nicely for this as well, or you can purchase a beverage muddler.

• Makes 2 quarts •

1 sprig fresh herbs or 2 drops natural extract (optional; see suggestions in the variations on page 82)

2 cups fresh or frozen fruits (any kind you like except bananas) or soft veggies (such as cucumbers)

2 quarts fresh, clean drinking water

Place a sprig of fresh herbs (if using) in the bottom of the dry container; use the handle of a wooden spoon or the flat end of a kitchen mallet to gently bruise the herbs (do not crush or pulverize) to release their flavor.

Add the desired fruits or veggies to the container. Use the handle of a wooden spoon or the flat end of a kitchen mallet again to gently press and twist the fruit/veggies just enough to release some of the juices. Do not crush or pulverize the fruit/veggies into pieces. If using frozen fruits/veggies, allow them to thaw before pressing.

Fill the container with water, stir, cover, and refrigerate.

You can drink the water immediately, but the best method is to leave the container in the refrigerator to let the flavors infuse overnight. The infusion time allows you to get the most flavorful and nutritious water. The infusion will stay fresh for up to 3 days. When you're ready to drink, you'll want to strain the infusion by pouring it through a fine-mesh strainer or cheesecloth to avoid getting bits of fruit/veggies or herbs in your glass. You can either strain the whole batch at once into a different container or strain each time you pour a glass.

FLAVOR VARIATIONS

Below are some flavorful combinations you may want to try. The flavors in these waters are not explosive or sweet, just subtly infused to give a hint of flavor. While it may be tempting to sweeten these waters with a natural sweetener, please remember that this water is for hydration, so adding sweeteners is not recommended.

- Herbs: Mint and ginger are the most commonly used fresh herbs for making flavored water, but many other fresh herbs, such as basil, lavender, rosemary, sage, and tarragon, blend well with fruity flavors in a surprising way.

- Coconut water: If you want a nice tropical twist, you can replace some or all of the water with plain coconut water.

- Natural extracts: Mint or vanilla are great additional flavors that bump up the refreshing factor of the water.

- Orange: Slice 3 oranges into rounds, then cut in half and press in container.

- Triple Citrus: Slice 1 lemon, 1 lime, and 1 orange into rounds, then cut in half and press in container.

- Cucumber Mint: Press a handful of fresh mint sprigs and 1 large sliced cucumber in container; leave out the mint for plain cucumber water.

- Cranberry Orange: Press 1 cup fresh or frozen (thawed) cranberries and 2 oranges sliced into rounds in container.

- Lemon Ginger: Quarter 3 lemons, squeeze the juice into the jar with your hands, then drop the squeezed quarters into the container. Add 1 tablespoon grated fresh ginger. Press and twist with a wooden spoon to release some of the juices.

- Piña Colada: Press 2 cups pineapple chunks in container and fill with half coconut water and half regular water.

- Mint Apple: Press a handful of fresh mint sprigs and 2 cored and thinly sliced apples in container.

- Double Berry Sage: Press 1 sprig sage and 1 cup each blackberries and raspberries in container.

- Strawberry Rose: Press 1 cup fresh strawberries in container and add a teaspoon or more of organic rose water.

> ### SUPER QUICK VITAMIN WATER:
>
> *If you don't have time to make a big batch, you can still enjoy re-freshing flavored water on the spot when desired. I make a quick infusion by adding a few frozen berries into the stainless-steel water bottle I drink from throughout the day. As the frozen fruit melts, it releases its nice berry flavor. Another quick favorite is to press a few chunks of fresh watermelon in the bottom of a glass, then add a couple drops of mint extract, fill the glass with cold water and ice, stir, and enjoy. Ah, so refreshing!*

BANANA DATE SHAKE

Date shakes are a Southern California favorite, but they're loaded with ice cream and refined sugar. This version takes the classic date shake to a healthy new level.

• Makes 2 servings •

10 Medjool dates, pitted and coarsely chopped

1 cup coconut milk

2 bananas, frozen and cut into ½-inch slices

1 teaspoon pure vanilla extract, or ½ teaspoon vanilla powder

6 tablespoons organic whey protein concentrate (optional)

Place the dates and coconut milk in a blender; blend on high until smooth, about 30 seconds. Add the frozen banana slices, vanilla, and whey protein concentrate, if using, and blend until thick and frothy, about another 30 seconds.

FREEZING BANANAS

Frozen bananas come in handy for making smoothies, muffins, quick breads, shakes, and ice cream. There are several ways you can freeze ripe bananas:

+ Leave them in their peel and freeze whole
+ Peel first and freeze whole
+ Peel, slice into pieces, and freeze

In all cases, place them in a freezer-safe bag or container. Be aware that if you freeze bananas in their peel, the peel will turn black but the banana itself will be unaffected. I prefer to leave bananas in their peel while frozen, as it helps to protect them from freezer burn and loss of nutrients. When I need to use them, I quarter the frozen banana by first cutting it in half, then cutting each half down the middle lengthwise. Then I cut each quarter crosswise to get smaller pieces. The frozen cut pieces slip easily off the peel.

CARDAMOM ROSE LASSI

LASSI IS A MIDDLE EASTERN BEVERAGE MADE FROM YOGURT, CONSUMED REGULARLY FOR THE digestive and health benefits its probiotics provide. Homemade lassi makes a nourishing breakfast, snack, or post-workout recovery drink. It can be made with cow or goat milk yogurt. To ensure you are getting the full benefits of yogurt's probiotics, use organic grass-fed whole milk plain yogurt with live active cultures or raw milk yogurt when possible.

• Makes 1 serving •

1 cup organic plain whole milk yogurt

¼ cup cold water

¼ teaspoon organic rose water

Pinch of ground cardamom

Sweetener of choice (stevia, maple syrup, coconut nectar, raw honey), to taste

Combine all ingredients in a blender and blend until smooth. Serve in a glass filled three quarters full with ice.

LASSI VARIATIONS

- Fresh Mint Lassi: Omit the rose water and cardamom and add a few finely minced fresh mint leaves to the yogurt, water, and sweetener in the blender. Alternatively, you can steep sprigs of fresh mint in boiling water (see Fresh Mint Tea, page 79) and use ¼ cup of the tea, once it has cooled, instead of plain water.
- Mango Lassi: Omit the rose water and cardamom and add a handful of fresh or frozen mango chunks to the yogurt, water, and sweetener in the blender.

ICED MOLASSES MOCHA

BLACKSTRAP MOLASSES TAKES THE PLACE OF COFFEE IN THIS CREAMY, MOCHA-LIKE DRINK. IT'S great as is on the rocks, but the whole mixture can be blended into a luscious shake if desired. One tablespoon of blackstrap molasses provides 18 percent of the recommended daily value of calcium and 20 percent of the daily value of iron, in a highly absorbable form.

• Makes 1 serving •

1 tablespoon unsulphured blackstrap molasses	½ teaspoon pure vanilla extract
½ cup hot water	1 cup unsweetened almond milk

Add the molasses and hot water to a tall glass and stir until the molasses is dissolved. Fill the glass with ice, add the vanilla, and top off with the almond milk. Stir or shake until the molasses is well combined. You may need to add more ice to keep it cold. Drink immediately.

PROCESSED-FREE PEPPERMINT MOCHA

THE COFFEEHOUSE VERSION OF THIS SEASONAL FAVORITE CAN PACK A HIGH AMOUNT OF SUGAR, caffeine, and chemical additives. This better-for-you treat can be enjoyed any time of year. By using a caffeine-free herbal coffee, such as Dandy Blend or Teeccino, you'll get the benefits of dandelion root, a very therapeutic liver-cleansing herb. See Resources (page 280) for descriptions of some tasty options. Of course, organic coffee also works here.

• Makes 1 serving •

¼ cup light coconut milk	1 cup hot herbal coffee or organic coffee
1 teaspoon unsweetened cocoa powder	Liquid stevia extract, to taste (optional)
½ teaspoon peppermint extract	

Heat the coconut milk in a small saucepan over medium heat. Add the cocoa powder and peppermint and whisk to combine, until the cocoa is dissolved. Add the coconut milk mixture to the coffee in a mug and stir to combine. Sweeten, if desired. No whip!

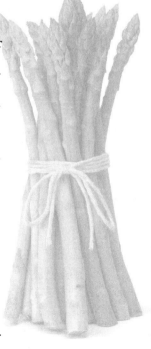

Power Juices and Green Smoothies

Freshly pressed vegetable juices and blended green smoothies are a delicious and easy way to get high amounts of raw vegetables and dark leafy greens into your body on a regular basis. When properly prepared, fresh juices and green smoothies can quickly shift your body chemistry from acidic to alkaline, leading to increased energy, better digestion, weight loss (or weight gain if needed), and an overall sense of well-being. The juice recipes in this section range from the one-ingredient Ultimate Carrot Juice (page 93)—a simple juice with enormous power to cleanse the liver, clear arteries, improve eyesight, and fight cancer—to the Supercharged Green Juice (page 96), a strong alkalizing juice that combines the strength of a variety of green vegetables, fruits, and herbs that can be rotated to switch up the nutrients, flavors, and health benefits. I've included a variety of smoothie recipes to please the palates of children and grown-ups alike, starting with the sweet tropical notes of banana and mango in the Beginner's Delight Green Smoothie (page 104) and the ultra-indulgent flavors in the Mint Chocolate Bliss Smoothie (page 109). For those who prefer smoothies with more savory vegetable tones, I offer the Zesty Savory Green Smoothie (page 110), which includes the zing of ginger and lime combined with the cool sweetness of carrots and cucumbers.

In this chapter, you'll find general instructions for making the best juices and great smoothies, every time, followed by my favorite juice and smoothie recipes. Regularly consuming these super-nutritious drinks is one of the tastiest pathways to health!

Drinking Your Greens: An Overview

Even if you love eating vegetables and greens, it is nearly impossible to consume the large quantities our bodies require for optimal health. It takes some serious chewing (which requires time, strong jaw muscles, and a near perfect set of teeth) and a strong, healthy digestive system to adequately break down the cellular structure of raw produce to a liquefied form in order to maximize absorption of their nutrients. Even when vegetables and fruits are chewed well, only a fraction of their nutrients are actually released. The results of a 2002 Swedish in-vitro study showed that only 3 percent of the total beta-carotene content is released from a raw carrot chewed in a typical manner. When pulped, 21 percent of the beta-carotene is released.[1] In juiced or pulverized (blended) form, it is possible to assimilate nearly all of the nutrients from fruits and vegetables.

Juicing is a process that extracts, or squeezes, water and nutrients out of vegetables and fruits, leaving the pulp and fiber behind. This is different from blending, which pulverizes vegetables and fruits while retaining the pulp and fiber. With both methods, the fast spinning blades of the juicer or blender break down and "chew" vegetables and fruits much faster and more thoroughly than your own teeth, allowing for easier, faster, and higher nutrient absorption compared with when you chew the vegetables and fruits yourself. Additionally, both methods make it easier to take in larger quantities and a wider variety of fruits and vegetables than when you eat them in their whole form.

Basic Equipment

To prepare fresh juices and smoothies, you will need some special equipment. At the very least, a standard blender will be needed for making smoothies (two of the juice recipes in this chapter, Cool and Collected Cucumber Juice, page 94, and Simply Skinny Watermelon Juice, page 99, require only a standard blender). For best results with the smoothie recipes, however, a high-powered blender that can pulverize and liquefy whole fruits and veggies is highly recommended. Lastly, a juicer is required for preparing fresh fruit and vegetable juices, though a couple of the recipes (Ultimate Carrot Juice, page 93, and Root Veggie Ginger Juice, page 95) can be made in a high-powered blender if you don't have a juicer. Recommendations for blenders and juicers can be found in Resources (page 282–283).

Green Superfood Drink Powders

If you don't have a juicer or blender, don't despair. You still can benefit from the alkalizing power of vegetable juices by supplementing with a green superfood drink powder. This is the second best way to get more nutrients from greens into your body. Green superfood drink powders contain highly concentrated, carefully dehydrated green alkalizing vegetables, herbs, grasses, algae, sea vegetables, and other important superfoods. Stirring a scoop of green superfood powder into a glass of water or nondairy milk and drinking it one to three times a day can assist you in achieving and maintaining an alkaline body chemistry. A scoop of green superfood drink powder is also a great addition to your smoothies.

You'll find suggestions for alkalizing green superfood drink powders in Resources (page 282).

Fresh Vegetable Juices: Basics

While juicing is an easy way to consume a larger and more varied amount of vegetables than you might normally eat in a day, it is important to understand that juices are powerful foods that require careful consumption and should not be taken to the extreme. So before you dive into making fresh juices, there are some important things to keep in mind:

JUICE VEGETABLES FREQUENTLY—FRUITS NOT SO MUCH: With a few exceptions, fruits are best eaten whole or blended into smoothies, not as extracted juices. When you consume a fruit or vegetable juice, the nutrients—including the sugars—are released into your bloodstream almost immediately. This is very advantageous with vegetable juices, as they contain high amounts of easily absorbed nutrients and very minimal sugar. However, a fruit juice can contain anywhere from double to quadruple the amount of sugar contained in an equivalent amount of vegetable juice. That high amount of sugar can quickly spike your blood sugar and, if consumed too frequently, can wreak havoc on your health.

On the other hand, when fruits are eaten whole (or blended into smoothies), they take about 30 minutes to digest, and their fiber ensures that the sugar contained in them is taken into the bloodstream gradually over that time, preventing blood sugar spikes. For this reason, fruit juices should be considered an occasional treat (in the same way that sweet desserts are occasional treats), not a part of your daily routine.

An exception to this rule is lemon and lime juice, which may be consumed frequently and in larger quantities if desired, as they are very low in naturally occurring sugar and do not negatively impact blood sugar levels.

This doesn't mean that you can't ever juice an apple with your vegetables, only that if you do, limit it to only one apple per glass of vegetable juice. Ideally, however, you should not juice fruits with vegetables, which brings me to my next point . . .

PROPER JUICE COMBINATIONS: The fundamental rule of juicing is this: Do not combine fruits with vegetables, because it can cause difficult digestion. Vegetables contain complex carbohydrates (starches) that require different enzymes for digestion than the simple carbohydrates (sugars) in fruits. When you combine the two, it hampers your body's ability to easily absorb the nutrients. However, there are some exceptions to this rule.

- Apples: Apples have a longer digestive time than other fruits and can be juiced with vegetables. The sweet flavor of apples can help offset the taste of some of the vegetables. But remember, too much fruit juice can spike blood sugar levels, so the goal is to minimize using apples to sweeten your juice and eventually get to the point where you no longer need to add them at all.
- Lemons and limes: Although they are fruits, their sugar content is nearly zero, so they can be combined with vegetable juices.
- Dark green leafy vegetables: These can be combined with either fruits or other vegetables. Greens do not contain the same type of starch as other types of vegetables and do not create difficult digestion when combined with fruits. So fruits and greens can be combined, but it is not recommended to combine fruits with any other types of vegetables.
- Herbs and spices may be combined with either vegetable juices or fruit juices. Parsley, cilantro, basil, and garlic

taste great juiced with vegetables, while the flavors of mint and ginger go very well with both fruit and vegetable juices.

RAMP UP SLOWLY, THEN YOU CAN JUICE DAILY: If you are new to juicing, start out by gradually introducing juices into your routine. One cup (8 fluid ounces) of juice several times a week is a good starting point. If drinking fresh vegetable juices causes you to feel tired or like you have the flu, it means you are taking in too much juice. Sometimes people think the juices are making them sick, when it is actually an indication that their body is getting a well-needed cleansing. If this happens, you should cut your juice intake in half and drink plenty of extra water to help flush out the toxins more quickly.

Beginner juices should consist of more familiar and basic vegetables such as carrots, celery, cucumber, and lettuces. When you're ready to ramp up to more powerful produce, introduce beets, fennel, broccoli, ginger, garlic, and dark green leafy vegetables like kale, dandelion greens, parsley, beet greens, chard, spinach, and others. Once you have ramped up to daily juicing, you can increase the volume to at least a quart (32 ounces), but not all at one time. For example, you can drink a 16-ounce juice in the morning and another 16 ounces in the afternoon or evening. Drinking a quart of fresh juice will ensure that you surpass the recommended daily intake of vegetables.

GREEN JUICES: Due to their high amount of chlorophyll, the cleansing properties of juices made from dark green leafy vegetables are much more powerful than any other vegetable juice, so the gradual ramp-up is especially important when juicing vegetables such as beet greens, carrot greens, cabbage, chard, collard greens, dandelion greens, kale, lettuces, mustard greens, spinach, broccoli, and others.

Start by using just one large handful of small green leaves (such as spinach) or a few large leaves (such as kale or chard) with your other vegetables and gradually increase the quantity. Ultimately, you never want more than half of the total volume of your juice to be green juice (even a quarter of the total volume is sufficient). Also, it is not advised to drink juices made from only greens. Aside from the fact that their taste is quite strong, they can cause loose bowel movements. Greens are best juiced with at least two or three other types of vegetables.

ROTATE THE GREENS: You may think that juicing kale every day is a great idea, especially since it has earned the reputation of being one of the healthiest greens on the planet. But no matter how healthy they are, all dark green leafy plants contain defensive compounds called alkaloids to protect themselves from being eaten to extinction by animals in the wild.

When large amounts of alkaloids from the same plant species are consumed over a period of many weeks, they can build up in the body, causing unpleasant symptoms. So we just need to be mindful not to consume too much of a good thing day after day for long periods of time. Some people juice a different type of green each day. Others

switch the greens weekly. The point is not to go for months at a time using the exact same greens for your juices.

DRINK JUICE ON AN EMPTY STOMACH: Ideally, the best time to drink fresh juice is when your stomach is empty—at least twenty to thirty minutes before a meal or two hours after a meal. Your body will get the maximum nutrients from your juice when there is nothing else in your stomach to interfere with the absorption. If you like juicing first thing in the morning, it's best to drink the juice first, wait fifteen to twenty minutes, and then eat breakfast.

JUICES ARE NOT MEAL REPLACEMENTS: A common mistake many people make when they begin juicing is to drink juice in place of eating a meal. This is not recommended, as juiced vegetables lack important components that make up a complete meal—namely fiber and natural fats. Juices are more like live vitamin supplements and should be consumed as such. Additionally, drinking vegetable juice before a meal helps to "program" your taste buds to want more vegetables and reduces cravings for sweets and carbs.

YOU STILL NEED TO EAT VEGETABLES: Even though juicing is a great way to meet your vegetable quota for the day, you still need to eat vegetables. Fiber from raw and lightly cooked vegetables acts as an intestinal broom, keeping the walls of the intestines clean, strong, and healthy. Therefore, you should still strive to eat a good amount of raw and cooked vegetables daily in addition to any vegetable juices you may want to consume.

Remember to chew: Many people drink fresh juices the same way they drink water and other beverages—by downing them quickly without chewing. However, juices are foods that require enzymes from saliva to deliver the nutrients to your cells. Therefore, even though the blades of the juicer or blender do all of the masticating for you, you still need to chew your juice a few times to generate saliva. Swish the juice around in your mouth or move your jaw up and down for a couple of seconds before swallowing. It may seem strange at first to chew a juice, but it's an important part of digestive health. Without good digestion, nutrients are not properly absorbed.

Sugar-sensitive individuals need to use caution: If you have diabetes or candida, or are otherwise sensitive to sugar, you may need to avoid juicing vegetables and fruits with higher sugar contents. Some of my clients who are diabetic cannot handle even small amounts of apple, carrot, or beet juices, so please be cautious when selecting your ingredients for juicing. It may be best to stick with cucumbers, celery, ginger, parsley, greens, limes, lemons, and other low-sugar juices. If the juices need a little sweetness, you can add a few drops of stevia. It may be helpful to monitor your blood sugar after drinking juices to determine how much and what types of juice you can tolerate.

Clean, varied, seasonal, organic, and local: Juicing extracts concentrated nutrients and water from produce; therefore, the juicing process can extract concentrated pesticides, herbi-cides, parasites, and other contaminants as well. As much as possible, choose locally grown organic produce for juicing and use the Environmental Working Group's Dirty Dozen and Clean 15 lists for strategizing your produce budget (see pages 18–19).

Apples and carrots can be staple ingredients for juicing, but it's a good idea to regularly switch out the other vegetables you juice in order to get a wide range of nutrients. Different vegetables in varying combinations have different health properties benefitting different parts of the body. So if you juiced cucumbers and celery this week, try radishes and parsnips next week, beets and watercress the following week, and so on.

Even if you're using organic produce, you still need to make sure it's clean by washing it thoroughly. Unless otherwise specified in the juice recipes, leave the peels on all vegetables and fruits.

Drink immediately or properly store your juice: As soon as your freshly made juice gets exposed to air, the enzymes and nutrients begin to degrade (oxidize), so you have to drink or properly store the juice within fifteen minutes of preparation.

To keep the air out of your stored juice, use glass jars with tight-fitting lids (such as mason jars). Fill the jars to the very top with juice, almost spilling over. The juice should form a slight dome shape at the top of the jar. Next, hold the disk sealer just over the top of the jar and press down. A small amount of juice will spill down the sides of the jar. Screw on the metal lid to lock the disk tightly in place.

Always keep stored juice in the refrigerator because harmful bacteria can begin to grow if it becomes warm. The amount of time a juice can be stored depends on the type of juicer used to extract the juice. Juices made with a masticating or centrifugal juicer can be stored for up to twenty-four hours, while juices made with cold-press juicers can be stored for up to seventy-two hours (see Resources, pages 282–283, for juicer types and recommendations). Once you open the jar of juice and expose it to air, drink it within fifteen minutes.

RECYCLE THE PULP: Instead of discarding or composting the leftover pulp from juicing, why not put it to good use? Consider adding the pulp to pancakes, quick breads, or muffin recipes. It can also be added to soups, stews, broths, marinara sauce, and lasagna. If you have a dehydrator, it makes great crackers. You can also feed it to your pets.

The following juice recipes will give you some ideas to get started with juicing, but you really have a blank canvas when it comes to filling your juice glass with alkalizing goodness. The possibilities are truly endless. Enjoy!

ULTIMATE CARROT JUICE

RAW CARROT JUICE IS ONE OF THE MOST DELICIOUS ALKALINE-FORMING VEGETABLE JUICES, AND IT can be made with either a juicer or a high-powered blender. Carrot juice boasts an impressive list of health benefits, which is why it is often called the "miracle juice." It is loaded with live enzymes and antioxidant compounds called carotenes that fight cancer, improve eyesight, and cleanse toxins from the liver. It is also an excellent source of vitamins A, C, E, and K and most of the B vitamins. And that's not all: It is also rich in the alkaline-forming mineral calcium, which helps to strengthen the bones and teeth. Miracle juice, indeed!

• Makes about 8 ounces •

6 large carrots, ends and greens removed

Run the carrots through your juicer and collect the juice in a bowl or glass. If using a blender, cut the carrots into small pieces and add ½ cup purified water to the blender to help liquefy the carrots. Blend on high until puréed, adding more water if necessary. Strain the juice using a hand strainer, cheesecloth, or nut-milk strainer bag, squeezing to extract as much juice as possible from the pulp. Drink immediately.

VARIATIONS

Carrots juice well with apples and practically all other vegetables. Below are a couple more variations on carrot juice. A juicer is recommended for these juices, but a high-powered blender can also be used.

- Carrot Beet Green Juice: 1 green apple, cored, ¼ large red beet with greens and stalks (or ½ small beet), 4 large carrots with greens
- Carrot Ginger Green Juice: 4 large carrots with greens, ¼-inch piece peeled fresh ginger, 1 green apple, cored

COOL AND COLLECTED CUCUMBER JUICE

THERE ARE FEW DRINKS MORE REFRESHING AND NOURISHING THAN A COOL GLASS OF CUCUMBER juice. Cucumbers are high in silica, a trace mineral known as the "beauty mineral" for its ability to strengthen connective tissues of the skin, hair, and nails. Cucumbers also contain electrolytes (calcium, magnesium, potassium), vitamins and antioxidants (vitamins A and C), and lots of water (96 percent by weight), which means they yield a high amount of hydrating, alkalizing, and liver-izing juice.

• Makes about 16 ounces •

1 cucumber

2 celery stalks

1 lime, peeled

Handful of fresh mint leaves

1 apple, cored

Run all ingredients through your juicer and collect the juice in a bowl or glass. If using a blender, cut the cucumbers into chunks and add ½ cup purified water to the blender to help liquefy the ingredients. Blend on high until puréed, adding more water if necessary. Strain the juice using a hand strainer, cheesecloth, or nut-milk strainer bag, squeezing to extract as much juice as possible from the pulp. Pour over ice and drink immediately.

ROOT VEGGIE GINGER JUICE

GROWN BENEATH THE EARTH, ROOT VEGETABLES OFFER A WIDE ARRAY OF BENEFITS: GINGER AND fennel aid digestion; red and gold beets are packed with unique phytonutrients called betalains that help cleanse toxins from the liver; and parsnips add a nice creamy texture to vegetable juices and provide high levels of potassium.

• Makes about 16 ounces juice •

1 (½-inch) piece fresh ginger, peeled	2 parsnips
2 red or golden beets	½ fennel bulb and stalk
4 carrots	Handful of fresh curly parsley leaves

Run all ingredients through your juicer and collect the juice in a bowl or glass. Drink immediately.

BEGINNER'S GREEN JUICE

IF YOU'RE NEW TO JUICING GREENS, THIS RECIPE WILL GIVE YOU A SWEET START! THE APPLES AND cucumbers lend a pleasing taste, and the juice is packed with the important nutrients from dark leafy greens.

• Makes about 16 ounces •

¼ bunch spinach (about 1 cup chopped, packed in cup)	1 apple, cored
1 cucumber	1 sprig fresh mint

Run all ingredients through your juicer and collect the juice in a bowl or glass. Drink immediately.

SUPERCHARGED GREEN JUICE

THE GREENS AND HERBS IN THIS JUICE CAN BE ROTATED SO THAT YOU CAN HAVE DIFFERENT GREEN juices throughout the week.

• Makes about 16 ounces •

1 bunch any green of your choice (collards, chard, spinach, kale, dandelion; about 2½ cups chopped, packed tightly in cup)

Handful of fresh herbs of your choice (basil, parsley, cilantro, mint)

1 cucumber

2 carrots

2 asparagus spears

1 lime, peeled

1 apple, cored

Run all ingredients through your juicer and collect the juice in a bowl or glass. Drink immediately.

LIVER-IZING GREEN JUICE

DANDELION GREENS CLEANSE THE LIVER BY REMOVING TOXINS AND FLUSHING OUT STORED FAT; turmeric reduces fat, purifies the blood, and is believed to be a cleanser for all organ systems in the body. This juice is powerful, so please make sure to drink plenty of water throughout the day to aid in the flushing and removal of released toxins.

• Makes about 16 ounces •

½ bunch dandelion greens (1½ cups chopped, packed tightly in cup)

3 carrots

1 cucumber

½ lemon, peeled

1 (¼-inch) piece fresh turmeric

Run all ingredients through your juicer and collect the juice in a bowl or glass. Drink immediately.

LICORICE LETTUCE JUICE

CRISP ROMAINE LETTUCE IS A NUTRITIOUS LEAFY GREEN RICH IN PROTEIN, CALCIUM, OMEGA-3 fatty acids, and of course, chlorophyll. Lettuce juice hydrates at the cellular level and cleanses fats and toxins from congested cells. Fennel contains a variety of essential oils that lend a beautiful licorice flavor to the juice. The most powerful essential oil in fennel is anethol, which has been shown to reduce inflammation, prevent cancer, and protect the liver from harmful toxins.

• Makes about 16 ounces •

4 large dark green outer romaine leaves (about 2 cups chopped)

4 carrots

½ fennel bulb and stalk (about 1 cup chopped)

1 apple, cored

Run all ingredients through your juicer and collect the juice in a bowl or glass. Drink immediately.

"V"ITALITY-8 JUICE

THE BENEFITS OF THE NUTRITIVE VEGETABLES CONTAINED IN THIS FAMILIAR-TASTING JUICE ARE truly amazing. Tomatoes, which are technically fruits, are loaded with cancer-fighting lycopene; carrots provide beta-carotene and are superb for increasing vitality and vigor; celery tames a sweet tooth and reduces acidity; beets improve blood circulation; parsley inhibits tumor formation, particularly in the lungs; spinach maintains healthy blood vessels and improves vision; lettuce helps calm the nervous system and improves sleep; and watercress supports kidney function and reduces fluid retention. Nothing in a bottle can compare!

• Makes about 16 ounces •

4 Roma tomatoes, or 2 large vine-ripened tomatoes (use firm tomatoes for juicing)	¼ cup packed fresh curly parsley leaves

4 Roma tomatoes, or 2 large vine-ripened
   tomatoes (use firm tomatoes for juicing)

3 carrots

2 celery stalks

¼ large or ½ small beet

¼ cup packed fresh curly parsley leaves

2 large dark green outer romaine leaves
   (about 1 cup chopped, packed in cup)

½ cup packed watercress

1 cup packed fresh spinach

Run the tomatoes through your juicer and collect the juice in a bowl or glass. If the tomato juice still contains some seeds and pulp, strain it through a fine-mesh strainer for a smoother juice. Run the remaining ingredients through the juicer and collect in the same bowl or glass with the tomato juice. Drink immediately.

ALTERNATIVE BLENDER METHOD:

This juice can also be made in a high-powered blender. Cut the tomatoes, carrots, celery, and beet into chunks and add to the blender. Add the parsley, romaine, watercress, spinach, and ½ cup purified water to help liquefy the ingredients. Blend on high until puréed, adding more water if necessary. Strain the juice using a fine-mesh strainer, cheesecloth, or nut-milk strainer bag, squeezing to extract as much juice as possible from the pulp. Drink immediately.

PUMPED-UP PUMPKIN JUICE

THE BRIGHT ORANGE COLOR OF PUMPKIN FLESH IS THE DISTINGUISHING MARK THAT THIS SEASONAL gourd is loaded with beta-carotene and other carotenoids. The best pumpkins for juicing are the small, sweet varieties such as pie pumpkins and kabocha, a type of winter squash commonly known as "Japanese pumpkin." Pumpkins are high in soluble fiber, which results in a creamy, smoothie-like juice. Among its many therapeutic benefits, pumpkin juice lifts depression, lowers cholesterol, boosts the immune system, and protects the respiratory system from infections and asthma attacks. The combination of pumpkin juice and carrot juice pumps up the power of the carotenoids to fight off cancer, improve eyesight, and keep the skin wrinkle-free.

• Makes about 10 ounces •

½ to 1 whole pie pumpkin or kabocha squash, peeled, seeded, and cut into chunks (about 4 cups of chunks)

3 large carrots

1 apple, cored

1 (¼-inch) piece fresh ginger, peeled

Pinch of pumpkin pie spice (page 45 or store-bought)

Run all ingredients except spices through your juicer and collect the juice in a bowl or glass. Sprinkle with spices. Serve over ice, if desired, and drink immediately.

SIMPLY SKINNY WATERMELON JUICE

THIS FAVORITE SUMMER FRUIT CAN BE BLENDED INTO A SWEET, REFRESHING BEVERAGE OFFERING impressive health benefits. As its name implies, watermelon juice is mainly water (92 percent) and very low in natural sugar (8 percent), making it an excellent drink for hydration, cleansing, and detoxification. Additionally, research indicates that the antioxidants and amino acids in watermelon juice aid in reducing belly fat accumulation, lower cholesterol, improve insulin sensitivity, and reduce muscle soreness after workouts.[2]

• Makes about 32 ounces •

4 cups ripe watermelon chunks, seeded

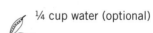 ¼ cup water (optional)

Place the watermelon chunks into a blender. Blend the watermelon for about 30 seconds, or until it is completely liquefied. Add the water to thin out the juice if it is too thick. Pour the juice directly into glasses filled with ice and drink immediately or place the juice in containers or ice cube trays and freeze. Watermelon-juice ice cubes add a nice touch to iced tea, especially mint tea.

VARIATIONS

- Add the juice of a lime and a handful of fresh mint leaves to blend with the watermelon.
- Add 1 teaspoon freshly grated ginger, 1 teaspoon freshly grated lemongrass, the juice of a lime or lemon, and a few grains of sea salt to blend with the watermelon.

Green Smoothies

Fresh juices and green smoothies each have their own unique virtues, though green smoothies may be more appealing to many people for several reasons. First, a green smoothie can serve as a snack or a complete meal in itself. Second, because all of the fiber and pulp are retained, you can safely consume several servings of fruit in one green smoothie without spiking your blood sugar. Also, the additional fiber from the greens helps slow the absorption of the fruit sugar even more. As with juicing, a large salad's worth of greens can be consumed in a smoothie, but the delicious flavors of the fruits overpower the bitter flavors of the greens, so you don't really taste them at all.

Many of the same guidelines I present for juicing on pages 89–93—proper combinations, rotating the greens, drinking on an empty stomach, remembering to chew, and the importance of organic and seasonal variety—also apply to green smoothies. Here are some additional tips and recipes that will let you experience for yourself the amazing health benefits of green smoothies.

YOU CAN DRINK A QUART OR MORE OF GREEN SMOOTHIES DAILY: To begin, you may want to start with 16 ounces (2 cups) per day. Over time, you can increase the amount and drink what is comfortable for you to consume in a day. Most people consume 1 or 2 quarts (4 to 8 cups) of green smoothie per day, but you shouldn't consume more than 1 quart at a time.

You can prepare a large amount of green smoothie, drink some immediately, and then keep the rest in the refrigerator to consume later. When properly stored in an airtight container with minimal airspace, such as a mason jar, green smoothies can be stored in the refrigerator for up to two days. However, depending on what ingredients you use, water separation may occur and you may need to shake or re-blend it before drinking.

KISS YOUR SMOOTHIE (KEEP INGREDIENTS SIMPLE AND SWEET): A basic green smoothie is made with just fruit, greens, and water—two to four different fruits and one to two different greens is a good guideline.

The ideal ratio of fruit to greens in a smoothie is about 60:40—60 percent fruit and 40 percent greens. If this ratio of fruit to greens makes a smoothie that tastes too "green," you can start with more fruit and less greens. For more sweetness without adding extra fruit, you can add a few drops of liquid stevia extract or better yet, a piece of a fresh stevia leaf (more green!).

As far as adding ingredients other than fruit, greens, and water, keep those to a minimum as well. Too many add-ins or multiple types of fats and proteins can slow down the digestion and interfere with the assimilation of nutrients. Replacing all or part of the water with coconut water is very beneficial and doesn't compromise digestion. Replacing half of the water with coconut milk, almond milk, or other nut milks is also acceptable.

A high-quality organic whey protein concentrate or plant-based protein powder can be added to green smoothies. Organic yogurt or kefir is another protein option, but don't use more than one of these in the same smoothie.

The same goes for healthy fats. Ground nuts or seeds, nut or seed butters, and beneficial oils such as flaxseed oil and coconut oil are great additions, but choose only one or two types of fat for your smoothie and keep the amount to only 2 tablespoons per pint (16 ounces) of smoothie. Also, keep in mind that many commercially available plant-based protein powders already contain seeds and healthy fats, so the addition of more is not necessary.

As a general guideline, if you feel bloated, gassy, or otherwise uncomfortable after consuming a green smoothie, consider keeping the number of ingredients to a minimum.

SAVORY GREEN SMOOTHIES FOR THE SUGAR SENSITIVE: If you have sugar sensitivities (diabetes, candida, hypoglycemia, or other conditions) then you may have to stick with low glycemic fruits such as apples, berries, lemons, and limes. Another option is to omit the sweet fruits in your smoothies and replace them with vegetables such as bell peppers, broccoli, red cabbage, cauliflower, celery, cucumber, tomatoes, zucchini, and others. Sweet potatoes and pumpkin can also be included in savory smoothies, as they are both known for their blood sugar–stabilizing properties. The key to making a great savory green smoothie is to add part of an avocado

for the creamy consistency and a piece of lemon or lime for zest. When making savory green smoothies, remember to always respect proper food combinations. The only fruits that combine well with vegetables are lemons, limes, apples, and avocados. For example, to make a savory green smoothie following proper food combinations, you could use greens, herbs, garlic, celery, avocado, tomato, or other vegetables, but you wouldn't also add a banana or a pear to the smoothie.

DRINK YOUR SMOOTHIE BY ITSELF: For the same reasons as drinking juices on their own, green smoothies are best consumed when you have nothing else in your stomach. Also, drink your smoothie by itself, not as part of a meal with other food. Wait about forty minutes after you've finished your smoothie to eat a meal or a snack. To give your digestive system a proper break, wait at least two to three hours after eating a meal before having another green smoothie.

DRINK YOUR SMOOTHIE SLOWLY: Quickly gulping down smoothies dumps too much food into your digestive system too fast, so drink your green smoothie slowly and give each mouthful a few good chews before swallowing.

How to Make the Best Green Smoothie

The combinations of fruits and greens are endless for making green smoothies, but there is an art to making them great. You have to use a strategic combination of fruits with greens to make sure your smoothie turns out sweet and creamy every time.

Fiber: The strategy is to make sure you have the right balance of soluble fiber to insoluble fiber.

Apples, blueberries, raspberries, blackberries, citrus, melons, pineapples, and greens are all high in *insoluble* fiber (the type known as "roughage" that does not dissolve in water). When you blend a combination of these ingredients with water, you will produce a horrible green mess!

The key to making green smoothies that look and taste great is *soluble fiber*. Fruits with high amounts of soluble fiber include avocados, bananas, dates, kiwis, mangos, papayas, peaches, pears, plums, prunes, strawberries, and the creamy, soft meat of a young coconut. Combining one or more of these creamy, high-soluble fiber fruits with greens and fruits that are high in insoluble fiber will make a delicious green smoothie every time.

Frozen fruit: Frozen fruit also adds creaminess to green smoothies and gives them a little bit of a chill. However, you should avoid consuming *very cold* smoothies, like the kind that give you brain freeze or make your stomach feel sore. Foods that are too cold can slow down your digestion and make it harder for your body to absorb nutrients. To avoid making smoothies that are too cold, a good general rule is to use more fresh fruits than frozen and to run your blender a little longer to help bring up the temperature.

Greens: Different greens have different levels of flavor. If you are new to making green smoothies, start with the milder-flavored greens like spinach or romaine lettuce. Moderately flavored greens include celery, kale, Swiss chard, and collards. More strongly flavored greens include arugula, dandelion greens, mustard greens, beet greens, radish greens, and bok choy. Microgreens or any type of sprouts can also be used for some of the greens. If you drink green smoothies on a regular or daily basis, it is important to rotate the types of greens you use. See page 91 for a detailed explanation of the importance of rotating greens.

Liquid: Water is the best liquid for a green smoothie, but you can replace some of it with coconut water, herbal tea, nut milk, or coconut milk. I recommend using half water and half other liquid to make the total volume of liquid called for in the recipe.

Add-ins: Finally, you may include fresh herbs and a few add-ins to your smoothies. Some of my favorites are fresh mint, basil, parsley, cilantro, sage, ginger, garlic, turmeric, and green superfood powders.

Other add-ins such as cinnamon, vanilla, chia seeds, freshly ground flaxseeds, cacao (nibs and powder), maca, bee pollen, and rose water can add different flavors and benefits to your smoothie. Keeping simplicity of ingredients in mind, however, it is best to select only a few add-ins per smoothie and vary what you add on different days.

Basic 60:40 Green Smoothie Recipe

Here is a guideline for making a basic green smoothie. Select the specified amounts from each column, place in your blender, and blend on high for one to two minutes, or until all ingredients are completely liquefied. This recipe makes about 1 quart (4 cups), which can be cut in half or doubled, depending on your needs.

With the exception of avocados, fruit servings are equal to either one whole fruit or 1 cup, whichever is larger. Avocados are the exception; use no more than a quarter of a large or half of a small avocado per quart of smoothie. As fruits come in different sizes with varying water content, you may need to adjust the amounts of fruit slightly to get the desired texture. Smoothies are an art, so feel free to experiment with what works best!

• Makes 1 quart (4 cups)—2 servings •

Greens/Fresh Herbs	Water	Soluble Fiber Fruits	Insoluble Fiber Fruits
2 cups, tightly packed (if using fresh herbs, use smaller amounts of them combined with larger amounts of leafy greens)	2 cups	2 servings or 2 cups, depending on type of fruit	2 servings or 2 cups, depending on type of fruit
Greens Beet greens Bok choy Chard leaves, stems removed Collard leaves Dandelion greens Kale, stems and ribs removed Lettuces Microgreens Radish greens Rapini (broccoli rabe) Romaine lettuce Spinach Spring mix **Fresh herbs** Basil Cilantro Dill Mint Parsley		Apricot Avocado* Banana Coconut meat (scooped from a young coconut) Date Kiwifruit Mango Papaya Peach Pear Plum Prune Strawberry *use no more than ¼ to ½ avocado per quart of smoothie	Apple Blackberry Blueberry Cantaloupe Cherry Cranberry Fig Goji berry Grape Grapefruit Lemon Lime Lychee Minneola Orange Passion fruit Persimmon Pineapple Pomegranate Pomelo Raspberry Starfruit Tangelo Tangerine Watermelon

BEGINNER'S DELIGHT GREEN SMOOTHIE

This is a great starter smoothie that the whole family will love. It's sweet, creamy, and loaded with tropical flavors. If you're not a fan of bananas, you can use more mango instead.

• Makes 1 quart •

½ large head romaine lettuce, or
    1 whole heart of romaine, chopped
2 cups water
1 large peach, pitted

1 large banana
1 mango, peeled and pitted
    (or 1 cup frozen chunks)

Add the lettuce and water to the blender and blend on high until all leafy chunks are gone. Add in the fruits and blend again.

BANANA BERRY MANGO GREEN SMOOTHIE

This rich, creamy smoothie is packed with colorful nutrition. Mangos are a super fruit high in soluble fiber as well as vitamins A, B6, C, E, and K. They are also a good source of potassium, protein, and omega-3 fatty acids. Any green you choose will add a healthy dose of chlorophyll to flush out toxins and boost your immune system. If you rotate the greens and the berries in this smoothie, you can drink it every day! Using one or all of the add-ins will boost the nutritional value even higher and keep sugar cravings at bay.

• Makes about 1 quart •

- ½ to 1 cup water
- ½ cup unsweetened nut milk or coconut milk
- 2 tightly packed cups greens (any type)
- 1 medium fresh or frozen banana
- 1 cup fresh or frozen mango chunks
- 1 cup fresh or frozen berries (blueberries, raspberries, blackberries, etc.)

Place ½ cup water and the remaining ingredients into a blender and blend on high for 1 to 2 minutes, or until all ingredients are completely liquefied, stopping to add more water if necessary. Drink immediately.

OPTIONAL ADD-INS

- 1 scoop protein powder of your choice (see Resources, page 275)
- 1 tablespoon raw cacao nibs
- 1 teaspoon bee pollen granules

PARSLEY GINGER PEAR SMOOTHIE

PARSLEY IS ONE OF THE WORLD'S SEVEN-MOST POTENT DISEASE-FIGHTING HERBS, OFFERING health-protective properties that rival those of many green leafy vegetables. It contains high levels of beta-carotene, vitamin B12, folate, chlorophyll, calcium, more vitamin C than citrus fruits, and more vitamin K than kale, spinach, and collard greens. Adding a handful of parsley to any green smoothie is a great way to boost your intake of its impressive nutrients.

• Makes about 1 quart •

- 2 cups water
- 2 cups packed fresh baby spinach
- 1 large handful fresh curly parsley
- 2 pears, cored
- 1 apple, cored
- 1 (¼-inch) piece fresh ginger, peeled and minced (or grated)

Place all ingredients into a blender (along with some ice, if desired) and blend on high for 1 to 2 minutes, or until all ingredients are completely liquefied, stopping to add more water if necessary. Drink immediately.

CHERRY CHIA VANILLA SMOOTHIE

THERE'S MORE THAN MEETS THE EYE, AND THE TASTE BUDS, IN THIS SWEET, CREAMY SMOOTHIE. Anthocyanins, the same compounds that give cherries their bright red hue, are powerful antioxidants that have been scientifically proven to be just as effective as aspirin and ibuprofen in relieving the pain and inflammation of arthritis. They're also packed with a number of cancer-fighting compounds. The darker the cherry, whether sweet or sour, the higher the concentration of antioxidants.

• Makes 1 serving •

1 cup unsweetened nut milk of your choice

1 ounce unsweetened cherry juice (optional)

2 cups tightly packed greens (any type)

1 banana

½ cup frozen pitted dark cherries

1 tablespoon chia seeds

1 teaspoon pure vanilla extract, or ½ teaspoon vanilla powder

Liquid stevia extract, to taste

Place all ingredients into a blender and blend on high speed for about 2 minutes, or until all ingredients are smooth and creamy, stopping to add more liquid if necessary. Drink immediately.

PEACHY ROMAINE GREEN SMOOTHIE

ROMAINE LETTUCE IS A HIGHLY NUTRITIOUS LEAFY GREEN WITH A MILD FLAVOR THAT IS NICELY masked by fruit. You can add an entire heart of romaine to a fruit smoothie and not impact the taste at all, so it's the perfect leafy green for kids and green smoothie beginners. One head of romaine is packed with protein, calcium, omega-3s, and more vitamin C than an orange.

• Makes about 1 quart •

1 cup water or unsweetened nut milk

½ large head romaine lettuce, or 1 whole heart of romaine, chopped

1 banana

2 peaches, pitted

1 tablespoon chia seeds

Place the water and romaine into a blender and blend on high until the romaine is completely liquefied. Add the remaining ingredients and blend again on high until smooth and creamy. Drink immediately.

TROPICAL COLADA KALE SMOOTHIE

THIS CREAMY SMOOTHIE COMBINES ALL THE FLAVORS OF THE TROPICS WITH THE NUTRITIONAL power of kale. The skin of the kiwifruit contains fiber and flavonoids, as well as omega-3 fatty acids, so toss the whole fruit into the blender without peeling.

• Makes about 1 quart •

1 cup coconut milk

1 cup water

1 cup tightly packed chopped Lacinato kale leaves (stems and ribs removed)

¼ cup loosely packed fresh mint leaves

2 fresh or frozen bananas

1 cup fresh or frozen pineapple chunks

2 kiwis, sliced

Place all ingredients into a blender (along with ½ cup ice, if desired) and blend on high speed for about 2 minutes, or until all ingredients are completely liquefied, stopping to add more liquid if necessary. Drink immediately.

HOLIDAY PIE GREEN SMOOTHIE

FEATURING PUMPKIN PURÉE (OR BAKED SWEET POTATO) AND HOLIDAY SPICES, THIS TASTY DRINK is a super-nutritious way to keep your blood sugar levels in check. Pumpkin contains two major compounds—trigonelline and nicotinic acid—that are effective in lowering blood sugar levels by improving insulin resistance and suppressing the onset of diabetes. These powerful compounds also inhibit the accumulation of triglycerides in the blood, a danger that often accompanies diabetes.[3] Sweet potatoes are also known for their ability to improve blood sugar levels, even in people with type 2 diabetes. Health benefits aside, this smoothie is a delicious comfort food you can enjoy any time of year.

• Makes about 1 quart •

½ cup coconut milk

½ cup water

1 cup tightly packed fresh spinach or spring mix

½ cup pumpkin purée (page 70 or store-bought) or mashed baked sweet potato

¼ avocado, peeled

¼ teaspoon ground cinnamon

1 teaspoon pumpkin pie spice (page 45 or store-bought)

½ teaspoon pure vanilla extract

⅛ teaspoon liquid stevia extract, or more to taste

Place all ingredients into a blender (along with a few ice cubes, if desired) and blend on high speed until smooth and creamy, about 1 minute. If the smoothie is too thick, add more water and blend again to thin it out. Adjust sweetness and spices to taste. Drink immediately.

MINT CHOCOLATE BLISS SMOOTHIE

When you're in the mood for a treat, this smoothie is your ticket to bliss without the sugar overload. The greens lend their color, but the flavors of mint and chocolate are all over this creamy, dense creation.

• Makes about 1 quart •

1 cup coconut milk or unsweetened nut milk

1 cup water

2 cups packed fresh spinach

¼ cup fresh mint leaves, or ¼ teaspoon mint extract

½ avocado, peeled

2 tablespoons unsweetened cocoa powder

1 tablespoon raw cacao nibs or 70 percent cacao dark chocolate chips (see Resources, page 280)

3 drops liquid stevia extract, or more to taste

Place all ingredients into a blender (along with a few ice cubes, if desired) and blend on high speed until smooth and creamy, about 1 minute. If the smoothie is too thick, add more water and blend again to thin it out. Adjust sweetness to taste. Drink immediately.

BEGINNER'S SAVORY GREEN SMOOTHIE

Savory green smoothies are sometimes called blender salads, and their taste is slightly salty, spicy, or zesty, rather than sweet. Savory smoothies are perfect for diabetics and those who want to keep their sugar intake low. Use this recipe as a template for making savory smoothies, adding other vegetables and switching out herbs and spices to create a drink that suits your tastes. The key to a creamy savory smoothie is the avocado, so make sure you always have a ripe one on hand. Ice cubes are optional, but they add a nice chill.

• Makes about 1 quart •

4 Roma tomatoes

2 cups tightly packed fresh spinach

3 celery stalks, cut into 1-inch pieces

1 cup packed fresh curly parsley, bottom stems removed

2 to 3 fresh basil leaves

½ avocado, peeled

1 garlic clove, finely minced

Juice of ½ lemon

Pinch of sea salt or kelp (optional)

1 to 1½ cups water

Place all ingredients in the order listed into a blender (along with 6 to 8 ice cubes, if desired) and blend on high speed until smooth and creamy, about 1 minute. If the smoothie is too thick, add more water and blend again to thin it out. Adjust salt to taste. Drink immediately.

ZESTY SAVORY GREEN SMOOTHIE

THIS SAVORY DRINK GETS ITS ZEST FROM GINGER AND CAYENNE, TWO STRONG ALKALINE-FORMING and liver-cleansing herbs that also help to improve digestion. Several compounds in ginger, including gingerols, are similar to cayenne's capsaicin, and both help to reduce the pain and inflammation of arthritis.

• Makes about 1 quart •

3 large collard greens, stems removed, coarsely chopped

½ small cucumber, cut into chunks

1 carrot, sliced into ½-inch coins

½ cup packed fresh cilantro, bottom stems removed

½ avocado, peeled

1 (1-inch) piece fresh ginger, peeled

⅛ teaspoon cayenne pepper (optional)

Juice of 1 lime

Pinch of sea salt or kelp (optional)

1 to 1½ cups water

Place all ingredients in the order listed into a blender (along with 6 to 8 ice cubes, if desired) and blend on high speed until smooth and creamy, about 1 minute. If the smoothie is too thick, add more water and blend again to thin it out. Adjust salt to taste. Drink immediately.

Outside-the-Cereal-Box Breakfasts

While I've categorized these recipes as breakfast fare, they can be enjoyed at any time of day. Some, like Soft-Boiled Eggs on Avocado Toast (page 122) and Red Pepper Quiche with Sweet Potato Crust (page 124), are satisfying enough to stand in for lunch or dinner; others, like Seasonal Fruit Salads (page 112) and Pumpkin-Spiced Quinoa Granola (page 121), make great snacks or desserts. It's important to not limit yourself to any specific type of food for any meal just because it's the cultural norm. In fact, eating processed-free means breaking norms and eating outside the "box." For example, one of my favorite breakfasts is Hearty Vegetable Miso Soup (page 219). That may sound *way* outside the box to you, and it would have to me several years ago, but as my taste buds have become more accustomed to eating vegetables, I crave them now more than ever. A plate of chopped spring mix with slices of avocado and tomato, topped with warm cooked quinoa, poached eggs, and herbed goat cheese, makes a great breakfast too. On the other hand, I sometimes splurge and enjoy my Banana Waffles or Pancakes (page 126) for dinner, paired with Sweet Potato Morning Glory (page 116). As you create and personalize your processed-free meals, I invite you to be imaginative and reassess what types of foods you're willing to consider eating for breakfast.

SEASONAL FRUIT SALADS

A SALAD CONSISTING OF THREE OR FOUR DIFFERENT FRUITS MAKES A WONDERFULLY NOURISHING and cleansing breakfast. The fruits you choose for this salad will be determined by the season and your locale. These are a few of my favorite seasonal fruit combinations.

• Each salad makes 2 servings •

SPRING/SUMMER FRUIT SALAD

1 cup blackberries

1 cup cherries, pitted and halved

1 large peach, cut into chunks

20 raw walnut halves (about 2 ounces)

½ teaspoon organic rose water (optional)

Dollop of organic sugar-free vanilla yogurt (page 67 or store-bought; optional)

Place the fruit and walnuts in a medium bowl. Sprinkle the rose water over the fruit, if using, and toss to coat. Divide equally to make 2 servings.

FALL/WINTER FRUIT SALAD

2 blood oranges, peel and pith removed, cut into segments

½ pomegranate, seeded

2 pears, cored and cut into thin wedges

1 banana, sliced

8 fresh mint leaves, chopped

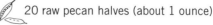 20 raw pecan halves (about 1 ounce)

Place all ingredients together in a medium bowl. Squeeze the juice from one of the orange segments over all of the ingredients and toss to coat. Divide equally to make 2 servings.

BLOOD ORANGES

BLOOD ORANGES ARE SO NAMED FOR THEIR dark crimson-colored flesh. These unique oranges get their distinctive pigment from the presence of anthocyanins, the same class of compounds that give blueberries their "super antioxidant" properties and intense color. Anthocyanins are not found in other citrus fruits, which is why blood oranges have much higher antioxidant levels than other varieties of oranges and why you'll want to opt for them when they're in season. Anthocyanins have anti-inflammatory properties, prevent cancer, diabetes, and bacterial infections, prevent the accumulation of LDL (bad) cholesterol, and reduce the risk of heart disease. Blood oranges are also high in vitamins A and C, folic acid (vitamin B9), and calcium. They are typically in season from December through March, or January through May, depending on the area of the country they are cultivated in.

FRESH COCONUT VANILLA "YOGURT"

THIS DELIGHTFUL VERSION OF COCONUT YOGURT IS NOT FERMENTED, SO IT DOESN'T CONTAIN any probiotics, but it is loaded with alkalizing mineral electrolytes from the coconut's water and antioxidants from the coconut meat. It has a creamy, thick consistency similar to Greek yogurt and only takes a few minutes to whip together. Once you get the hang of cracking open the coconut, this may become one of your favorite breakfast staples. Serve with a sprinkling of Pumpkin-Spiced Quinoa Granola (page 121) and fresh fruit.

• Makes 1 serving •

¼ to ½ cup coconut water from a young
   Thai coconut

1 cup coconut meat from a young
   Thai coconut

½ teaspoon pure vanilla extract or ¼ teaspoon
   vanilla powder

Open the coconut with a cleaver or large chef's knife (see page 65 for instructions). Pour the coconut water into a glass and set aside. Scoop out the soft white coconut meat and add 1 cup of it to a food processor or high-powered blender. If there is any coconut meat left, save the rest to use in smoothies or just to eat. Add ¼ cup of the coconut water and the vanilla and blend well. Continue adding coconut water until the "yogurt" reaches your desired consistency. Serve immediately. Store leftovers in an airtight container for up to 3 days.

FRUIT AND YOGURT CHIA PARFAIT

A CREAMY BLEND OF YOGURT AND CHIA SEEDS LAYERED WITH FRESH OR FROZEN FRUIT MAKES A scrumptious meal that satiates you for hours (and the chia seeds give you a protein and omega-3 boost!). These delights last for up to 3 days in the fridge, so plan ahead and make multiple parfaits to store in covered containers for a convenient grab-and-go breakfast for the whole family.

• Makes 1 serving •

¾ cup organic plain whole milk yogurt

1 teaspoon pure vanilla extract, or ½ teaspoon
   vanilla powder

3 drops liquid stevia extract or other natural
   sweetener, or more to taste

1 tablespoon chia seeds

½ banana, sliced

½ cup fresh or frozen berries

1 tablespoon unsweetened shredded coconut

1 tablespoon sliced raw almonds

In a bowl, combine the yogurt, vanilla, stevia, and chia seeds and stir. Cover the bottom of a tall pint-size glass container (such as a mason jar) with a third of the fruit. Top with half the yogurt mixture and another third of the fruit, then layer in the remaining yogurt and the fruit. Top with the coconut and sliced almonds. Refrigerate overnight, covered. Parfaits keep for up to 3 days in the refrigerator.

LICKETY-SPLIT BANANA BOWL

SWITCH UP YOUR MORNING ROUTINE BY HAVING DESSERT FOR BREAKFAST. THIS BANANA-SPLIT makeover takes just minutes to put together in the morning. Organic Greek yogurt is thick and creamy like ice cream, but any yogurt will do. A half cup of fresh berries or other fruit can be used in place of the fruit jam. Feel free to swap out the other toppings to suit your tastes.

• Makes 1 serving •

1 banana

½ cup organic plain Greek-style yogurt

2 tablespoons raw fruit jam (page 164) or 100 percent fruit preserves

1 tablespoon unsweetened shredded or flaked coconut

1 tablespoon chopped raw almonds, pecans, or other nuts

Peel and cut the banana in half lengthwise and place the halves in a bowl. Top with the yogurt along the length of the banana. Drizzle the jam on top of the yogurt, then sprinkle with the coconut and nuts. Serve immediately.

SWEET POTATO MORNING GLORY

THE SWEET POTATO COMES FROM THE SAME PLANT FAMILY AS SEVERAL GARDEN FLOWERS CALLED morning glories, and what better way to start your day than with this glorious vegetable? The topping suggestions are open to your imagination, but please don't skip the healthy fats (i.e., raw nuts), as they are needed by your body to get the optimal absorption of the beta-carotene in the sweet potatoes.

• Makes 1 serving •

1 small sweet potato or yam, or ½ large one, washed and dried (about 4 or 5 ounces)

1 cup organic plain whole milk yogurt

1 tablespoon pure maple syrup

1 tablespoon chopped raw pecans or other nuts

¼ teaspoon ground cinnamon

Preheat the oven to 375°F. Pierce the skin of the sweet potato a few times with a fork. Place the sweet potato on a parchment-lined baking sheet and bake until tender when pierced with a paring knife, about 40 to 50 minutes. Remove the sweet potato from the oven and let it cool enough to handle.

Slice the sweet potato across the top with a knife, then squeeze the potato slightly so the flesh rises out of the skin.

Spoon on the yogurt, drizzle with syrup, and sprinkle with nuts and cinnamon. Serve warm.

NOTE:

One or more sweet potatoes can be baked ahead of time and kept refrigerated for about 5 days. To warm a prebaked sweet potato, place it in a 375°F oven or toaster oven for 5 minutes.

COCONUT CURRANT BREAKFAST MUESLI

MUESLI IS A TRADITIONAL SWISS BREAKFAST CEREAL THAT IS LIKE A RAW VERSION OF GRANOLA. It is typically made with uncooked rolled oats, fresh or dried fruit, and nuts and seeds and is served with nut milk. You can make a large batch of this cereal and store it in an airtight glass jar or sealed container in your pantry for up to three months. To serve muesli you need to plan ahead, as it needs some time to soak overnight. Once you've soaked your portion, enjoy muesli with some fresh fruit in the morning.

• Makes 10 (½-cup) servings •

MUESLI

2 cups uncooked rolled oats

1 cup raw nuts of your choice (almonds, cashews, pecans, walnuts, etc., or a mixture)

½ cup unsweetened coconut flakes or shredded coconut

½ cup raw sunflower seeds

¼ cup currants or raisins

5 dates, pitted and chopped, or 5 dried apricots, chopped

1 teaspoon ground cinnamon

1 teaspoon vanilla powder (optional but divine; see note)

FOR SERVING

A few frozen berries (optional)

½ cup unsweetened nut milk of your choice, plus more as needed

1 teaspoon freshly squeezed lemon juice

Fresh fruit, for garnish (optional)

Natural sweetener (such as liquid stevia extract or pure maple syrup), to taste (optional)

Place all the muesli ingredients in a bowl and toss gently to combine. Transfer to a storage container.

To serve: Prepare the muesli the night before you'd like to serve it. Measure out your desired portion into a serving dish or a container that can be taken with you as a grab-and-go breakfast. For some extra flavor and sweetness, toss in a few frozen berries, if desired. Pour enough nut milk over the muesli just to cover it and the berries. Add the lemon juice and stir to combine everything. Cover the container and place it in the refrigerator overnight or for at least 6 hours. In the morning, it's ready to eat. Add some fresh fruit and a small amount of natural sweetener, if desired.

NOTE: *If you don't have vanilla powder, you can add a drop or two of vanilla extract to the mixture along with the milk and lemon juice.*

CINNAMON QUINOA PORRIDGE WITH BLUEBERRIES AND ALMONDS

THE COMFORTING AROMA OF CINNAMON AND QUINOA COOKING IN THE MORNING IS WELCOME IN both cold and warm weather. Quinoa makes a high-protein porridge that is lighter in texture and heavy on satisfaction. Packed with calcium, copper, iron, and potassium, quinoa has an alkaline-forming edge over other types of porridge. The blueberries add antioxidants and vitamin C, while the almonds provide additional fiber and alkalinity. What a wonderful way to start the day!

• Makes 4 servings •

1 cup unsweetened almond milk or light
   coconut milk

1 cup water

1 cup organic white quinoa, soaked
   and rinsed

1 teaspoon ground cinnamon

2 cups fresh or frozen blueberries

⅓ cup chopped raw almonds

Combine the milk, water, quinoa, and cinnamon in a medium saucepan. Bring to a boil over high heat. Reduce the heat to medium low; cover and simmer 15 minutes, or until most of the liquid is absorbed. Turn off the heat; let stand, covered, for 5 minutes. Stir in the blueberries. Transfer to 4 bowls and top with the chopped almonds. Leftover porridge can be stored in the refrigerator for up to 3 days and can quickly be reheated on the stovetop with some additional almond milk. It can also be frozen for up to 1 month.

VARIATIONS

- Instead of adding the blueberries after cooking, you can core and dice 2 apples and add them to the cooking pot for a nice cooked apple quinoa porridge.

- Use red quinoa instead of white quinoa; replace the blueberries with blackberries; and replace the almonds with pecans or walnuts.

BAKED OATMEAL WITH SWEET POTATO AND APPLES

THIS WARM AND SLIGHTLY SWEET OATMEAL IS THE IDEAL COMFORT FOOD ON CHILLY MORNINGS, but it can be enjoyed anytime. Soaking the oats overnight with lemon juice neutralizes the phytates in the oats and increases the bioavailability of their nutrients. If using presoaked and dried or sprouted oats, you can skip the soaking step.

• Makes 1 (13 x 9-inch) pan, about 8 (1-cup) servings •

1½ cups rolled oats

1½ cups warm water

3 tablespoons freshly squeezed lemon juice, organic cultured buttermilk, or liquid whey

1 cup coconut milk

⅓ cup virgin coconut oil, melted, plus more for the baking dish

2 cups peeled and diced sweet potatoes

1 apple, cored and diced

½ cup unsweetened coconut flakes or shredded coconut

½ cup raw pecan halves

2 tablespoons ground cinnamon

1 tablespoon pure vanilla extract

1 cup raisins

 ¼ teaspoon liquid stevia extract, or ¼ cup coconut sugar, raw honey, or other sweetener (optional)

Place the oats in a large glass or ceramic bowl and pour in the warm water and lemon juice. Stir gently, cover with a kitchen towel, and let soak for 8 hours or overnight (no more than 24 hours).

After soaking, drain the oats in a colander and place them back in a clean mixing bowl.

Preheat the oven to 350°F. Coat a 13 x 9-inch baking dish with coconut oil or organic butter.

Add the remaining ingredients to the oats in the bowl and stir to combine. Place the mixture in the prepared baking dish. Bake for 35 to 40 minutes, or until the sweet potatoes are tender and the mixture is firm. Serve warm. The oatmeal can be stored in the refrigerator for up to 4 days or frozen for up to 1 month.

CREAMY PUMPKIN OAT BRAN

A BOWL OF CREAMY COOKED OAT BRAN CONTAINS TWICE THE AMOUNT OF FIBER, HALF THE AMOUNT of calories, and higher amounts of antioxidants, protein, and calcium than the same-size bowl of oatmeal. The addition of puréed pumpkin and spices lends wonderful flavor and increases the antioxidant content and blood sugar–stabilizing properties of this warming bowl of goodness. Soaking the oat bran overnight helps with digestion, but this recipe can always be made without the soaking step. See note on page 133 for instructions on how to soak oat bran.

• Makes 2 (¾-cup) servings •

⅔ cup raw oat bran

2 cups water

½ cup pumpkin purée (page 70 or store-bought)

2 tablespoons unsweetened nut milk

2 teaspoons ground cinnamon or pumpkin pie spice (page 45 or store-bought)

4 to 6 drops liquid stevia extract, or 1 teaspoon pure maple syrup

2 tablespoons chopped raw pecans

Place oat bran and water in a saucepan and bring it to a boil over medium-high heat while stirring. Reduce the heat to low, stir in the pumpkin purée, nut milk, cinnamon, and stevia, and simmer for 3 to 5 minutes, or until thick and creamy, stirring frequently. Remove from the heat, transfer to two bowls, and sprinkle each bowl with the pecans. Serve immediately.

VARIATIONS

- Creamy Oat Bran can be served without the addition of the pumpkin. I often cook the oat bran with just the water until it's thick and creamy, then add in a pinch of cinnamon, a few drops of stevia or maple syrup, and the pecans. Then I top it with an over-easy egg.

- Try this recipe with rolled oats or steel cut oats too! Just replace the oat bran with the preferred type of oat and adjust the cooking time accordingly.

PUMPKIN-SPICED QUINOA GRANOLA

MOST COMMERCIALLY PREPARED GRANOLA IS MADE WITH HIGH AMOUNTS OF SUGAR AND UNHEALTHY oils. Making your own granola is easier than you think, and you can customize the ingredients to suit your tastes. Soaked rolled oats are better for digestion, but unsoaked versions work too. Serve with almond milk or yogurt and fresh fruit.

• Makes 11 (⅓-cup) servings •

¼ cup uncooked quinoa (soaked, rinsed, and patted dry)

2 cups rolled oats (preferably soaked and dried; see page 41)

½ cup raw almonds

½ cup chopped raw pecans

½ cup raw pepitas

½ cup raisins

¼ cup pure maple syrup or other liquid sweetener (such as brown rice syrup or raw honey)

½ cup pumpkin purée (page 70 or store-bought)

6 tablespoons virgin coconut oil, melted

1 teaspoon pure vanilla extract

2 teaspoons pumpkin pie spice (page 45 or store-bought)

Pinch of sea salt

Preheat the oven to 325°F. Spread the quinoa out on a parchment-lined baking sheet. Toast in the oven for 10 minutes, stirring halfway through to toast evenly.

Remove the quinoa from the oven and pour it into a large mixing bowl. Add the oats, nuts, pepitas, and raisins.

Reduce the oven temperature to 300°F.

In a second mixing bowl, combine the maple syrup, pumpkin purée, coconut oil, vanilla, pumpkin pie spice, and salt. Pour the pumpkin mixture over the quinoa mixture and stir to combine. Spread the granola onto a parchment-lined baking sheet and bake for 20 minutes, or until golden. Let cool completely, then store in an airtight container in the refrigerator for up to 2 weeks.

SOFT-BOILED EGGS ON AVOCADO TOAST

EGG YOLKS ARE A GOOD SOURCE OF CAROTENOIDS SUCH AS LUTEIN AND ZEAXANTHIN, WHICH HELP keep your eyesight sharp. With the healthy fats of the avocado and the nutritional power of the greens, protecting your eyesight has never been so delicious!

• Makes 2 servings •

2 large eggs

2 slices sprouted grain bread (page 142 or store-bought)

1 avocado

2 handfuls spring mix, baby greens, or watercress leaves

Sea salt and freshly ground black pepper

2 tablespoons salsa (optional)

Fill a medium saucepan about two-thirds full with water and bring it to a boil. Use a large spoon to gently lower the eggs into the pot of boiling water. There should be enough water to completely cover the eggs. Set a kitchen timer for 6 minutes.

While your eggs are cooking, toast the bread.

Slice the avocado in half, remove the pit, and scoop out each half onto a slice of toast. Mash the avocado with a fork, then top each half with a small handful of greens.

When the eggs are ready, drain the hot water from the pan and fill it with cold running water from the sink. Run the cold water over the eggs for 1 minute. This will stop the cooking but will not make the inside of the egg cold.

Carefully crack and peel each egg (slip a teaspoon under the egg shell to help you carefully remove the shell), then place it on a slice of the avocado toast. Cut each egg in half to allow the yolk to run over the greens. Season with salt and pepper and top with salsa, if desired. Serve immediately.

EGG PRESERVER

YOU CAN EXTEND THE SHELF LIFE OF fresh eggs by applying a thin coat of virgin coconut oil to the unbroken egg shell. Liquefy the coconut oil (but don't make it hot), dip the egg into the oil or brush on a coat of oil over the egg surface, and then store in a cool place. The oil creates a seal that keeps oxygen from penetrating the eggs. Eggs prepared this way are reported to maintain their grade A status freshness for 4 weeks longer than non-coated eggs.[1]

POWER PROTEIN SCRAMBLE

Eggs and other animal-protein foods always need to be paired with vegetables to balance their acid-forming tendency. You can whip up different versions of this fluffy egg creation, depending on what vegetables you have on hand and even top it with salsa for a spicy southwestern version. Serve with cooked quinoa, brown rice, or sprouted grain toast or tortillas, if desired.

• Makes 2 servings •

4 large eggs

2 tablespoons coconut milk

2 tablespoons virgin coconut oil

½ medium red onion, chopped

4 garlic cloves, minced

2 cups chopped fresh spinach

¼ teaspoon sea salt

¼ teaspoon freshly ground black pepper

2 Roma tomatoes, chopped

1 ounce organic white Cheddar or other favorite cheese (preferably raw), grated

2 tablespoons chopped fresh curly parsley, plus a few parsley sprigs for garnish

Crack the eggs into a bowl and add the coconut milk. Whisk the mixture until well combined. Set aside.

Heat the coconut oil in a skillet over medium-high heat. Add the onions and cook for 2 minutes, using a spatula to stir the onions in the oil. Lower the heat to medium, add the garlic, stir, and cook for 1 minute. Add the spinach and cook just until lightly wilted, stirring constantly, about 30 seconds.

Give the eggs another quick whisk and pour them over the vegetables in the skillet. Sprinkle with the salt and pepper, then add the tomatoes but don't stir. Let the eggs set for about 30 seconds, then use the spatula to scrape the eggs from the edge of the pan to the center, forming large, soft curds. Continue cooking and scraping until the eggs are no longer wet.

Turn off the heat but leave the skillet on the burner. Sprinkle the eggs with the grated cheese, then sprinkle on the chopped parsley. Cover the pan and let sit until the cheese melts, about 1 minute.

Divide the eggs evenly between 2 plates, garnish with fresh parsley sprigs, and serve immediately.

RED PEPPER QUICHE
WITH SWEET POTATO CRUST

THIS QUICHE, PACKED WITH POWERFUL LIVER-CLEANSING FOODS, MAKES A GREAT WARM OR COLD meal at any time of day, especially served with a green salad. A good timesaving strategy is to double the recipe and make two quiches—one to eat now and one to freeze for an easy meal another time.

• Makes 4 servings •

2 medium sweet potatoes, baked, or 1½ cups canned sweet potato purée

1 red bell pepper, halved

1 tablespoon virgin coconut oil, plus more for the pan

1 medium yellow onion, chopped

2 garlic cloves, minced

½ cup chopped fresh basil

1 cup chopped fresh spinach

8 large eggs

¼ cup coconut milk

Sea salt and freshly ground pepper

Fresh curly parsley sprigs, for garnish

Preheat the oven to 350°F and situate a rack in the center. Coat a 9-inch pie pan (deep-dish works best) with coconut oil.

If using baked sweet potatoes, remove the peels and slice the flesh into thin slices. Cover the bottom and the sides of the prepared pie pan with the slices to create a "crust." Alternatively, if you are using canned sweet potato purée, spread the purée over the bottom and up the sides of the pie pan to create the crust. Set aside.

Slice one half of the red bell pepper into long, thin strips. Set aside. Dice the other half to use in the next step.

Place the tablespoon of coconut oil in a skillet over medium heat. Sauté the diced bell pepper, onion, and garlic until the peppers are soft, about 5 minutes. Add the basil and spinach and cook just until slightly wilted, 1 to 2 minutes. Remove from the heat.

Whisk the eggs and coconut milk together in a large bowl, season with salt and pepper, and whisk again to combine.

Spread the cooked vegetables over the bottom of the prepared pie pan. Pour the egg mixture over the vegetables. Place the thin slices of red bell pepper on top of the egg, radiating outward from the center to look like a pinwheel. Place the pan on the center rack of the oven and bake for 20 to 30 minutes, or until the center of the quiche is set. Remove from the oven, let cool slightly, then cut into 4 equal pieces. Serve with fresh parsley sprigs.

VARIATIONS

You can add more or different veggies, such as broccoli, asparagus, or carrots; just remember to lightly cook them before adding to the quiche. If the veggies are not cooked first, your quiche may become too watery.

COLLARD GREENS AND SWEET POTATO FRITTATA

THE COMBINATION OF EGGS, COLLARDS, SWEET POTATOES, AND BELL PEPPERS MAKES THIS AN excellent liver-cleansing meal. Health benefits aside, this frittata makes a delightful warm breakfast or brunch for the cool winter mornings.

• Makes 4 servings •

3 tablespoons virgin coconut oil

1 cup chopped yellow onion

4 garlic cloves, minced

1 medium sweet potato, thinly sliced

1 teaspoon sea salt, divided

1 red bell pepper, sliced

1 cup sliced cremini mushrooms

2 teaspoons dried rosemary

½ teaspoon dried sage

2 cups chopped collard greens (stems removed)

8 large eggs

Freshly ground black pepper

5 ounces goat cheese (plain or herbed), crumbled

¼ cup chopped fresh curly parsley, for garnish

Heat the oil in a large skillet over medium heat. Toss in the onions, garlic, and sweet potatoes. Cook, stirring frequently, for about 3 minutes, then reduce the heat to low, add ½ teaspoon salt, and cover. Cook 10 minutes more, or until the potatoes are tender.

Stir in the bell pepper, mushrooms, and herbs. Cover and cook about 3 minutes, stirring intermittently.

Stir in the greens and cook another minute, or until the leaves are wilted but still bright green. Remove the skillet from the heat.

Break the eggs into a large bowl, add the remaining ½ teaspoon salt, and whisk together. Season with black pepper and add the goat cheese. Stir until evenly distributed.

Add the egg mixture to the skillet and return to the burner over medium heat. Cook, undisturbed, for 3 to 4 minutes, or until the bottom of the eggs have firmed.

Cover and cook about 5 minutes more, or until the frittata is firm in the center. Remove from the heat and run a spatula around the edge to loosen the frittata. Slide or invert onto a large, round plate. Sprinkle the chopped parsley on top and cut into wedges. Serve hot, warm, or at room temperature.

BANANA WAFFLES OR PANCAKES

WAFFLE AND PANCAKE RECIPES CALLING FOR REFINED WHITE FLOUR CAN BE CONVERTED INTO super-healthy versions by using whole grain flour instead. I prefer to use sprouted spelt flour, but the recipe works with regular whole wheat, white whole wheat, or whole spelt flours. Top waffles or pancakes the traditional way with pure maple syrup or give your taste buds a treat and try brown rice syrup or coconut nectar.

• Makes 12 (4-inch) pancakes or waffles •

1 cup plus 2 tablespoons sprouted spelt flour
    (you can also use whole spelt flour, white
    whole wheat flour, or whole wheat flour)
1 teaspoon ground cinnamon
2½ teaspoons aluminum-free baking powder
¼ plus ⅛ teaspoon sea salt
¾ cup coconut milk or unsweetened
    almond milk

2 large eggs
1 banana
1 teaspoon pure vanilla extract
2 tablespoons virgin coconut oil or organic
    butter, melted, plus more for coating the
    waffle iron or pan

Combine the flour, cinnamon, baking powder, and salt in a mixing bowl. Stir to combine well. Place the milk, eggs, banana, vanilla, and coconut oil into a blender and blend until smooth.

Add the blender ingredients to the flour mixture and stir to combine well, until you have a smooth, pourable batter.

To make pancakes: Heat a griddle or large skillet (cast iron works best) over medium heat until hot. Add enough coconut oil to cover the bottom. When the oil is hot, pour in ¼ cup of batter for each pancake. Cook for 2 to 3 minutes, or until golden brown on the bottom and bubbles appear on top of the pancakes. Flip and continue cooking until the other side is golden brown, about 1 to 2 minutes. Repeat with the remaining batter, adding more oil as needed. Serve immediately.

To make waffles: Preheat the waffle iron and coat with coconut oil, if needed. Pour batter onto the hot waffle iron and cook until golden brown.

Leftover pancakes and waffles can be frozen individually and then reheated in the toaster for quick breakfasts, dinners, or snacks.

VARIATIONS

- Fold 1 cup fresh or frozen blueberries into the batter to make blueberry banana pancakes.
- Fold ½ cup granola into the batter to make granola banana pancakes.

GLUTEN-FREE BUCKWHEAT PANCAKES

MOST COMMERCIAL BUCKWHEAT PANCAKES ARE NOT GLUTEN-FREE, AS THEY ARE TYPICALLY MADE from a blend of mostly refined white flour and a small amount of buckwheat flour. This recipe uses just buckwheat flour to make delicious fluffy pancakes that taste just like the conventional version. Buckwheat flour is rather dense, so the secret to these fluffy pancakes is to separate the egg yolk from the white and to use an electric mixer or whisk to firm up the egg white before adding them to the batter.

• Makes 10 (4-inch) pancakes •

1 large egg, separated	¼ teaspoon sea salt
1 cup buckwheat flour (preferably sprouted)	1¼ cups organic cultured buttermilk (see note)
1 teaspoon aluminum-free baking powder	¼ teaspoon liquid stevia extract (optional)
¼ teaspoon baking soda	½ teaspoon pure vanilla extract
2 teaspoons ground cinnamon	Virgin coconut oil or organic butter, for the pan

Place the egg white into a bowl. Add the egg yolk and all other ingredients except for the coconut oil to a blender and blend, scraping the sides as necessary, until you have a smooth, pourable batter. If the mixture is too thick, add more milk to thin it out. It should flow relatively slowly but easily drop from a spoon.

Use an electric mixer to whisk the egg white until soft peaks form and it is relatively firm, like a meringue. Gently fold the egg white into the pancake batter with a rubber spatula until just combined. Do not overmix, otherwise you will lose the fluffiness of the pancakes.

Heat a griddle or large skillet (cast iron works best) over medium heat until hot. Add enough coconut oil to cover the bottom. When the oil is hot, pour in ¼ cup of batter for each pancake. Cook for 2 to 3 minutes, or until golden brown on the bottom and bubbles appear on top of the pancakes. Flip and continue cooking until the other side is golden brown, about 1 to 2 minutes. Repeat with the remaining batter, adding more oil as needed. Serve immediately.

Leftovers can be frozen individually and then reheated in the toaster for quick breakfasts, dinners, or snacks.

> **NOTE:**
>
> To make your own buttermilk, place 1 tablespoon plus ¾ teaspoon freshly squeezed lemon juice or raw organic unfiltered apple cider vinegar in a liquid measuring cup. Add enough almond milk or other milk to bring the liquid up to the 1¼-cup line. Let it sit for 5 minutes to curdle, then stir to mix well before using.

FLUFFY COCONUT FLOUR PANCAKES

COCONUT FLOUR IS A UNIQUE AND DEEPLY NUTRITIOUS TYPE OF FLOUR THAT IS RICH IN PROTEIN, fiber, and beneficial fat. That combo makes it exceptionally filling, so you'll be satisfied with just a few of these fluffy pancakes. Because it comes from a coconut and not a grain, coconut flour is very low in carbohydrates, making it a great choice for diabetics and those following grain-free and gluten-free lifestyles.

A balanced breakfast would include five of these small pancakes, plus ½ cup of yogurt and a cup of fresh fruit. A small amount of pure maple syrup can be drizzled on top of the pancakes, if desired.

• Makes 10 small (2-inch) pancakes •

3 tablespoons coconut flour

3 large eggs, at room temperature

2 tablespoons unsweetened applesauce

1 teaspoon ground cinnamon

1 tablespoon organic butter or virgin coconut oil, melted, plus more for the pan

¼ cup coconut milk or unsweetened almond milk

1 teaspoon pure vanilla extract

¼ teaspoon baking soda

¼ teaspoon raw organic unfiltered apple cider vinegar

Stir together the coconut flour and eggs until a smooth paste forms. Stir in the applesauce, cinnamon, butter, milk, and vanilla until smooth. Let the batter "soak" for 5 minutes before adding in the baking soda and vinegar. Mix to combine.

Heat a griddle or skillet over medium-high heat and coat with butter. Make small pancakes by dropping the batter by tablespoons onto the griddle or skillet. Spread with a spoon, if necessary, but don't make them too big; you should be able to get 10 pancakes out of the batter. Cook until the edges and center start to look opaque, about 2 to 3 minutes. Flip and continue cooking until the other side is golden brown, about another 2 to 3 minutes. Repeat with the remaining batter, adding more butter as needed. Serve immediately.

Leftovers can be frozen individually and then reheated in the toaster for quick breakfasts, dinners, or snacks.

Breads, Muffins, Tortillas, and More

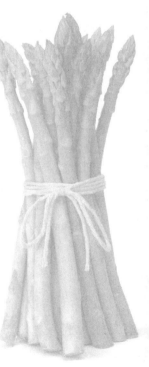

8

This chapter features an eclectic set of baked goods using a variety of ingredients ranging from sprouted flours for traditional bread recipes to oat bran, coconut flour, and almond meal to make flourless or gluten-free recipes. In the spirit of full disclosure, breads and baked goods are really more like treats for me rather than regular fare, so my tinkering in the kitchen with creating baked goods has been very select. The recipes I offer here are those that have become my tried-and-true favorites. In fact, my Blueberry Banana Flourless Oat Bran Muffins (page 132) are a new variation on the commercial variety that I sold in natural food markets for many years. I have recently made the switch to using organic sprouted grain flours instead of the traditional whole wheat or whole spelt flours, but they can be used interchangeably in the recipes if you don't have access to sprouted flours. Whole Grain Pumpkin Bread (page 135), Whole Grain Flour Tortillas (page 140), and Seasoned Spelt Pizza Crust (page 146) can be made with either sprouted or unsprouted whole grain flours. I also offer a recipe for making your own Super Sprouted Bread (page 142), using two different approaches to yield a highly nutritious sandwich bread. I've learned that the secret to making great-tasting bread products is experience. So if at first you don't succeed with baking a great loaf of bread, try again.

BLUEBERRY BANANA FLOURLESS OAT BRAN MUFFINS

MOIST, FLAVORFUL, AND FILLING, THESE MUFFINS ARE PERFECT FOR BREAKFAST OR AFTERNOON snacks. They're dairy-free and have the potential to be gluten-free if you use certified gluten-free oat bran. For an egg-free muffin, try the chia seed egg replacer described in the variations below. Soaking the oat bran overnight helps with the absorption of its nutrients, but the recipe can be made without soaking.

• Makes 12 muffins •

2¼ cups oat bran, preferably soaked overnight (see note)

2⅛ teaspoons aluminum-free baking powder

1 tablespoon ground cinnamon

½ teaspoon sea salt

3 egg whites

1 cup unsweetened almond milk or other milk

1 large banana, mashed (about ½ cup)

2 tablespoons virgin coconut oil, melted, plus more for the pan as needed

1 teaspoon pure vanilla extract, or ½ teaspoon vanilla powder

½ teaspoon liquid stevia extract

½ cup raw honey or coconut nectar

1 cup fresh blueberries

Preheat the oven to 400°F. Line a standard 12-cup muffin pan with paper muffin cups or coat with coconut oil or organic butter.

Place the oat bran, baking powder, cinnamon, and salt in a large mixing bowl. Whisk together until well combined.

Place the egg whites, milk, banana, coconut oil, vanilla, and stevia in a separate mixing bowl. Whisk until the mixture becomes somewhat frothy.

Add the oat bran mixture to the wet ingredients and mix with a wooden spoon or rubber spatula. Next add the honey and mix again until well combined. The batter should become lighter in texture. Fold in the blueberries.

Divide batter evenly into the muffin cups and bake until the muffins are golden on top and a toothpick inserted into the middle comes out clean, about 20 minutes. Let cool 10 minutes in the pan, then transfer to a wire rack to cool completely. Enjoy immediately or refrigerate in a sealed container for up to 1 week. To freeze, wrap each muffin individually with waxed paper, then store in a freezer-safe container for up to 1 month.

NOTE:

Soaking oat bran overnight prior to making this recipe is preferred to neutralize the phytates and improve the absorption of the bran's minerals. To soak, place the oat bran in a small bowl and cover with warm water. Add 1 tablespoon freshly squeezed lemon juice, raw organic unfiltered apple cider vinegar, or liquid whey. Let soak overnight or up to 24 hours. Rinse oat bran in a fine-mesh strainer and then use in the recipe.

VARIATIONS

- Egg-Free Muffins: You can use what is called a "chia seed gel" as an egg replacer in this recipe. Place 3 tablespoons of chia seeds in a small bowl or measuring cup and add 9 tablespoons of water. Stir to make sure the chia seeds are completely mixed with the water. Let the mixture sit for 15 minutes or longer, until the seeds have set and formed a "gel." Add the chia seed gel to the recipe in place of the egg whites.

- Banana Spice Muffins: Omit the blueberries. Keep the cinnamon and also add ½ teaspoon ground cardamom and ½ teaspoon ground ginger.

- Pumpkin Pecan Muffins: Omit the blueberries. Replace the banana with ½ cup pumpkin purée. Replace the cinnamon with 1 tablespoon plus 1 teaspoon pumpkin pie spice (page 45 or store-bought). Fold in 1 cup chopped raw pecans to the batter.

- Add cream cheese filling to any variety: Make the Honey Lemon Cream Cheese Frosting or Filling recipe on page 265. Fill muffin cups halfway with batter, place 1 rounded teaspoon cream cheese filling in the center of each muffin, then top with more batter to finish filling the muffin cups. Baking time remains the same.

MILK SWAP

UNSWEETENED ALMOND MILK, COCONUT milk, or unsweetened rice milk can be used interchangeably in this recipe and my other muffin recipes. Flavors will vary slightly depending upon which type of milk you use. Because coconut milk is very thick, I recommend using only half the amount called for in the recipe and adding an equivalent amount of water to get a thinner consistency.

BERRY SCRUMPTIOUS SCONES

THESE LIGHT AND FLUFFY LITTLE SCONES ARE PERFECT FOR BREAKFAST, LUNCH, OR SNACKS. Though regular blueberries will work in this recipe, wild blueberries have double the amount of antioxidant power packed into their compact size. Serve these with yogurt, with quiche or other egg dishes, or as a complement to green salads.

• Makes 6 scones •

Virgin coconut oil, for the pan as needed

1 cup almond meal (page 71 or store-bought)

2 tablespoons coconut flour

¼ cup coconut sugar, unrefined whole cane sugar, or date sugar

2 teaspoons aluminum-free baking powder

¼ teaspoon sea salt or Himalayan pink salt

2 large eggs

1½ teaspoons pure vanilla extract

½ cup fresh or frozen wild blueberries

Preheat the oven to 375°F. Line a baking sheet with parchment paper or coat with coconut oil.

In a large mixing bowl, sift together the almond meal, coconut flour, sugar, baking powder, and salt.

In a separate mixing bowl, whisk together the eggs and vanilla. Add the egg mixture to the flour mixture and mix together with a rubber spatula until well combined. Fold in the blueberries.

Drop 6 equal-size mounds of batter onto the prepared baking sheet. Bake for 15 to 18 minutes, or until the scones are lightly browned. Let cool 10 minutes on the pan, then transfer to a wire rack to cool completely. Enjoy immediately or refrigerate in a sealed container for up to 1 week. Scones may be frozen for up to 1 month.

WHOLE GRAIN PUMPKIN BREAD

ONE OF MY EARLIEST BAKING MEMORIES IS MY MOTHER'S DECEMBER TRADITION OF MAKING loaves of pumpkin bread to give as holiday gifts. I've carried on this holiday tradition but upgraded the recipe to make the bread a true gift of health. Both sprouted and unsprouted flour work in this recipe, and you can use either white whole wheat or whole spelt flour.

• Makes 1 (9 x 5-inch) loaf •

2 cups whole spelt flour or white whole wheat flour (preferably sprouted)

1½ teaspoons ground cinnamon

¾ teaspoon ground ginger

¼ teaspoon ground nutmeg

¼ teaspoon ground cloves

1 teaspoon baking soda

¼ teaspoon aluminum-free baking powder

½ teaspoon sea salt

¾ cup unrefined whole cane sugar or coconut sugar

½ cup virgin coconut oil, plus more for the pan

3 large eggs

1 teaspoon pure vanilla extract

3 cups shredded fresh pumpkin or pumpkin purée (page 70 or store-bought)

1 cup chopped raw pecans or walnuts

½ cup golden raisins (optional)

Preheat the oven to 350°F. Coat a 9 x 5-inch loaf pan with coconut oil.

Sift the flour, spices, baking soda, baking powder, and salt together in a large mixing bowl. In a separate bowl, mix the sugar, coconut oil, eggs, and vanilla. Add the sugar mixture to the flour mixture and combine. Fold in the pumpkin, pecans, and raisins, if using. Once the ingredients are all incorporated, pour the batter into the prepared pan.

Bake for 1 hour and 15 minutes, or until a knife inserted into the middle comes out clean. If not done, bake another 10 minutes and check again for doneness. Let cool in the pan for 15 minutes, then transfer to a wire rack to cool completely. Pumpkin bread can be stored in a tightly sealed container in the refrigerator for up to 1 week and in the freezer for up to 3 months.

SUGAR-FREE BANANA BREAD

'VE MADE OVER A CLASSIC FAVORITE INTO SOMETHING TRULY SPECTACULAR AS WELL AS NUTRITIOUS. Sprouted grain flour is ideal for this recipe, but it works just as well with white whole wheat flour or whole spelt flour. The bananas and dates provide the sweetness, along with a nice dose of heart-healthy potassium, magnesium, and fiber.

• Makes 1 (9 x 5-inch) loaf •

Virgin coconut oil, for the pan

2 large eggs

1 teaspoon pure vanilla extract

2 cups whole spelt flour or white whole wheat flour (preferably sprouted)

½ teaspoon baking soda

1 teaspoon aluminum-free baking powder

½ teaspoon ground allspice

¼ cup ground flaxseeds

1 teaspoon sea salt

¼ cup finely chopped pitted Medjool dates

3 to 4 very ripe bananas, peeled and mashed (about 2 cups)

½ cup raw walnut pieces

Preheat the oven to 350°F. Coat a 9 x 5-inch loaf pan with coconut oil.

Whisk the eggs and vanilla in a small bowl. Set aside.

In a large mixing bowl, combine the flour, baking soda, baking powder, allspice, flaxseeds, and salt. Add the dates, banana, walnuts, and whisked eggs with vanilla. Stir until a firm dough forms.

Transfer the dough to the prepared pan. Bake for 50 to 60 minutes, or until a knife inserted into the center comes out clean. Let cool in the pan for 10 minutes, then transfer to a wire rack to cool completely. Banana bread can be stored in a tightly sealed container in the refrigerator for up to 1 week and in the freezer for up to 3 months.

ROSEMARY-TOPPED FLOURLESS CORNBREAD

THIS MOIST GOLDEN BREAD IS MADE FROM 100 PERCENT WHOLE GRAIN CORNMEAL—NO FLOUR whatsoever. Rosemary adds a nice flavor accent that blends well with the sweet honey and butter. Be sure to use organic stone-ground whole grain cornmeal to get the full nutritional benefit; degermed cornmeal (the type most supermarkets carry) has had the nutritious germ of the grain removed. See Resources (page 276) for recommended brands.

• Makes 1 (8-inch) pan •

1¾ cups organic stone-ground whole grain yellow cornmeal (medium grind)

2 teaspoons aluminum-free baking powder

1 teaspoon sea salt

2 large eggs

1 tablespoon raw honey

1 cup coconut milk plus 1 cup water, mixed together to make 2 cups diluted coconut milk

2 tablespoons organic butter or virgin coconut oil, melted, plus more for the pan

1 cup frozen organic corn kernels, thawed (optional)

2 sprigs fresh rosemary, or 1 tablespoon dried rosemary, finely chopped

Raw honey, for serving (optional)

Organic butter, for serving (optional)

Preheat the oven to 400°F. Grease an 8-inch baking dish with butter.

In a large mixing bowl, add the cornmeal, baking powder, and salt. Stir together until combined, then make a well in the center of the mixture. In a separate bowl, beat the eggs with the honey, milk, and butter. Pour the wet ingredients into the well of the dry ingredients and stir until just combined. Add the corn, if using, and stir to combine thoroughly.

Pour the batter into the prepared baking dish and use a spatula to spread it evenly. Sprinkle the rosemary evenly over the top. Bake for 20 to 25 minutes, or until a knife inserted into the center comes out clean. Allow to cool for 10 to 15 minutes, then cut into 9 equal pieces. Serve warm with a small amount of honey and butter, if desired. Store leftovers in a sealed container for up to 3 days or freeze for up to 1 month.

SPROUTED SPELT BUTTERMILK BISCUITS

THESE QUICK AND EASY BISCUITS ARE REMINISCENT OF THE FLUFFY WHITE-FLOUR VERSIONS, only better. Spelt is an ancient variety of wheat that is less allergenic and easier to digest, especially when sprouted. The buttermilk in this recipe can be substituted with any nut milk (coconut, almond, etc.) acidified with vinegar or lemon juice, to make these biscuits suitable for dairy-free or vegan diets.

• Makes 10 large or 20 small biscuits •

2¼ cups sprouted spelt flour

½ teaspoon baking soda

1½ teaspoons aluminum-free baking powder

¾ teaspoon sea salt

6 tablespoons virgin coconut oil, chilled and solid, plus more for the pan (unchilled)

¾ cup organic cultured buttermilk, or ¾ cup unsweetened nut milk plus 1 tablespoon raw organic unfiltered apple cider vinegar or freshly squeezed lemon juice

Preheat the oven to 450°F if making smaller biscuits or 425°F if making larger ones. Generously coat a baking sheet with coconut oil.

If using the nondairy buttermilk substitute, measure the nut milk into a 1-cup measuring cup and add the vinegar. Let stand until curdled, about 5 minutes.

Combine the flour, baking soda, baking powder, and salt in a large mixing bowl. Using a pastry cutter or a fork and knife with a cutting motion, cut the chilled coconut oil into the flour mixture until the chilled oil is the size of small peas.

Add the buttermilk or buttermilk substitute, then lightly mix with a wooden spoon or rubber spatula to just barely combine the ingredients. Do not overmix.

Turn the dough out onto a lightly floured surface and roll or pat it into a ½-inch-thick rectangle. Cut into 20 2-inch biscuits with a knife or 2-inch biscuit cutter, or use a 3 ⅝-inch biscuit cutter to make 10 large biscuits. Place the biscuits onto the prepared baking sheet about 1 inch apart for crusty sides or touching for soft sides.

Bake for 8 to 10 minutes, or until the biscuits are golden brown. If making larger biscuits, bake for 3 to 5 minutes longer. Transfer to a wire rack to cool slightly. Serve warm.

Biscuits can be stored in a sealed container in the refrigerator for up to 1 week or in a freezer-safe container in the freezer for up to 1 month.

WHOLESOME CORN TORTILLAS

O THER THAN THE ORGANIC SPROUTED CORN TORTILLAS SOLD IN NATURAL FOOD MARKETS, IT IS dif-ficult to find corn tortillas without chemical additives. The good news is that it's easy to make your own. You can use masa harina, the traditional corn flour used to make tortillas and tamales, or regular corn flour (not to be confused with cornmeal). You can typically find corn flour made from non-GMO corn in natural food markets or online. If you want to go the extra step and use organic sprouted corn flour, you can purchase it from To Your Health Sprouted Flour Company (see Resources, page 275, and for recommended brands of masa harina and corn flour, see page 276).

• Makes 14 to 16 tortillas •

2 cups organic masa harina (corn flour, not cornmeal) or sprouted corn flour

1 teaspoon sea salt

1¼ cups plus 2 to 3 tablespoons hot water

Mix the masa harina with the salt in a large mixing bowl. Make a well in the center and gradually add the water, a teaspoon at a time, mixing until the dough comes to a spongy wet consistency. The dough should be wet enough to stick together, but not so sticky that it stays on your hands. If you add too much water, simply add a bit more flour to the mix. Knead the dough for a minute or so to fully combine the ingredients, then remove the dough from the bowl. Divide it into 14 to 16 equal-size balls, each about the size of a golf ball. As the balls are formed, place them in the bowl and cover the bowl with a towel in order to keep the moisture in the dough.

Take one of the dough balls and lay it between layers of waxed paper or a resealable plastic bag cut in two. Press flat with a rolling pin or using a tortilla press. If the dough sticks to the waxed paper, roll it in a little bit of flour to dry it out.

Heat a dry skillet, griddle, or *comal* (a side-less cast-iron skillet) over medium-high heat. Place the pressed tortilla on the hot surface and cook for 40 seconds to 1 minute on each side. Place the cooked tortilla in a folded towel to keep it warm and soft while you cook the rest.

Repeat with the remaining balls of dough.

Enjoy the tortillas fresh and warm, or store tightly sealed in the refrigerator for up to 1 week or the freezer for up to 1 month (to store in the freezer, place pieces of parchment paper between each tortilla and then place the stack in a resealable plastic bag). Reheat by placing back on a hot skillet.

WHOLE GRAIN FLOUR TORTILLAS

FRESHLY MADE FLOUR TORTILLAS ARE WARM, SOFT, AND CHEWY AND HAVE SO MUCH MORE FLAVOR than the store-bought varieties. This recipe has been modified from one of my family's traditional tortilla recipes that included white flour and lard. To get the unique taste of a white flour tortilla and the appearance of a whole wheat tortilla, I use a combination of half white whole wheat flour and half traditional whole wheat flour. If you don't have both types of flour, you can use just one type for the full volume. Whole spelt flour can also be substituted. Sprouted varieties of these flours can also be used in the same amounts.

• Makes 22 to 24 tortillas •

2 cups whole wheat flour (preferably sprouted)

2 cups white whole wheat flour (preferably sprouted)

1½ teaspoons sea salt

1½ teaspoons aluminum-free baking powder

¼ cup virgin coconut oil, organic butter, or palm shortening, at room temperature but still in solid form

1 to 1½ cups warm water, divided

In a large mixing bowl, combine the flours, salt, and baking powder. Cut in the coconut oil. Add ½ cup water and knead the mixture into a dough. Add 1 teaspoon additional water at a time, kneading after each addition, to form a smooth dough. It should be soft, smooth, and elastic. Cover the bowl with a towel and let the dough rest for 20 minutes.

Remove the dough from the bowl and divide into small, golf ball–size balls. You should be able to get 22 to 24 balls out of the dough. As the balls are formed, place them in the bowl and keep them covered with the towel to prevent them from drying out.

Flatten and roll out a dough ball with a rolling pin or tortilla press into a 10-inch circle, lightly patting with additional flour to keep it from sticking to the counter, rolling pin, or press. If it shrinks back excessively, let it rest for an additional 5 minutes before rolling.

Heat a dry skillet, griddle, or *comal* (a side-less cast-iron skillet) over medium-high heat.

Place the tortilla on the hot surface. Cook for about 1 minute, or until bubbles appear on the top, then flip the tortilla over and cook about 30 seconds more.

Place the finished tortilla on a plate lined with a clean dish towel to absorb moisture. Fold the dish towel over the top of the tortilla to seal in freshness.

Repeat with the remaining balls of dough.

Cooked tortillas may be stored in a sealed container and kept refrigerated for up to 1 week or frozen for up to 1 month (to store in the freezer, place pieces of parchment paper between each tortilla and then place the stack in a resealable plastic bag). Reheat by placing back on a hot skillet.

LAVENDER-SPICED ALMOND PULP CRACKERS

THESE TASTY LITTLE CRACKERS HAVE A LIGHT AND CRISPY TEXTURE THAT MAKE THEM PERFECT for snacking with bean dips, mashed avocado, or cheese. They can also be crumbled on top of salads to replace croutons. The main ingredient is the nutritious almond pulp left over from making almond milk (page 62), but you can use almond meal instead (see note).

• Makes about 100 (1-inch) square crackers •

1 cup almond pulp, squeezed dry and firmly packed into the measuring cup

2 tablespoons virgin coconut oil, melted

½ teaspoon Herbamare or sea salt

2 garlic cloves, minced, or ¼ teaspoon garlic powder

2 tablespoons chopped fresh lavender

Preheat the oven to 350°F. Tear off 2 baking sheet–size pieces of parchment paper (the size will depend on the size of your baking sheet) and set aside with your baking sheet. If your baking sheets are small, you may need to use 2 of them (and 4 pieces of parchment).

Make sure that your almond pulp is squeezed to near dryness (it may still feel moist but should not be dripping wet). Place all ingredients into a large mixing bowl and stir together to combine. Using your hands, roll the dough into a ball.

Place the ball of dough between the 2 sheets of parchment paper and use a rolling pin to roll out the dough until it is ⅛ inch thick and has spread close to the edges of the parchment paper.

Carefully peel off the top sheet of parchment to reveal your smooth dough. Use a silicone spatula to smooth the edges and shape the dough into a rectangle. Pick up the bottom piece of parchment with the dough and place it onto the baking sheet.

Score the dough with a knife or pizza cutter into 1-inch squares. For a true "cracker look" and to help release moisture, you can press the prongs of a fork into the dough to make small holes on each square.

Bake the crackers for 20 to 25 minutes, then remove from the oven and flip each square over (they should come apart easily due to the scoring). Place the crackers back in the oven and bake for another 15 minutes. Allow to cool on the baking sheet (they will become more crispy as they cool). Enjoy immediately or store in a tightly sealed container. The crackers will keep for several days in the refrigerator.

VARIATIONS

The lavender can be replaced with other herbs and spices for some different flavor variations, such as rosemary, chives, oregano, smoked paprika, taco seasoning, and even some Parmesan cheese or nutritional yeast. The possibilities are endless!

NOTE:

If using almond meal instead of almond pulp, you will need to add 1 to 2 teaspoons of water to the ingredients.

SUPER SPROUTED BREAD, TWO WAYS

COMPANIES MAKING SPROUTED GRAIN BREAD PRODUCTS USE TWO DIFFERENT APPROACHES— dry and wet—once the grains are sprouted. These two approaches can also be used to make homemade sprouted grain breads. The dry method uses grains that have been sprouted, then dried and milled into flour. You can purchase whole grains that have already been sprouted and dried, then freshly mill them into flour yourself just before making the bread, or you can purchase sprouted grain flour in natural food markets or online (see Resources, page 275). The wet method involves sprouting the grains yourself over the course of a few days, then immediately blending them into a dough while they are still wet. The wet approach is a little more involved, and definitely more temperamental, but the result is the most nutritious bread on this earth.

I call my version of sprouted grain bread using the dry method Real Wonder-ful Sandwich Bread, which can be made either in a bread machine or by kneading with your hands. The recipe can be doubled.

REAL WONDER-FUL SANDWICH BREAD

• Makes 1 (2-pound) loaf •

1½ cups warm water

3 tablespoons raw honey or coconut nectar

2¼ teaspoons, or 1 (¼-ounce) package, active dry yeast

¼ cup virgin coconut oil, melted, plus more for the bowl and pan

4 cups (16 ounces) sprouted wheat flour or sprouted spelt flour, or a combo of both

1½ teaspoons sea salt or Himalayan pink salt

Make sure all ingredients are brought to room temperature before mixing the dough.

METHOD FOR KNEADING BY HAND:

Proof the yeast by placing the warm water and honey in a glass measuring cup. Sprinkle the yeast on top and let it sit for 5 minutes, or until the yeast bubbles slightly. Add the coconut oil.

Combine the flour and salt in a large bowl, then add the yeast mixture. Mix until a cohesive ball of dough forms. The dough may be wetter and stickier than other bread doughs you've worked with.

Remove the dough from the bowl and knead it on a lightly floured surface for about 8 minutes, or until it is smooth and elastic.

Alternatively, you can use an electric mixer with a dough hook to combine everything and knead the dough.

Clean the bowl and grease it with coconut oil. Return the dough to the bowl. Cover the bowl with a dish towel and let the dough rise in a warm place until it's puffy, about 1½ to 2 hours. The dough will not rise as much as other types of bread dough, so don't expect it to double in size. The blended-up particles of bran and sprouted grains create tiny channels in the dough that allow the carbon dioxide gas released by the yeast to escape, and therefore the gas is not trapped inside the dough like it is with other bread doughs. (When you poke your finger into it, it should not spring back.) Most of the leavening in this bread happens during the second rise, after the dough has been formed and placed in a loaf pan.

Grease an 8½ x 4½-inch loaf pan with coconut oil or butter.

Turn the dough out onto a clean counter, punch it down, then form the round ball into a flattened rectangular shape about ½ inch thick, with the long side being about the length of your loaf pan. Starting at one of the long ends of the rectangle, roll the dough up jelly-roll style to form a bread loaf.

Pinch the seam to hold the loaf together, then place it seam-side down into the prepared pan. Cover the dough with a towel and set it in a warm place to let the dough rise again for another 1 to 1½ hours, or until it has risen and crested above the top of the pan. It is during this second rising period that the yeast will do most of its leavening.

Preheat the oven to 350°F. Bake the bread for 35 to 38 minutes. Baking times will vary depending on the oven, the weather, and the size of the loaf. The bread is done when an instant-read thermometer placed into the middle of the loaf reads 190°F. Remove the bread from the oven, turn it out of the pan onto a wire rack, and allow it to cool completely before slicing.

Since this bread does not have any preservatives in it, it is best kept stored in a resealable plastic bag in the refrigerator for up to 1 week. Store in a freezer-safe bag in the freezer for up to 3 months. If you are going to freeze it, I recommend slicing it first so you can take out only the number of slices you need each time.

METHOD FOR USING A BREAD MACHINE:

Place the water, honey, and oil in a bread maker and add the flour, salt, and yeast on top, ending with the yeast.

Program for the basic rapid cycle and press start.

FLOURLESS SPROUTED GRAIN BREAD

I'VE HAD NUMEROUS REQUESTS FROM *SCIENCE OF SKINNY* READERS WHO WANT A RECIPE FOR THE "flourless" type of bread sold in stores. This is that recipe! The wet method for making sprouted grain bread is more challenging than the dry method. It takes several days to sprout the grains, and you need to rinse them several times a day while they are sprouting, keeping a close watch to make sure they don't sprout too much. I have spent a fair amount of time getting this recipe right, and I hope that if you are up for the challenge, you will take it on yourself. Once you taste the freshness of this bread, you won't want to go back to buying the frozen (or previously frozen) store-bought loaves. The recipe can be doubled.

• Makes 1 (2-pound) loaf •

3¼ cups wheat berries or spelt berries

1½ teaspoons salt, divided

2 tablespoons warm water

2 tablespoons raw honey

2¼ teaspoons, or 1 (¼-ounce) package, active dry yeast

Virgin coconut oil or organic butter, for the pan

SPROUT THE GRAINS:

Place the grains in a large glass bowl and add 4 cups of water. Soak the grains for about 18 hours. Drain and rinse the grains using a fine-mesh strainer. Rinse and clean the soaking bowl.

Place a clean paper towel in the bottom of the clean bowl and put the rinsed grains on top of it. Cover the bowl with plastic wrap and let it sit on the counter at room temperature. Every 6 to 8 hours, transfer the grains to the strainer and rinse well, replace the paper towel in the bowl, put the grains on top of it, and cover again with plastic wrap. Do this until you see tiny little sprouts forming on the grains. The sprouts should not be too long, just little tails. Be very careful to only sprout the grains until the tiny sprout is just beginning to show and the grain itself is tender.

This sprouting process can take from 12 to 36 hours and will vary with the temperature and humidity of your kitchen. Keep a close eye on your grains as they are sprouting to make sure you stop the process before the sprouts get too long. If the sprouts are too long, the dough will end up too gooey and won't bake properly.

Once your grains have sprouted, you are ready to move on to the next step. However, if at this point you don't have time to finish making the bread, you can put the sprouted grains in a bowl with a clean paper towel, cover with plastic wrap, and refrigerate to slow their sprouting rate down. You can leave them like this in the refrigerator for 2 to 3 days.

PURÉE THE GRAINS:

Remove the excess moisture from the grains by patting them with dry paper towels. If you have left your grains in the refrigerator for any amount of time, rinse and drain them again before patting them dry.

Begin by placing half of the sprouted grains into the bowl of a food processor with an S-shaped blade. Sprinkle ¾ teaspoon salt over the grains and run the food processor until the mixture forms a ball of dough, stopping if necessary to scrape the sides of the bowl and push the mixture back down onto the blades. Process again until the ball thickens to the point where it won't mix any further and the blades just spin underneath. This takes about 1 to 1½ minutes. Transfer the purée to a clean space on your kitchen counter and repeat the process with the remaining sprouted grains and remaining ¾ teaspoon salt. Add the second batch to the first batch on the counter, then knead the dough for a minute or so to ensure that the salt is evenly distributed throughout the entire mixture. Place the dough in a large mixing bowl.

Alternatively, you can use a high-powered blender to purée the grains, but you may need to purée in smaller batches. Just remember to divide up the salt according to how many batches you purée.

ADD THE YEAST AND KNEAD THE BREAD DOUGH:

Proof the yeast by placing the warm water and honey in a glass measuring cup. Sprinkle the yeast on top and let it sit for 5 minutes, or until the yeast bubbles slightly. Add the yeast mixture to the sprouted grain purée in the bowl and mix everything together very well with your hands. The dough may be wetter and stickier than other bread doughs.

Once the dough is well mixed, turn it out onto a clean counter and knead for no less than 20 minutes. The long knead time allows the yeast to become more active and draws the gluten proteins out of the wheat, dispersing them into the dough. As you are kneading, the dough will change in texture, going from wet and sticky to a more normal texture of bread dough.

Alternatively, you can use an electric mixer with a dough hook to combine everything and knead the dough.

LET THE DOUGH RISE:

After kneading, clean the bowl, place the dough into the clean bowl, and form it into a ball. Cover the bowl with a towel and let it rise in a warm place for 1½ to 2 hours. The dough will not rise as much as other types of bread dough, so don't expect it to double in size. The blended-up particles of bran and sprouted grains create tiny channels in the dough that allow the carbon dioxide gas released by the yeast to escape, and therefore the gas is not trapped inside the dough like it is with other bread doughs. (When you poke your finger into it, it should not spring back.) Most of the leavening in this bread happens during the second rise, after the dough has been formed and placed in a loaf pan.

LET THE DOUGH RISE AGAIN:

Grease an 8½ x 4½-inch loaf pan with coconut oil or butter.

Turn the dough out onto a clean counter, punch it down, then form the round ball into a flattened rectangular shape about ½ inch thick, with the long side being about the length of your loaf pan. Starting at one of the long ends of the rectangle, roll the dough up jelly-roll style to form a bread loaf.

Pinch the seam to hold the loaf together, then place it seam-side down into the prepared pan. Cover the dough with a towel and set it in a warm place to rise again for another 1½ to 3 hours, or until it has risen above and crested the top of the pan. It is during this second rising period that the yeast will do most of its leavening. This process takes longer due to the dense and heavy nature of the dough and the carbon dioxide from the yeast escaping through the tiny channels created by the particles of blended-up grains and bran.

BAKE THE BREAD:

Preheat the oven to 350°F. Bake the bread for 60 to 65 minutes. Baking times will vary depending on the oven, the weather, and the size of the loaf. The bread is done when an instant-read thermometer placed into the middle of the loaf reads 190°F. Remove the bread from the oven. When cool enough to handle, turn it out of the pan onto a wire rack and allow it to cool completely before slicing.

Since this bread does not have any preservatives in it, it is best kept stored in a resealable plastic bag in the refrigerator for up to 1 week. Store in a freezer-safe bag in the freezer for up to 3 months. If you are going to freeze it, I recommend slicing it first so you can take out only the number of slices you need each time.

SEASONED SPELT PIZZA CRUST

THERE ARE MANY WAYS TO MAKE A TASTY PIZZA BUT ONLY A FEW WAYS TO MAKE A TASTY CRUST that is also healthy. Pizza crust made with spelt flour tastes amazing, is easy to make, and ups the health factor by leaps and bounds.

This recipe can be doubled so you can freeze the extra dough to thaw and bake at a later time. You can also divide the dough into smaller portions to make individual-size pizzas. Add your favorite toppings and you're good to go. For my favorite pizza, I use a tomato basil marinara sauce, steamed broccoli, fresh basil leaves, goat cheese, and a sprinkle of pine nuts.

• Makes 1 thick or 2 thin pizza crusts •

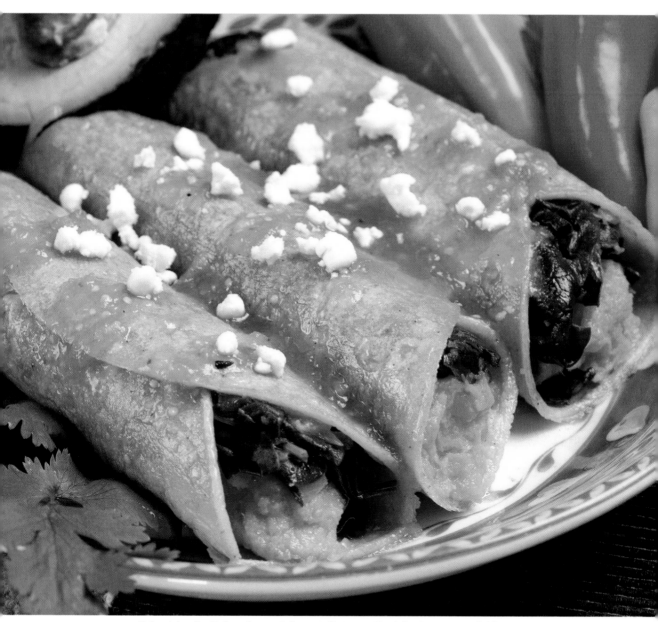

Salsa Verde Spinach and Sweet Potato Enchiladas, page 249

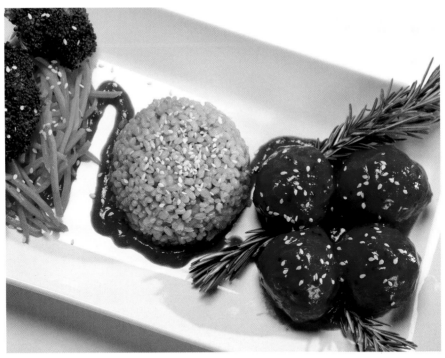

Apricot Sweet and Sour Meatballs, page 233

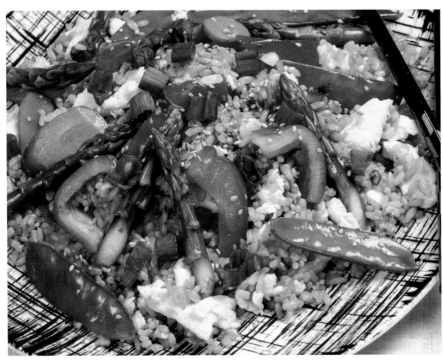

Veggie Egg Fried Rice, page 245

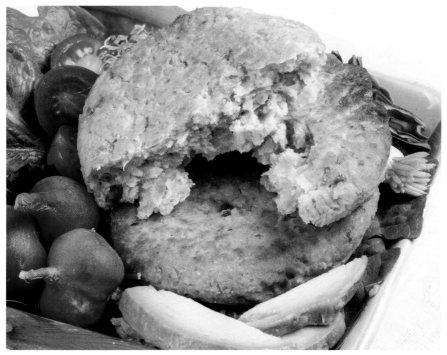

Chickpea Garden Patties, page 243

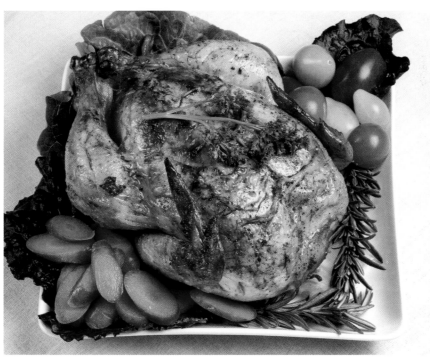

Coconut Oil Garlic-Roasted Chicken, page 234

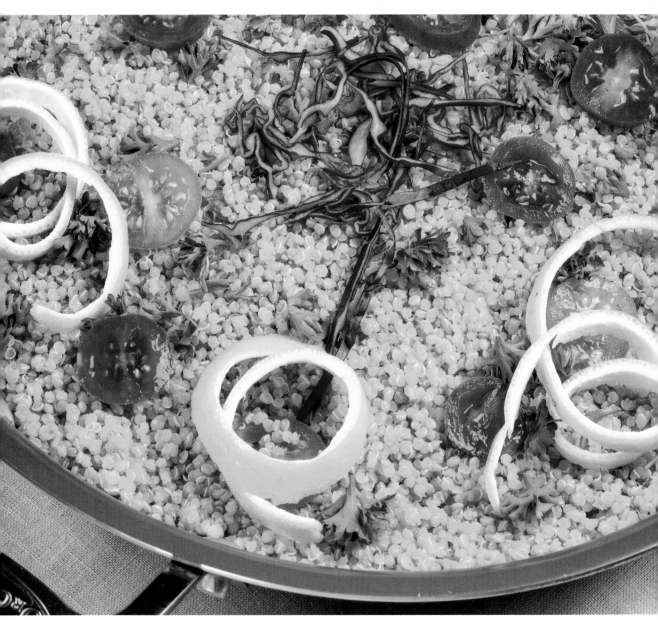

Lemon Turmeric Quinoa, page 225

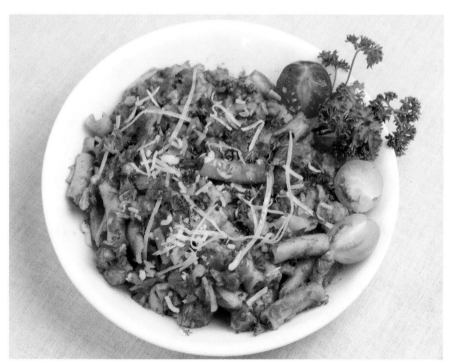

Pasta e Fagioli, page 236

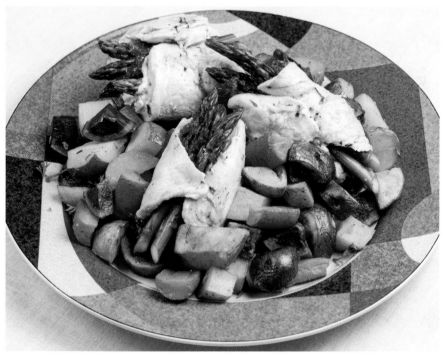

Asparagus and Sun-Dried Tomato–Stuffed Chicken, page 232

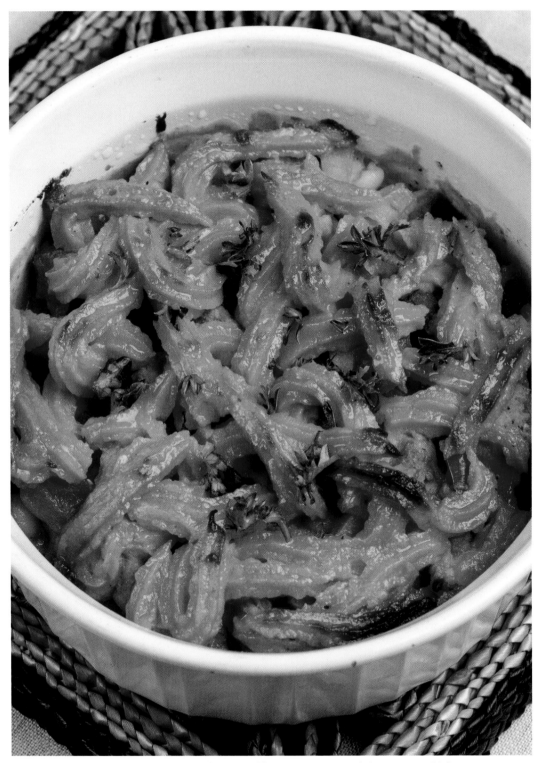

Sweet Potato and Ground Turkey Shepherd's Pie, page 238

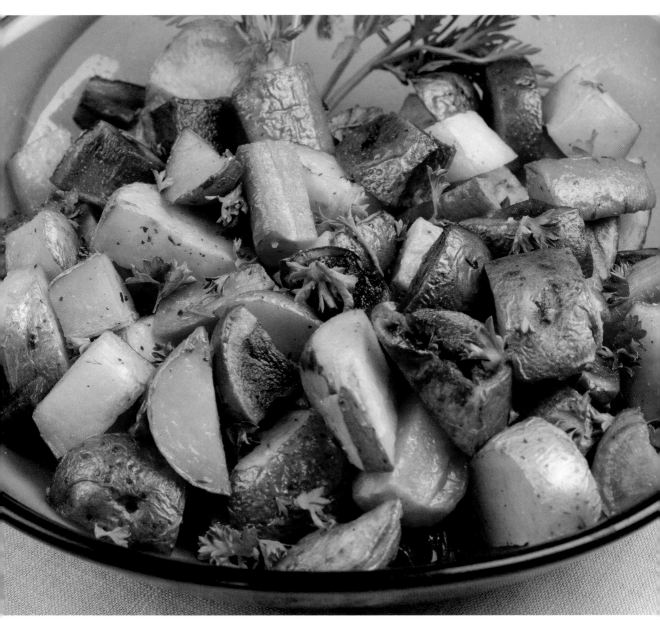

Roasted Tricolor Taters and Carrots, page 209

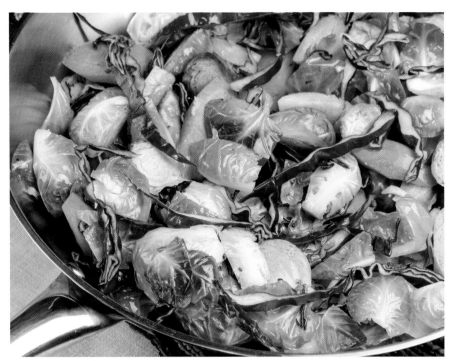

Carrot, Brussels Sprout, and Purple Cabbage Sauté, page 208

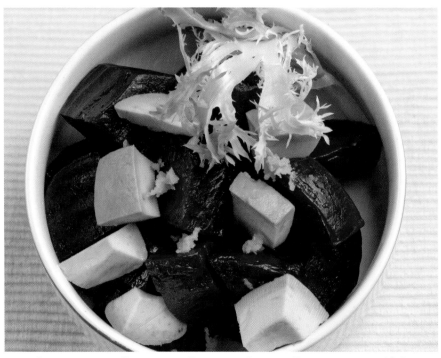

Avocado and Beets with Balsamic Orange Dressing, page 194

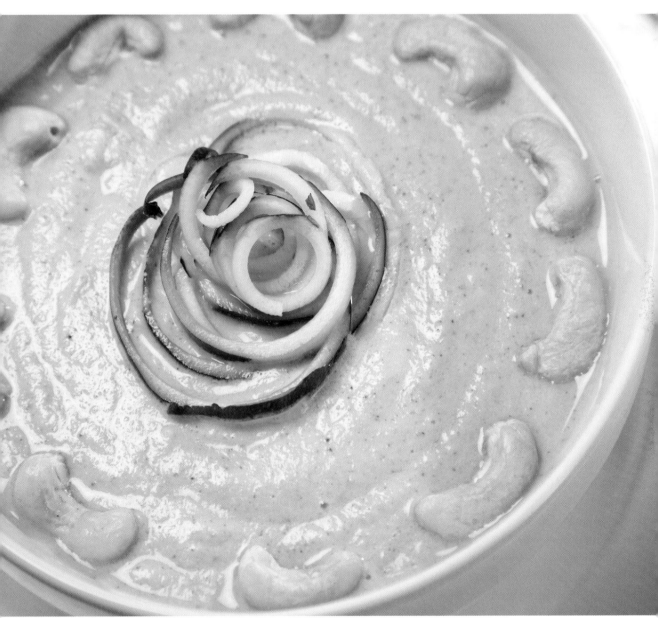

Creamy Zucchini Cashew Soup, page 217

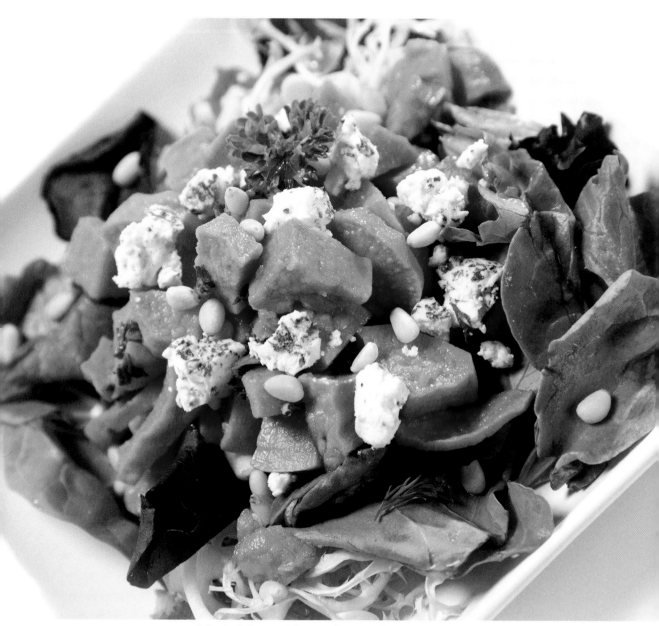

Maple Mustard Sweet Potato Salad, page 193

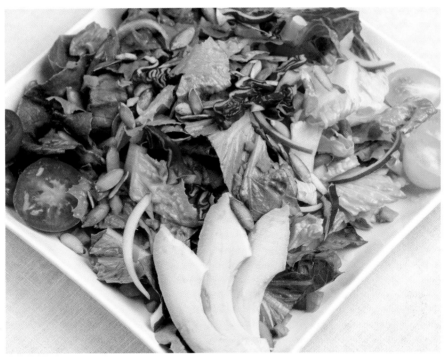

Mexican Caesar Salad with Cilantro Pepita Dressing, page 197

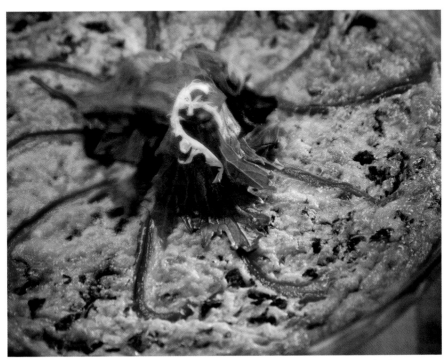

Red Pepper Quiche with Sweet Potato Crust, page 124

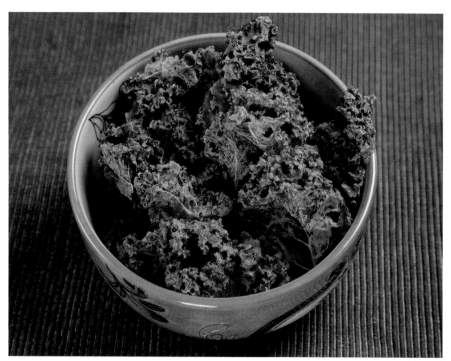

Zesty Nacho Kale Krunch, page 188

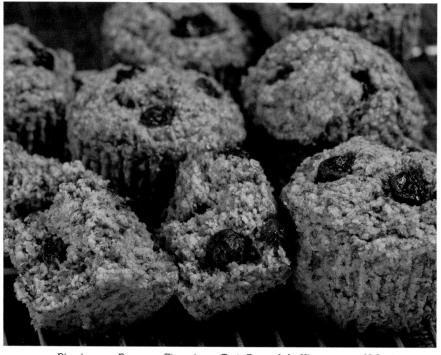

Blueberry Banana Flourless Oat Bran Muffins, page 132

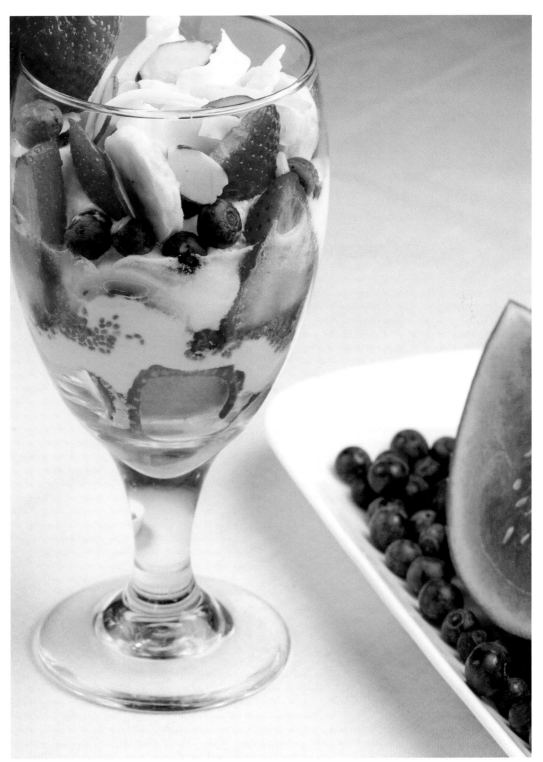

Fruit and Yogurt Chia Parfait, page 114

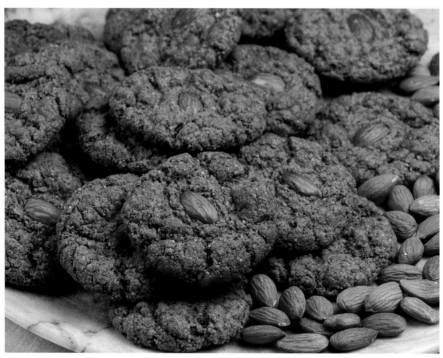

Grain-Free Almond Spice Cookies, page 253

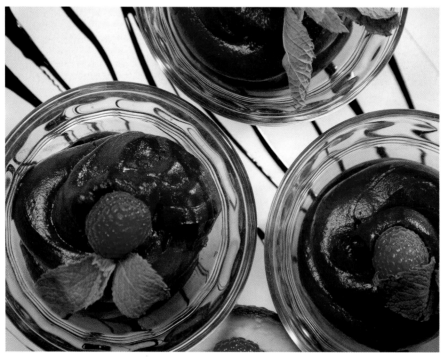

Choco-cado Mousse, page 259

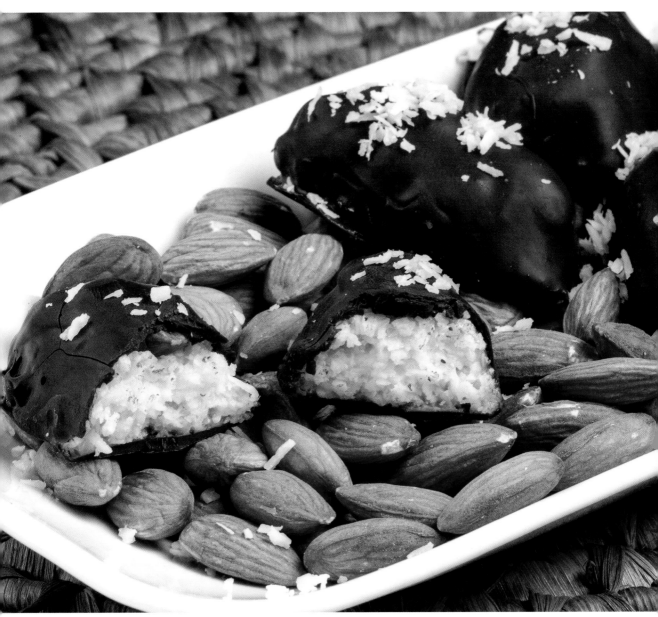

Joyful Chocolate Almond Bars, page 264

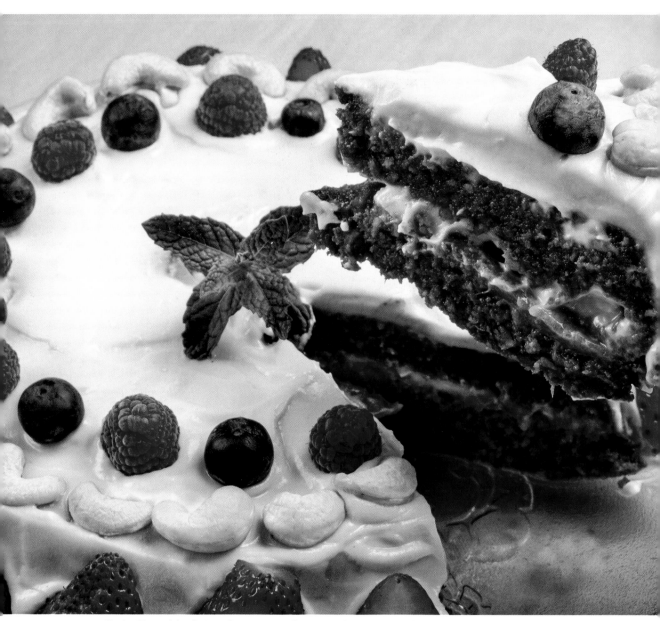

Grain-Free, No-Bake Chocolate Orange Cake with Cashew Frosting, page 266

1½ cups warm water

1½ teaspoons raw honey

1½ teaspoons active dry yeast

3 tablespoons virgin coconut oil, melted, plus more for the bowl and pan

3 cups whole spelt flour or sprouted spelt flour

1½ teaspoons sea salt or Himalayan pink salt

½ teaspoon garlic powder

2 tablespoons chopped fresh herbs (such as basil and oregano), or 2 teaspoons dried Italian seasoning

Proof the yeast by placing the warm water and honey in a glass measuring cup. Sprinkle the yeast on top and let it sit for 5 minutes, or until the yeast bubbles slightly. Add the coconut oil to the yeast mixture. Combine the remaining ingredients in a large bowl, add the yeast mixture, and mix well. Remove the dough from the bowl and knead for 5 to 8 minutes, or until it feels smooth and springy.

Alternatively, you can use an electric mixer with a dough hook to combine everything and knead the dough.

Let the dough rest while you clean the bowl and grease it with coconut oil.

Form the dough into a ball and place it in the greased bowl. Turn the dough so it is evenly coated with the oil. Cover it with a towel and place it in a warm place, away from drafts. Let the dough rise for 30 to 45 minutes, or until it has doubled in size.

Preheat the oven to 475°F. Grease a baking pan with coconut oil and preheat it or preheat a pizza stone.

Turn the dough out onto a floured surface. Punch it down and break up the large bubbles. To make thin crust, divide it into two even-size balls. (At this point you can freeze the dough for future use by carefully wrapping it in waxed paper and then placing it in a resealable freezer-safe bag or container. It will keep frozen for up to 3 months. When you are ready to use it, take it out of the freezer, let it thaw at room temperature, and then follow the remaining steps.)

Roll the dough out to the desired size and thickness.

To prebake your crust, place it on the preheated baking pan or pizza stone; carefully press the dough to the edges of the hot pan. Poke the dough with a fork (known as "docking") about every inch so that the crust does not bubble while prebaking.

Bake for about 8 to 10 minutes. Remove the prebaked crust from the oven. (At this point you can freeze the prebaked crust for future use: Let it cool to room temperature and then wrap it in waxed paper and place it in a resealable freezer-safe bag or container. It will keep frozen for up to 3 months. When you are ready to use it, take it out of the freezer, let it thaw at room temperature, and then follow the remaining steps.)

Top with your favorite pizza toppings.

Place the pizza back in the oven and bake for 5 to 10 more minutes, or until the toppings are cooked to the desired state. Remove from the oven and slice into pieces. Enjoy immediately!

METHOD FOR USING A BREAD MACHINE:

Place the water, honey, and oil in the bread machine. Add the flour, salt, garlic powder, herbs, and yeast on top, ending with the yeast. Program the machine for pizza dough and press start. When ready, remove the dough from the machine, then roll into the desired size and bake according to the above instructions.

Salad Dressings, Condiments, Sauces, and Such

9

t has been many years since my refrigerator door was jammed full of salad dressing bottles and jars of condiments. Once I started making food choices based on the quality of ingredients, my purchases of such items gradually dropped off and I began learning how to make my own versions of them. I discovered that the best dressings and sauces are the homemade ones—not just because they taste amazing, but because they are made with nourishing, healthy foods that heal, rather than nutrient-depleting ingredients that steal.

While there are some commercially available condiments that I use (I've listed my trusted brands in Resources, page 278), not all of them are widely available. For that reason, I've included an eclectic assortment of my favorite homemade creations. Recipes include the well-loved classic Better-for-You-Buttermilk Ranch

Dressing (page 153) and Creamy Cashew Ranch Dressing (page 155; a modern non-dairy spin on the classic). You'll also find Sugar-Free Orange Cranberry Sauce (page 165) for the holidays, Naturally Sweetened Tangy Barbecue Sauce (page 162) for the outdoor grill days, and Awesome Hoisin Sauce (page 163) for quick stir-fry days. You'll never have to buy another packet of Taco Seasoning Mix (page 168) after you discover how easy it is to make your own, and Shortcut Organic Ketchup (page 158) may become your new refrigerator staple.

SWEET SKINNY HERB VINAIGRETTE

THIS SWEET AND TANGY VINAIGRETTE IS MY STAPLE SALAD DRESSING. I TYPICALLY DOUBLE OR triple the recipe so that I have enough on hand to last several weeks. In addition to the health benefits offered by unfiltered apple cider vinegar, garlic, and lemon juice, the herbs pack surprising additional benefits of their own. Parsley, basil, oregano, and thyme all contain various antioxidants that provide anti-inflammatory, antiviral, and cancer-fighting properties. When combined, they make a powerful health-promoting seasoning blend.

• Makes 1½ cups •

1 cup extra-virgin olive oil

½ cup raw organic unfiltered apple cider vinegar

1 tablespoon freshly squeezed lemon juice

¼ teaspoon liquid stevia extract

2 garlic cloves

3 teaspoons chopped fresh curly parsley, or 1 teaspoon dried

3 teaspoons chopped fresh basil, or 1 teaspoon dried

3 teaspoons chopped fresh oregano, or 1 teaspoon dried

3 teaspoons chopped fresh thyme, or 1 teaspoon dried

½ teaspoon Herbamare, sea salt, or Himalayan pink salt

Place all ingredients in a blender and blend on high speed to combine thoroughly.

Let the blender run for about 2 minutes for a creamy-type Italian vinaigrette. It can be used on any salad or as a marinade. Store in the refrigerator for up to 3 weeks.

> **NOTE:**
>
> *If you don't have the individual dried herbs on hand, you can use 3 teaspoons of Italian seasoning or Bragg Sprinkle (a salt-free seasoning blend of 24 organic herbs and spices found in the spice aisle of natural food markets).*

ZESTY TOMATO ITALIAN DRESSING

THIS DRESSING RECIPE WAS INSPIRED BY THE POPULAR HOUSE SALAD DRESSING AT NELLO'S pizzeria, a family-run Italian eatery in the Phoenix, Arizona, area. At a private dinner with the owner, I boldly asked for the "secret" ingredient in the dressing. Once revealed, I knew that I could make a dressing with the same amazing flavor using healthier oils and no sugar. Can you guess what the "secret" ingredient is?

• Makes about 2 cups •

1 cup extra-virgin olive oil

½ cup raw organic unfiltered apple cider vinegar

½ cup pizza sauce (I use the Eden Foods organic pizza sauce that comes in a glass jar)

1 tablespoon freshly squeezed lemon juice

¼ teaspoon liquid stevia extract

3 garlic cloves

¼ teaspoon sea salt

Place all ingredients in a blender and blend on high speed to combine thoroughly.

Let the blender run for about 2 minutes. Store the dressing in the refrigerator for up to 3 weeks.

GREEN GODDESS DRESSING

THE ORIGINAL GREEN GODDESS DRESSING WAS MADE WITH LOADS OF FRESH HERBS, MAYONNAISE, sour cream, and anchovies. In my version, I've replaced the mayo and some of the other ingredients with healthier fats and bumped up the herbs. This creamy dressing is wonderful over baby greens or soft lettuces such as butter lettuce, as a replacement for mayo in chicken, tuna, or salmon salad, served as a veggie dip, or drizzled on cooked vegetables.

• Makes 1½ cups •

1 garlic clove

2 small avocados, peeled, pitted, and mashed (about 1 cup)

¼ cup water

¼ cup extra-virgin olive oil

2 tablespoons raw organic unfiltered apple cider vinegar

2 tablespoons freshly squeezed lemon juice, or more to taste

½ cup packed fresh curly parsley leaves

½ cup packed fresh basil

¼ cup loosely packed fresh tarragon leaves

2 tablespoons finely chopped fresh chives

2 tablespoons chopped fresh dill

½ teaspoon sea salt or Himalayan pink salt

¼ teaspoon liquid stevia extract or other natural sweetener, or more to taste

Place all ingredients in a blender or food processor and blend until smooth and creamy, scraping down the sides as needed. Adjust the salt, lemon juice, and sweetener to taste. Store the dressing in the refrigerator for up to 1 week.

TAHINI MISO DRESSING WITH ORANGE AND GINGER

THIS VERSATILE DRESSING CAN BE USED AS A DIP FOR RAW VEGGIES, DRIZZLED OVER COOKED vegetables or whole grains, and as a dressing for slaws and leafy lettuce salads. Tahini is made from ground sesame seeds, which are a great source of calcium, protein, and fiber, in addition to their healthy, great-tasting oil. Miso, made from fermented soybeans, is also a great source of protein, beneficial probiotics, and antioxidants. The addition of fresh orange juice, ginger, and parsley put this dressing into the superfood category.

• Makes about ¾ cup •

¼ cup tahini

1 tablespoon white miso paste

1 tablespoon freshly grated orange zest

¼ cup freshly squeezed orange juice

1 tablespoon finely minced curly fresh parsley

1 teaspoon finely grated fresh ginger

2 tablespoons water, plus more as needed

In a small bowl, whisk together the tahini, miso, orange zest, and orange juice into a smooth paste. Whisk in the parsley and ginger, then add the water gradually, whisking until the dressing reaches the desired consistency. It may need more than 2 tablespoons.

Store in the refrigerator for up to 1 week. The dressing will thicken as it sits, so you may need to add more water or orange juice to thin it out.

BETTER-FOR-YOU BUTTERMILK RANCH DRESSING

OF ALL THE REQUESTS I'VE RECEIVED FOR HEALTHIER FOOD OPTIONS, NONE HAS BEEN MORE frequent than the one for the beloved ranch dressing. This reinvention of the classic omits the unhealthy oils and all the chemical additives, leaving you with a fresh burst of satisfying real flavor. Use this dressing in all the favorite ways you know and love. See my note for how to make a quick buttermilk substitute.

• Makes about 1½ cups •

1 garlic clove

½ teaspoon sea salt or Himalayan pink salt

1 cup organic plain Greek-style yogurt

¼ cup chopped fresh flat-leaf parsley

1 tablespoon minced fresh dill

2 tablespoons minced fresh chives

½ teaspoon freshly ground black pepper

1 tablespoon freshly squeezed lemon juice (the juice from about 1 lemon)

½ teaspoon onion powder

1 teaspoon sweet paprika

1 teaspoon dried mustard

½ cup organic cultured buttermilk (more or less for desired consistency)

Make a garlic paste by mashing the clove with the side of a large knife, sprinkling the salt on top, then using a fork to mash together into a paste.

In a bowl, whisk together the garlic paste, yogurt, parsley, dill, chives, pepper, lemon juice, onion powder, paprika, and dried mustard. Whisk in the buttermilk, adding more or less to reach the desired consistency. Adjust seasonings to taste as needed.

Transfer to an airtight container and chill for 1 to 2 hours before using, thinning with more buttermilk if needed. Store in the refrigerator for up to 1 week.

NOTE:

If you can't find organic buttermilk, or if you don't want to buy an entire carton of buttermilk when you only need ½ cup, you can quickly make a buttermilk substitute in less than 10 minutes using regular milk or unsweetened nondairy milk (coconut, almond, or other nut milk) and lemon juice or apple cider vinegar. Simply measure out ½ cup of your preferred milk and stir in ½ tablespoon freshly squeezed lemon juice or raw organic unfiltered apple cider vinegar and let the mixture stand at room temperature for 5 to 10 minutes. When it is ready, the milk will have curdled. Use this substitute (including the curdled bits) in the recipe. To make larger amounts of buttermilk substitute, use the ratio of 1 cup milk to 1 tablespoon lemon juice or apple cider vinegar.

CREAMY CASHEW RANCH DRESSING

THIS DAIRY-FREE VERSION OF EVERYONE'S FAVORITE SALAD DRESSING USES SOAKED, BLENDED cashews to stand in for the dairy components of traditional ranch dressing. In addition to lending creaminess, cashews are chock-full of magnesium, a mineral that lowers blood pressure, helps prevent heart attacks, diminishes the frequency of migraines, and reduces the severity of asthma. Cashews also contain proanthocyanidins, compounds that prevent cancer cells from multiplying. The only downside to this recipe is that it can't be thrown together on a whim—the cashews need to soak for two hours, so plan ahead!

• Makes about 1¼ cups •

1 cup raw cashews

¼ cup coconut milk or unsweetened almond milk

½ teaspoon raw organic unfiltered apple cider vinegar

1 garlic clove, minced

1 tablespoon finely chopped fresh chives

1 tablespoon finely chopped fresh curly parsley

1 tablespoon finely chopped fresh oregano

1 tablespoon finely chopped fresh dill

2 tablespoons nutritional yeast or finely grated Parmesan cheese

⅛ teaspoon sea salt

Put the cashews in a bowl and add water to cover them. Cover the bowl and let soak for 2 hours at room temperature.

Drain the cashews and rinse under cold water. If needed, the cashews can be soaked a day ahead of time, then drained, rinsed, and placed in a container in the refrigerator until ready to use.

Place the soaked cashews in a blender with just enough fresh cold water to cover them. Blend on high for several minutes until very smooth. (If you're not using a high-powered blender such as a Vitamix, which creates an ultra-smooth, creamy texture, strain the cashew cream through a fine-mesh sieve. Rinse the blender and add the strained cream back in.)

Add the rest of the ingredients to the blender and blend on low speed for another minute, or until the dressing is smooth and creamy. Adjust the seasoning as needed. Store the dressing in the refrigerator for up to 3 weeks.

SALSA VERDE

Most bottled green salsa contains modified food starch and sodium benzoate. Here's a quick and easy recipe for making salsa verde without the added chemicals. Use it over enchiladas, tacos, and eggs.

• Makes 3 cups •

1½ pounds tomatillos, husks removed (about 11 to 12 medium-size tomatillos)

½ cup chopped white onion

2 jalapeño peppers, or 2 serrano peppers, stemmed, seeded, and chopped (see note)

½ cup packed fresh cilantro leaves

1 tablespoon freshly squeezed lime juice

3 garlic cloves

1 teaspoon sea salt

½ teaspoon freshly ground black pepper

Rinse the tomatillos well and place them in a medium saucepan. Add enough hot water to cover the tomatillos and bring to a boil. Simmer for 5 minutes. Remove the tomatillos from the water and place them in a blender or food processor with the remaining ingredients and process until smooth. Taste the salsa to test for heat; if more heat is desired, add seeds from the pepper and process again to combine. Store covered in the refrigerator for up to 1 week or freeze extra salsa for up to 5 months.

HANDLING HOT PEPPERS

THE SEEDS CONTAIN MOST OF THE HEAT in these peppers, so removing them cuts down on the heat factor. If you want more heat, you can keep some of the seeds to add to the salsa.

It's important to handle hot peppers carefully, as hot peppers (such as jalapeños and habaneros) contain compounds in their seed oils called capsaicinoids, which produce a painful burning sensation when they come into contact with skin and mucous membranes (such as your fingers, eyes, and tongue!). The molecules bind to pain recep-

tors, so the experience can be quite intense. Some people take the extra precaution of wearing rubber gloves when seeding and chopping hot peppers.

To easily remove the seeds and veins of hot peppers without having to touch the seeds, you can use a melon baller. First, slice the peppers in half the long way. Hold the stem end of the pepper down and use the melon baller to scrape out the seeds and membranes. When you're done handling the peppers, immediately wash your hands well with soap and water. It is still a good idea to avoid touching your eyes or mouth for a while after you've washed your hands.

ROASTED GARLIC SALSA

THE COMBINATION OF ROASTED GARLIC AND CHILE PEPPERS PACKS FLAVOR AND NUTRITIONAL benefits into everyone's favorite tomato-based dipping sauce. Made from vegetables, fresh lime juice, and vinegar, this salsa makes a perfect alkaline-forming complement to fish, poultry, beef, and grain dishes. And of course, it definitely goes great with baked tortilla chips!

• Makes 5 cups •

1 small yellow onion, quartered

1 to 2 jalapeño peppers, stemmed, seeded, and sliced (reserve seeds if you want to add more heat to the salsa)

2 roasted green chiles (Anaheim, Hatch, New Mexico, or poblano), stemmed, seeded, and sliced (page 75 or store-bought)

1 roasted garlic head (or more if you want a stronger roasted garlic flavor; page 76)

2 (14½-ounce) cans organic diced fire-roasted tomatoes, with juice

¼ cup freshly squeezed lime juice

¼ cup raw organic unfiltered apple cider vinegar

1 cup chopped fresh cilantro leaves

1 tablespoon ground cumin

1 tablespoon dried Mexican oregano

1 to 2 teaspoons sea salt or Himalayan pink salt

1 tablespoon freshly ground black pepper

Add the onion, jalapeños, and green chiles to the bowl of a food processor and squeeze in the cloves from the head of roasted garlic. Pulse until minced. Add the remaining ingredients and pulse again until the salsa is well blended and reaches the consistency of restaurant-style salsa. Adjust the salt to taste. For more heat, add as many reserved seeds as desired to bump up the heat level. Refrigerate the salsa for 4 to 6 hours or overnight to allow the flavors to meld.

Salsa may be refrigerated in an airtight container for up to 2 weeks. If 5 cups of salsa is more than you'll be able to use in 2 weeks, the recipe can be cut in half, or you can freeze the extra salsa for up to 5 months.

SHORTCUT ORGANIC KETCHUP

THIS SIMPLE RECIPE CAN BE WHIPPED TOGETHER IN LESS THAN 30 MINUTES. THE SWEETNESS comes from Medjool dates and blackstrap molasses, two alkaline-forming foods that contain special compounds that help slow down the absorption of their natural sugars. You can adjust the level of sweetness to your liking by adding or removing the number of dates.

• Makes about 2 cups •

1 cup water

3 Medjool dates, pitted and chopped into small pieces

3 (6-ounce) jars/cans organic tomato paste

½ cup raw organic unfiltered apple cider vinegar

1 tablespoon unsulphured blackstrap molasses

1 teaspoon garlic powder

1 tablespoon onion powder

1 teaspoon dried mustard

¼ teaspoon ground allspice

¼ teaspoon cayenne pepper (optional)

⅛ teaspoon ground cinnamon

⅛ teaspoon ground cloves

¼ teaspoon ground ginger

1 teaspoon sea salt or Himalayan pink salt

Pour the water into a liquid measuring cup or small bowl and add the dates. Let soak for 15 minutes to soften the dates. Once soft, pour them and the soaking water into a blender or the bowl of a food processor. Add all remaining ingredients and blend or process until smooth and well blended. Transfer the mixture to a saucepan and gently bring to a simmer, whisking occasionally. Remove from the heat, let cool, and transfer to an airtight container. Refrigerate for at least 2 hours or overnight to allow the flavors to meld. This ketchup will keep in the refrigerator for up to 2 weeks.

TRULY HEALTHY
ORGANIC MAYONNAISE

ACCORDING TO THE LEGENDARY COOK JULIA CHILD, THE KEY TO SUCCESS AT MAKING YOUR OWN mayonnaise is room temperature ingredients and a warmed mixing bowl or blender container. When making homemade mayonnaise, you'll want to use the highest-quality ingredients you can find—organic pastured eggs and organic oils. If you're concerned about using raw eggs, see the note on page 160.

It takes a little practice, but once you get the feel for it, you'll be making it all the time. And that's a good thing, because truly healthy organic mayonnaise is next to impossible to find in a store.

• Makes about 1½ cups •

1 whole organic pastured egg

2 organic pastured egg yolks

1 tablespoon freshly squeezed lemon juice

1 teaspoon dried or prepared mustard
  (yellow or Dijon)

½ teaspoon sea salt or Himalayan pink salt

¼ teaspoon freshly ground black pepper

⅛ teaspoon sweet paprika (optional)

½ cup virgin coconut oil, melted

½ cup organic extra-virgin olive oil

Allow all ingredients to come to room temperature. If your eggs are cold, you can place them in a bowl of warm water for 5 minutes to bring them up to room temperature. Combine the coconut oil and olive oil together in one measuring cup.

Mayonnaise can be hand-beaten (i.e., whisked), made in a blender, or made with an electric mixer or immersion blender. The best mixing bowls are glass, stainless steel, or ceramic.

Warm the mixing bowl or blender container by running it under hot water or filling it with hot water and letting it sit for a few minutes. When warmed, completely dry the bowl or blender. Add the whole egg and two egg yolks to the bowl or blender and beat with a wire whisk or blend for 1 to 2 minutes, or until the eggs are thick and sticky.

Add the lemon juice, mustard, salt, pepper, and paprika, if using. Beat or blend briefly for 30 seconds more.

The egg yolks are now ready to receive the oil. Turn the blender on the lowest speed, or start hand beating at a speed of two strokes per second, and then begin adding the oil very slowly, a drop at a time. As you are adding the oil, you must not stop beating or blending until the mixture has thickened. Don't be in a hurry; this will take several minutes.

After ⅓ to ½ cup of the oil has been incorporated, the sauce will thicken into a very heavy cream. If you've been beating by hand, you can take a short rest. If using the blender, just keep letting it run. Now add the rest of the oil in a slow, steady ¹⁄₁₆-inch-thick stream, blending or beating continuously until all the oil is used up and the mayonnaise is thick and creamy.

Use immediately or store refrigerated in a glass container for 3 to 4 days.

VARIATION

- Roasted Garlic Mayonnaise: Squeeze the cloves from one entire head of roasted garlic (page 76) and combine them with ½ cup of the mayonnaise. Mix the ingredients thoroughly in a bowl. Use this mayonnaise to enhance the flavor of chicken salad or tuna salad, deviled eggs, or potato salad.

> **NOTE:**
>
> *If you don't have pastured eggs, you should not make mayonnaise with raw eggs due to the slight, but real, possibility of salmonella contamination. To avoid that risk, you can gently cook the egg mixture prior to adding the oil. Slightly heating the eggs will destroy any pathogens.*
>
> *Add the whole egg and 2 egg yolks to the bowl or blender and beat with a wire whisk or blend for 1 to 2 minutes, or until the eggs are thick and sticky. Add the remaining ingredients except for the oil and beat or blend briefly for 30 seconds more. Transfer to a saucepan.*
>
> *Gently cook the egg mixture over a very low heat, stirring constantly, until the mixture forms bubbles in one or two places. Be careful not to heat it too much, as the egg yolks need to remain liquid and sticky, not cooked.*
>
> *Immediately remove the mixture from the heat and let it cool for 4 minutes.*
>
> *Pour the mixture back into the bowl or the blender. Add oil slowly to the mixture while beating or blending as described above.*

ZESTY FRESH MARINARA SAUCE

THE SECRET TO A TRULY AMAZING MARINARA SAUCE IS THE FRESH TOMATOES AND HERBS. WHILE most recipes call for sugar, I throw a fresh organic carrot into the pot to provide that all-important sweetness. Tomatoes are famously known for their high content of lycopene, a cancer-fighting antioxidant that is best absorbed into the body when the tomatoes have been cooked; however, tomatoes contain at least fourteen other known antioxidants, including beta-carotene and vitamins C and E. Use this marinara sauce to top your spaghetti squash, zucchini noodles, baked potatoes and other vegetables, whole grains, and anything else you can think of!

• Makes 4 to 5 cups •

5 pounds fresh, ripe tomatoes (any type)

2 tablespoons virgin coconut oil

2 tablespoons extra-virgin olive oil

3 medium yellow onions, diced

2 celery stalks, diced

1 large carrot, divided (cut the carrot in half—grate one half and leave the other half whole)

8 to 10 garlic cloves, minced

2 bay leaves

⅓ cup chopped fresh curly parsley, or 2 teaspoons dried

⅓ cup chopped fresh basil, or 2 teaspoons dried

2 sprigs fresh oregano, or 2 teaspoons dried

2 sprigs fresh thyme, or 1 teaspoon dried

2 sprigs fresh sage, or 2 teaspoons dried

1 sprig fresh rosemary, or 1 teaspoon dried

1 teaspoon sea salt

To easily remove the skins from the tomatoes, they need to be blanched in boiling water for 30 seconds and then immediately immersed in an ice water bath for a few minutes.

Prepare a pot of water that will hold 5 to 6 tomatoes at a time. Bring the water to a boil. Meanwhile, prepare an ice water bath of about the same size by filling a bowl halfway with water and half with ice.

Use a paring knife to remove the cores (the little dark spot on the top of the tomato where it was attached to the vine). Cut around the core at an angle, making a cone-shaped cut, and then pop out the core. Using the same paring knife, cut a very shallow "X" on the bottom of the tomatoes. This will make the actual peeling of the tomatoes easier later in the process.

Place 5 to 6 of the tomatoes into the boiling water for 30 seconds to a minute. The skins will wilt and look a bit cracked when they are ready. Remove the tomatoes from the boiling water with a slotted spoon and fully immerse them in the ice water bath immediately to stop the cooking process. Leave the tomatoes in the ice water bath for at least 5 minutes, then remove them. They should still be very firm, with the skin wrinkled and hanging off slightly. Repeat the process with another batch of 5 to 6 tomatoes.

Peel the skin off the tomatoes with your hands and discard. Remove any stubborn skins with a sharp knife. To remove the seeds, cut the tomatoes in half, then squeeze them over a fine-mesh strainer, catching any of the tomato juices in a bowl below the strainer. You may need to scrape some of the seeds out of the tomatoes with a spoon. Discard the seeds. Chop the tomato halves into smaller pieces and add to the bowl of tomato juice. Set aside.

Add the coconut oil and olive oil to a large stockpot and heat over medium. Sauté the onions, celery, and grated carrot for 5 minutes, then add the garlic and sauté another 2 to 3 minutes, or until the onions are translucent.

Add the tomatoes with juice, bay leaves, herbs, and salt. Stir to combine.

Reduce the heat to a low simmer and cook for 2 to 2½ hours, stirring occasionally, until cooked down but with still a bit of liquid in it. The sauce will thicken as it cools.

Add the remaining whole carrot half during the last 30 minutes of cook time to neutralize acidity.

When the sauce is done, remove the bay leaves, sprigs of herbs, and piece of carrot. If desired, you may purée the sauce in a blender to make it smooth. I like to purée half of the sauce and add it back to the chunky sauce for a nice consistency.

Enjoy the sauce immediately or store it refrigerated in glass jars with tight-fitting lids for up to 1 week. The flavors are more robust the next day. Freeze the sauce in freezer-safe containers for up to 1 year.

NATURALLY SWEETENED TANGY BARBECUE SAUCE

EVEN THE NATURAL, ORGANIC BOTTLED BARBECUE SAUCES HAVE TOO MUCH SUGAR FOR MY LIKING. This one is a perfect alternative. The ground dried chipotle peppers lend a naturally sweet, smoky flavor to the sauce. Toss it with leftover cooked chicken, crunchy carrots and chunks of avocado for a quick lunch, or use it as a sauce on Seasoned Spelt Pizza Crust (page 146), topped with black beans, organic corn, diced tomatoes, and mozzarella cheese.

• Makes 3 cups •

2 tablespoons virgin coconut oil

1 cup minced yellow onion

3 garlic cloves, minced

2 (8-ounce) jars/cans organic tomato sauce

1 (6-ounce) jar/can organic tomato paste, plus more if needed to thicken the sauce

2 tablespoons raw organic unfiltered apple cider vinegar

2 tablespoons freshly squeezed lemon juice

⅓ teaspoon ground chipotle pepper

⅛ teaspoon liquid stevia extract, or 1 tablespoon pure maple syrup

1 tablespoon unsulphured blackstrap molasses (optional)

1 tablespoon chili powder

1 teaspoon dried mustard

1 teaspoon smoked paprika

1 tablespoon chopped fresh curly parsley

1 teaspoon sea salt or Himalayan pink salt

¼ teaspoon freshly ground black pepper

Heat the oil in a large saucepan over medium heat. Add the onions and stir until tender, about 5 minutes. Add the remaining ingredients and whisk until smooth. Bring to a low boil, then reduce the heat to a simmer and cook for 30 to 45 minutes (or longer), or until nice and thick. Add more tomato paste if you need to thicken it further. Transfer to a glass storage container with a tight-fitting lid and refrigerate for up to 2 weeks or store in the freezer for 3 months.

AWESOME HOISIN SAUCE

I F YOU LIKE ASIAN FOOD, THEN YOU LIKE HOISIN SAUCE. USE THIS FOR ANY QUICK STIR-FRY. YOU can buy a commercially made Chinese 5-spice blend, but if you're feeling adventurous, I've included ingredients and directions for making it yourself.

• Makes about 1 cup •

½ cup reduced-sodium gluten-free tamari sauce

¼ cup natural creamy peanut butter or tahini

2 tablespoons raw honey or coconut nectar

4 teaspoons brown rice vinegar

2 garlic cloves, minced

4 teaspoons unrefined toasted sesame oil

1 teaspoon Chinese 5-spice blend (recipe follows)

Pinch of cayenne pepper or red pepper flakes (optional)

Pinch of freshly ground black pepper

Place all ingredients in a blender or food processor and blend until fully combined and smooth. Store covered in the refrigerator for up to 1 week.

CHINESE 5-SPICE BLEND

• Makes about ¼ cup •

2 whole star anise

2 teaspoons Szechuan peppercorns or regular peppercorns

1 teaspoon whole cloves

1 teaspoon fennel seeds

1 teaspoon coriander seeds

1 stick cinnamon, broken into a few pieces

In a dry skillet over medium heat, toast the anise, peppercorns, cloves, fennel, and coriander until fragrant, stirring the seeds occasionally with a spatula to prevent burning. Let cool.

Transfer to a spice grinder or coffee grinder and add the cinnamon stick pieces. Grind for 20 to 30 seconds, or until you have a fine powder.

Store the blend in an airtight container alongside your other spices. It will keep for several months.

RAW FRUIT JAM

MOST FRUIT JAMS AND PRESERVES ARE MADE BY COOKING THE FRUIT AND ADDING A LOAD OF sugar. This recipe takes advantage of the gelling property of chia seeds, which allows the fruits to be used in their raw form. With every bite, you'll get a boost of their amazing antioxidants, vitamins, and fibers. Add to that the omega-3 benefits from the chia seeds, and you've got a jam like no other. Apricot jam and blueberry-raspberry jam are two of my favorites, but feel free to experiment with your favorite fruits. The recipe calls for white chia seeds, which will be less visible in the final product. Black chia seeds will work in the recipe, but you will be able to clearly see them in the jam.

• Makes 4 cups •

APRICOT JAM
2 tablespoons white chia seeds
¼ cup water

4 cups fresh, ripe apricots, pitted and quartered
2 tablespoons raw honey or other natural sweetener (optional)

Soak the chia seeds in the water for 10 minutes. They will thicken and form a gel. Place the apricot quarters and honey, if using, in a blender and add the chia seed gel. Blend for 3 to 4 minutes, then transfer to a jam jar or other container and refrigerate for 1 to 2 hours to allow the jam to thicken and set. Store the jam in the refrigerator for up to 2 weeks. Freeze it for up to 6 months.

BLUEBERRY-RASPBERRY JAM

3 tablespoons white chia seeds

6 tablespoons water

¾ cup (6-ounce container) fresh blueberries

¾ cup (6-ounce container) fresh raspberries

2 tablespoons raw honey or other natural sweetener

2 teaspoons freshly squeezed lemon juice

½ teaspoon vanilla powder or pure vanilla extract

Soak the chia seeds in the water for 10 minutes. They will thicken and form a gel. Place the fruit and the remaining ingredients in a blender, then add the chia seed gel. Blend for 3 to 4 minutes, then transfer to a jam jar or other container and refrigerate for 1 to 2 hours to allow the jam to thicken and set. Store the jam in the refrigerator for up to 2 weeks. Freeze for up to 6 months.

SUGAR-FREE ORANGE CRANBERRY SAUCE

MY MOTHER ALWAYS MADE FRESH, WHOLE CRANBERRY SAUCE WITH SUGAR FOR OUR HOLIDAY MEALS. In my version, I swap the white sugar for stevia and add a whole orange for natural sweetness.

• Makes 2 cups •

1 (12-ounce) bag fresh cranberries (3 cups)

½ cup water

2 navel oranges, divided (peel 1 orange and cut into small bite-size pieces; juice and zest the other orange)

1 teaspoon liquid stevia extract, or more to taste (orange-flavored stevia works great here)

Note: The stevia can be replaced with 1 cup coconut nectar.

Place the cranberries, water, and orange juice in a saucepan over medium-high heat. Bring to a boil until the cranberries start to "pop," then reduce the heat to low and simmer gently for about 10 minutes, allowing the mixture to thicken.

Remove from the heat and add the stevia, orange pieces, and zest. Stir to mix.

Cool to room temperature. Cranberry sauce will thicken when chilled. It may be served warm or cold. Refrigerate any leftovers for up to 4 days.

ROSE WATER

ROSE WATER IS A VERSATILE CULINARY STAPLE USED IN VARIOUS CUISINES THROUGHOUT THE world. A small splash of rose water can completely transform the taste profile of fruit salads, sorbets, rice puddings, whipped cream, and beverages. Even grain dishes, curries, and meats are enhanced by the flavor of rose water. It is a suggested ingredient in several of the recipes throughout this book, including Vanilla Rose Yogurt with Peaches and Walnuts (page 69), Cardamom Rose Lassi (page 84), Seasonal Fruit Salads (page 112), and Choco-cado Mousse (page 259).

If you're new to using rose water in foods, I suggest starting lightly with small drops and increasing as desired. Although delightfully subtle in small amounts, its flavor can overpower and taste soapy if too much is used.

Rose water is produced by water distillation of fresh rose petals. The cooled vapor yields a clear water that contains the unique compounds that give roses their signature aroma and flavor. It is rich in antioxidants and is well known for its high content of vitamins A, B3, C, and E. Taken internally or applied externally, rose water has powerful antibacterial and anti-inflammatory properties as well.

Rose water can be purchased in specialty stores or online, but if you have fresh roses, it's easy to make your own rose water using a simple distillation process on your stovetop (here's your chance to do your own skinny science!). You can make about 2 cups of high-quality rose water in about twenty to forty minutes.

You'll need to have the following utensils and tools on hand: stockpot with lid; a small heavy object with flat surfaces, such as a brick, that can withstand the temperature of boiling water and will not move around in the pot while the water is boiling; and a heat-resistant glass or stainless-steel bowl, small enough to fit inside the pot (this will be referred to as the collection bowl in the instructions below); turkey baster; 2-cup or larger measuring cup.

• Makes 2 cups •

2 to 3 quarts fresh rose petals (see note)   Ice cubes
Distilled water

Lay the brick or other object flat on the bottom of the stockpot. Make sure it is centered. (There is nothing special about the brick—its purpose is merely to provide a raised, sturdy flat surface for the collection bowl to sit above the surface of the roses. Any similar object will work.)

Place the rose petals in the pot, arranging them evenly around the brick.

Pour in enough distilled water to just barely cover the rose petals. The water should come about halfway up the height of the brick.

Set the collection bowl on top of the brick. The rim of the bowl should not extend higher than the rim of the pot, but it should be high enough above the surface of the rose petals and water that none of the boiling water spills into it.

Cover the pot with the lid turned upside down so the rounded part and the handle are inside the pot.

Turn on the heat and bring the water to a rolling boil.

As soon as the water begins to boil, fill the well of the inverted stockpot lid with ice cubes, then lower the heat to a slow simmer.

As the steam rises inside the pot and comes into contact with the surface of the cold lid, it will condense and drip down into the collection bowl.

Continue gently boiling the rose petals and adding ice to the top of the inverted lid as needed to keep the lid cold at all times. You may have to remove melted ice from the inverted lid using a turkey baster.

Every 15 minutes or so, carefully lift the lid straight up off the pot so you can check to make sure there is still enough simmering water over the rose petals. If you need to add more water to the petals, carefully set the lid aside and remove the collection bowl. Add more water into the pot slowly to once again cover the rose petals. At this point you can transfer the collected rose water into a 2-cup or larger measuring cup so that you can see how much you have collected so far (you will be collecting a total of 2 cups).

Return the empty collection bowl to the pot, place the inverted lid with the ice back on the pot, and continue simmering to collect more rose water.

Repeat this step every 15 minutes, adding each successive collection of rose water to the measuring cup and replacing the simmer water if needed. It's time to stop when you have collected a total of 2 cups of rose water.

Store the rose water in a clean glass jar with a tight-fitting lid in the refrigerator for up to 1 month.

NOTE:

Since the rose water will eventually be added to your food, it's important that the rose petals you use have not been exposed to toxic chemicals. Most commercially grown flowers are heavily sprayed, and are even fed with systemic pesticides, so it's best to use roses that you know are chemical-free.

If you are not up for making your own rose water, it can be purchased in specialty stores and online. Be sure to look for pure organic food-grade rose water, which is clear (not colored) and made from real rose petals, as opposed to scented/flavored rose water with a pink color added. Check the Resources section (page 282) for recommended brands.

TACO SEASONING MIX

PACKAGED TACO SEASONING MIXES USUALLY CONTAIN MONOSODIUM GLUTAMATE (MSG) AND OTHER undesirable additives. This one tastes identical to the commercial variety, without the chemical ingredients. Try it on ground beef, ground turkey, chicken, and beans.

• Makes ½ cup •

4 tablespoons chili powder

1 teaspoon garlic powder

1 teaspoon onion powder

¼ teaspoon cayenne pepper

1 teaspoon Mexican oregano

2 teaspoons Spanish paprika

2 tablespoons ground cumin

4 teaspoons ground coriander

2 teaspoons sea salt

Mix all of the ingredients together in a small bowl until well combined. Store in an airtight container or spice jar.

Skinny Snacks and Finger Foods

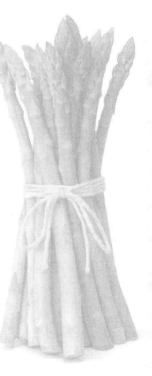

10

The best snacks are those you make yourself, and I have focused on incorporating skinny superfoods into fun and healthy snacks that can be eaten at home or packed to take to school, to the office, or on road trips. Many of these snacks, such as Banana, Nut Butter, and Hemp Seed Bites (page 170), Stuffed Dates, Three Ways (page 172), Avocado Caprese (page 182), and Cold Chicken, Zucchini, and Feta Sliders (page 183), are so simple to put together that they can hardly be called "recipes"—they are more like "snack ideas." Others, like Quinoa Pizza Bites (page 184) and Zesty Nacho Kale Krunch (page 188), take a little more time and planning but are well worth the effort. Once you try some of these wonderful finger foods, buying snacks that come in bags and boxes will hopefully become a thing of the past.

ORANGE AND DATE DELIGHT

MEDJOOL DATES ARE GREAT BY THEMSELVES, BUT WHEN COMBINED WITH THE SHARP FLAVOR OF oranges, the mix is exquisite—and makes a great lunchbox snack or dessert. Dates contain protein, fiber, antioxidants, a host of vitamins, and at least fifteen minerals, including selenium, a potent antioxidant shown to lower the risk of heart disease and cancer and that also plays a role in reducing allergies and inflammation.

• Makes 2 servings •

1 large juicy orange 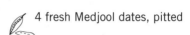 4 fresh Medjool dates, pitted

Peel the orange over a small bowl, catching as much juice as you can in the bowl. Slice the orange neatly into segments and place in the bowl.

Slice the dates crosswise into thin strips and scatter them over the orange segments. Toss with a spoon to make sure the juices coat the date slices. Enjoy immediately, or for a more intense flavor, cover and refrigerate for 1 hour. This mix will keep in the refrigerator for up to 3 days.

BANANA, NUT BUTTER, AND HEMP SEED BITES

SWEET, CREAMY, AND CRUNCHY—THESE BITE-SIZE MORSELS HAVE EVERYTHING YOU WANT IN A snack and more. They can be made in a matter of minutes and provide a punch of satisfaction that will please kids and grown-ups alike. Known for their healthy dose of protein, fiber, healthy oils, antioxidants, and minerals, hemp seeds provide a crunchy component that elevates the comfort-food combo of banana and nut butter to a whole new level of taste and nutrition.

My favorite variety of this snack is made with sunbutter (a.k.a. sunflower seed butter), but any nut or seed butter will do. Try it with almond butter, cashew butter, or peanut butter.

• Makes 1 serving •

1 banana

1 tablespoon nut or seed butter of your choice
(page 72 or store-bought)

1 tablespoon organic hemp seeds

Peel the banana and slice it in half lengthwise. Smear the nut or seed butter on the cut surface of half the banana and sprinkle the hemp seeds on top of the butter. Top with the other half of the banana, making a banana sandwich. Slice into bite-size pieces and enjoy this amazingly easy and tasty snack.

NO-BAKE CRISSCROSS CACAO PEANUT BUTTER COOKIES

THESE QUICK SNACKS WILL TAME YOUR SWEET TOOTH AND SATISFY YOUR CHOCOLATE CRAVINGS in a deliciously healthy way. I prefer peanut butter, but you can use your favorite nut or seed butter. This snack takes only ten minutes to prepare and is perfect for the lunchbox, kids' parties, potlucks, and road trips.

• Makes 15 to 18 cookies •

1 cup packed whole Medjool dates, pitted

½ cup crunchy natural peanut butter

1 teaspoon pure vanilla extract

1 cup raw almonds

¼ cup raw cacao nibs (see note)

Purée the dates in a food processor until a thick paste forms. Add the peanut butter, vanilla, almonds, and cacao nibs. Process until the almonds are well chopped but still course and are well incorporated into the mixture. The mixture should hold together when pressed between your fingertips. If it is too dry, add an additional tablespoon of nut butter.

Scoop out the cookie "dough" with a measured tablespoon or cookie scoop and form into balls.

Press each cookie with the prongs of a fork to flatten and make crisscross hatches. Enjoy immediately or place in an airtight container and keep chilled in the refrigerator until ready to eat. Cookies will keep for up to 1 week, but they probably will get eaten before then!

NOTE:

A chopped dark chocolate bar or dark chocolate chips can be used in place of the raw cacao nibs, if desired. See Resources (page 280) for recommended brands.

STUFFED DATES, THREE WAYS

Medjool dates are one of my favorite go-to treats when I'm craving something sweet. Every now and then, I like to change things up a bit and stuff them with something creamy. These three versions of stuffed dates make great appetizers or anytime snacks. They will keep for up to a week—if they last that long!

• Each recipe makes 12 stuffed dates •

NUT BUTTER CACAO–STUFFED DATES

2 tablespoons nut or seed butter of your choice (page 72 or store-bought)

1 tablespoon raw cacao nibs

12 Medjool dates, pitted

HONEY LEMON CREAM CHEESE–STUFFED DATES

⅓ cup organic Neufchâtel cream cheese, at room temperature

1 teaspoon raw honey

1 teaspoon freshly grated lemon zest

¼ teaspoon pure vanilla extract

12 Medjool dates, pitted

12 raw pecan halves, for garnish

SAVORY GOAT CHEESE–STUFFED DATES	1 garlic clove, crushed
⅓ cup goat cheese	12 Medjool dates, pitted
1 tablespoon chopped fresh curly parsley	12 raw pecan halves, for garnish

For each filling variety: Place the ingredients (except for the dates and pecans) in a small bowl and stir with a rubber spatula until well blended. Place about ½ teaspoon of the filling inside the pocket of each date. Smooth out the top of the filling. For the cream cheese and goat cheese varieties, top each stuffed date with a pecan half.

HEALTHY JELLO

WHEN MADE WITH REAL INGREDIENTS, "JELLO" CAN BE A SUPERFOOD THAT KIDS OF ALL AGES will love and benefit from. In addition to any fruits or nutrient-rich liquids that you may use to make the jello, the superfood status comes from gelatin—a unique nutrient consisting of amino acids that provide protein and a host of health benefits. Gelatin also significantly increases the absorption of vitamins and minerals from the other foods you eat it with.

To get the most benefit from your jello, it is important to use a high-quality gelatin product. I highly recommend the gelatins sold by Bernard Jensen and Great Lakes brands (see Resources, page 278). Both of these are grass-fed, hormone-free, all-natural kosher bovine gelatin.

• Makes 4 servings •

1¾ cups 100 percent fruit juice, divided (see note)	2 cups fruit (such as raspberries and blackberries, and sliced strawberries, bananas, oranges, peaches, pears, etc.)
1 tablespoon unflavored gelatin granules	
¼ cup boiling water	

Place ¼ cup of the juice in a 2-quart bowl. Sprinkle the granules of gelatin over the surface of the juice (do not dump them in a pile, as the granules in the middle won't dissolve). Let sit for a few minutes to allow the gelatin to moisten.

Add the hot (just boiled) water, then whisk to dissolve the gelatin. When the gelatin is completely dissolved, add the remaining 1½ cups of juice and mix well to combine.

Add the fruit and stir to coat it in the liquid gelatin mixture. Place the gelatin in the refrigerator to chill until set, at least 2 hours before serving. Store covered in the refrigerator for up to 1 week.

VARIATION

Here's a healthy variation of *Haupia* (pronounced "how-pee-yah"), a Hawaiian version of coconut milk jello cut into cute cubes and traditionally served as a dessert at luaus. If you don't want to use stevia, you can use ½ cup raw honey or coconut nectar instead.

½ cup water

3 tablespoons unflavored gelatin granules

2½ cups coconut milk

½ teaspoon liquid stevia extract (coconut-flavored stevia works great here)

Place the water in a 2-quart bowl. Sprinkle the granules of gelatin over the surface of the water (do not dump them in a pile, as the granules in the middle won't dissolve). Let sit for a few minutes to allow the gelatin to moisten.

Meanwhile, heat the coconut milk over medium heat in a saucepan. Bring to a simmer but do not boil. When the coconut milk begins to simmer, reduce the heat to low, add the gelatin mixture, and whisk to dissolve the gelatin. When the gelatin is completely dissolved, add the stevia and mix well to combine.

Pour the warm coconut milk–gelatin mixture into an 8-inch square pan. Let cool to room temperature, then cover with plastic wrap and refrigerate until firm, at least 2 hours. To serve, cut into 9 squares. Store covered in the refrigerator for up to 1 week.

> **NOTES:**
> - *You can use whatever type of juice you want for this recipe. Some of my favorites are Concord grape, apple, and cherry. This is an instance where I recommend using 100 percent fruit juice, either freshly juiced with your juicer or bottled with no sugar added, preferably organic.*
>   *Do not use fresh pineapple or fresh pineapple juice to make jello, as it contains an enzyme called bromelain, which breaks down the proteins in the gelatin, causing it to lose its gelling properties. Fresh kiwi, figs, guava, ginger, and papaya also contain enzymes that interfere with gelatin's gelling properties. Bottled juices have been heat pasteurized, which destroys the enzymes in the juices, making them suitable to use for jello, but not as nutritious as fresh juices.*
> - *Jello can be made without fruit juice—try using coconut water, kombucha, or even a favorite herbal tea. Sweeten as you like with stevia or other natural sweetener.*

FRUITY COCONUT POPSICLES

THESE POPSICLES ARE JUST LIKE THE SMOOTH AND CREAMY TREATS I ENJOYED AS A CHILD. You can combine coconut milk with any fruit, even avocado, for a variety of flavors and colors. These fruity frozen bars are perfect for after-school snacks or a great way to beat the summer heat, although they are fun to eat any time of year.

• Makes 6 to 8 popsicles, depending on size of popsicle mold •

1¾ cups coconut milk (about one 14-ounce can)

¼ teaspoon liquid stevia extract (flavored stevia works great here; see note for substitutions)

1 tablespoon pure vanilla extract or vanilla powder

1 tablespoon unsweetened shredded coconut (optional)

1 cup fresh or frozen fruit (optional)

Note: The stevia can be replaced with 3 tablespoons raw honey, coconut nectar, or pure maple syrup.

Mix all ingredients together in a bowl and pour into popsicle molds. Place in the freezer for 5 to 6 hours, or until frozen. When ready to serve, run warm water over the popsicle mold for 5 seconds to loosen the popsicles. Serve immediately.

VARIATIONS

Avocado Popsicles

2 ripe avocados

1¾ cups coconut milk (about one 14-ounce can)

½ teaspoon liquid stevia extract (flavored stevia works great here)

2½ teaspoons freshly squeezed lemon juice

1 teaspoon pure vanilla extract or vanilla powder

Add all ingredients to a food processor or blender and blend on high for 2 minutes, or until smooth and creamy. Spoon the mixture into popsicle molds and freeze for 2 hours, or until solid.

Orange Popsicles

1 cup orange juice

1 cup coconut milk

¼ teaspoon liquid stevia extract (orange-flavored stevia works great here)

¼ teaspoon orange extract

½ teaspoon pure vanilla extract

Whisk all ingredients together in a bowl. Pour the mixture into popsicle molds. Place in the freezer for 5 to 6 hours, or until frozen.

FAST FROZEN YOGURT

Y OU DON'T NEED AN ICE CREAM MAKER TO ENJOY THIS INSTANT FROZEN YOGURT. THE KEY IS TO start with frozen fruit and whirl it in a blender or food processor with plain yogurt. Though I've used bananas, mangos, and strawberries, you can use 3½ cups of whatever frozen fruit you have on hand. Try add-ins such as cacao nibs, chopped nuts, or chopped fresh mint leaves.

• Makes 4 servings •

1 cup organic plain whole milk yogurt

½ teaspoon liquid stevia extract (vanilla-flavored stevia works great here)

1 teaspoon pure vanilla extract

1 frozen banana, peeled and cut into bite-size pieces

1 cup frozen mango chunks

1½ cups frozen strawberries

Place all of the ingredients in a high-powered blender or food processor in the order listed. Process until creamy and firm, about 1 minute or so in a high-powered blender or 3 minutes in a food processor. The frozen yogurt should be the consistency of a soft-serve ice cream and firm enough to be served directly from the blender or food processor. If it is too liquid, add more frozen fruit and blend again to firm it up. Serve the frozen yogurt immediately or transfer it to an airtight container and store it in the freezer for up to 1 month.

ORANGE ALMOND ENERGY BARS

T HESE ENERGY BARS ARE SWEET, CHEWY, CHUNKY, AND CHOCK-FULL OF NOURISHING alkaline-forming foods. In this recipe I use the entire orange peel, not just the zest, as orange peels contain over 170 different phytonutrients that offer an impressive array of health benefits, including lowering cholesterol, averting several types of cancer, and relieving heartburn and digestive problems. Additionally, the peels of oranges contain nearly twice the amount of vitamin C as the flesh. Now that makes one powerful energy bar!

• Makes 1 (8-inch) square baking dish •

Peel from 1 orange, torn into small pieces

1½ cups packed pitted whole Medjool dates

⅓ cup raw cacao powder or unsweetened cocoa powder

1 cup almond meal (page 71 or store-bought)

½ cup unsweetened shredded coconut

¼ cup virgin coconut oil

1 teaspoon pure vanilla extract

1 teaspoon almond extract

Pinch of sea salt or Himalayan pink salt

1 heaping tablespoon (1 scoop) green superfood powder (optional)

1 cup raw whole almonds (preferably soaked and dried)

Place the torn orange peel in the food processor and process until it is very finely chopped. Add the dates and purée until a thick paste forms. Add the cacao powder, almond meal, shredded coconut, coconut oil, vanilla and almond extracts, salt, and green powder, if using. Process until all ingredients are well combined. Add the almonds and process again until the almonds are well chopped but still chunky and are well incorporated into the mixture.

Spread a large sheet of waxed paper on a work surface. Transfer the date mixture to the waxed paper and press the mixture into a ½-inch-thick rectangle. If desired, you can even out the edges by trimming with a knife. Wrap tightly in the waxed paper and chill for several hours or overnight.

Unwrap the chilled block and cut it into bars of the desired size. Refrigerate the bars in an airtight container for up to 1 week.

HIGH-PROTEIN GRANOLA BARS

THESE BARS ARE EXTREMELY DELICIOUS AND MAKE A GREAT ANYTIME SNACK. I OFTEN TAKE ONE with me to the movies. Their digestibility and nutrients are enhanced if the oats, nuts, and seeds have been soaked and dried; however, the bars are just as delicious using unsoaked raw ingredients. The protein comes from the nuts and seeds, with an additional boost from a protein powder.

• Makes 1 (11 x 9½-inch) baking dish •

DRY INGREDIENTS

2 cups rolled oats (preferably soaked and dried)

1½ teaspoons ground cinnamon

½ teaspoon sea salt or Himalayan pink salt

½ cup vanilla whey protein or hemp protein (optional)

2 tablespoons raw cacao powder or unsweetened cocoa powder (optional)

½ cup raw pepitas (preferably soaked and dried)

¼ cup raw sesame seeds (preferably soaked and dried)

1 cup raw cashews, chopped

1 cup raw almonds (preferably soaked and dried), chopped

2 tablespoons flaxseeds (preferably soaked and dried), ground

⅔ cup unsweetened flaked coconut

½ cup raisins, chopped dates, or dried cranberries

½ cup raw cacao nibs or dark chocolate chips (optional)

WET INGREDIENTS

2 teaspoons pure vanilla extract

½ cup virgin coconut oil, melted

½ cup raw honey, brown rice syrup, or coconut nectar

½ cup nut butter (page 72 or store-bought)

In a large bowl, combine the dry ingredients and mix well. In a separate bowl, add the vanilla to the coconut oil and whisk together, mixing well. Add in the honey and nut butter and whisk until the mixture is uniform in texture. Add the wet ingredients to the dry ingredients with a large spoon. Stir until all the dry ingredients are coated with the wet, mixing thoroughly. Transfer the mixture to an 11 x 9½-inch baking dish. Spread evenly and pat down. Cover the pan with plastic wrap and refrigerate several hours or overnight. To serve, slice into bars. Bars are best kept in the refrigerator until ready to be served and will keep for up to 1 week. Bars may be frozen for up to 1 month.

FOUR HUMMUS FAVORITES

CHICKPEAS, OTHERWISE KNOWN AS GARBANZO BEANS, ARE THE SIGNATURE INGREDIENT IN HUMMUS. They contain a high amount of soluble fiber as well as a unique mix of antioxidant phytonutrients that have been shown to protect against heart disease.

Hummus is a versatile dip: serve it with fresh veggies, use it as a spread on sandwiches, or serve it with roasted vegetables. Once you discover how simple it is to make, you'll never be satisfied with store-bought hummus again. Use the method for Classic Hummus as the guide for making the other varieties that follow.

• Each recipe makes about 4 cups •

CLASSIC HUMMUS

3 cups cooked chickpeas, or 2 (15-ounce) cans, drained and rinsed

Juice of 2 lemons (about ¼ cup)

¼ cup water, plus more as needed to achieve the desired consistency

2 tablespoons extra-virgin olive oil

2 tablespoons tahini

2 garlic cloves, minced

1 teaspoon ground cumin

¼ teaspoon sweet paprika

Pinch of sea salt, or more to taste

1 tablespoon chopped curly parsley, for garnish (optional)

Place the ingredients in the order listed into the bowl of a food processor or high-powered blender. Process until smooth, 1 to 2 minutes, stopping to scrape down the sides as necessary. If the hummus is too thick, add more water, a tablespoon at a time, and process again until the desired consistency is achieved. Taste and adjust salt, if needed. Transfer to a serving bowl or storage container. This hummus keeps in the refrigerator for up to 5 days.

ROASTED GARLIC HUMMUS

3 cups cooked chickpeas, or 2 (15-ounce) cans, drained and rinsed

Juice of 2 lemons (about ¼ cup)

¼ cup water, plus more as needed to achieve the desired consistency

2 tablespoons extra-virgin olive oil

2 tablespoons tahini

2 heads roasted garlic (page 76)

1 teaspoon ground cumin

¼ teaspoon sweet paprika

Pinch of sea salt, or more to taste

1 tablespoon chopped curly parsley, for garnish (optional)

ROASTED RED PEPPER HUMMUS

3 cups cooked chickpeas, or 2 (15-ounce) cans, drained and rinsed

2 roasted red bell peppers (preferably organic; page 75)

Juice of 1 lemon (about 2 tablespoons)

¼ cup water, plus more as needed to achieve the desired consistency

2 tablespoons extra-virgin olive oil

2 tablespoons tahini

1 teaspoon ground cumin

¼ teaspoon sweet paprika

2 garlic cloves, minced

Pinch of sea salt, or more to taste

1 tablespoon chopped curly parsley, for garnish (optional)

CILANTRO-LIME JALAPEÑO HUMMUS

3 cups cooked chickpeas, or 2 (15-ounce) cans, drained and rinsed

1 jalapeño pepper, stemmed, seeded, and chopped

1 cup loosely packed fresh cilantro leaves

Juice of 2 limes (about ¼ cup)

¼ cup water, plus more as needed to achieve the desired consistency

2 tablespoons extra-virgin olive oil

2 tablespoons tahini

3 garlic cloves, minced

1 teaspoon ground cumin

½ teaspoon ground coriander

Pinch of sea salt, or more to taste

PERFECT IN EVERY WAY GUACAMOLE

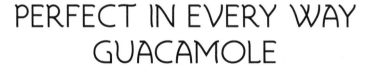

THERE IS NO OTHER SNACK FOOD THAT CAN BOAST A NUTRITION PROFILE AS IMPRESSIVE as guacamole. Every one of its ingredients are alkalizing and liver-izing, offering stunning health benefits in each bite. From stabilizing blood sugar levels, boosting the immune system, and lowering cholesterol and blood pressure to removing heavy metals from the body and promoting weight loss, guacamole is a food to include regularly in your meals and snacks.

See the note below for my chemistry secret to keeping your guacamole fresh and green for days.

• Makes 6 servings •

3 avocados

2 fresh garlic cloves, minced, or 4 roasted garlic cloves (page 76)

¼ cup minced red onion

Juice of 1 lime

¼ cup chopped fresh cilantro

½ jalapeño pepper, seeded and finely minced (optional)

Pinch of sea salt, or more to taste

1 Roma tomato, seeded and diced

Cut the avocados in half and remove the pits. Spoon the flesh of the avocados into a mixing bowl and mash with a fork, leaving some chunks. Add the garlic, onion, lime juice, cilantro, jalapeño, if using, and salt. Mix well with a rubber spatula. Fold in the diced tomato and taste. Adjust salt, if needed. Enjoy immediately.

NOTE:

Avocadoes oxidize quickly, so guacamole begins to turn brown after about an hour or so. If you want to save leftover guacamole, or if you want to make the guacamole a day ahead of time, there's a chemistry secret to keeping it fresh—create a barrier of water on the surface of the guacamole to prevent it from coming into contact with the air.

Here's what you do:

Place the guacamole into a food storage container that has a tight-fitting lid that seals out air (plastic wrap will not work). Rubbermaid or Pyrex food storage containers with snap-on lids work great for this.

Pack the guacamole tightly in the container with the back of a spoon, spreading to fill the entire size of the container and pressing out any pockets of air. Next, drizzle some room temperature water over the top of the guacamole until it covers the entire surface. Tilt the container slightly from side to side to allow the water to evenly cover the guacamole so there is no guacamole exposed to air. Don't worry, the guacamole is sturdy enough that it won't get soggy.

Seal on the lid and refrigerate the guacamole for up to 3 days. When ready to eat, remove the lid and gently pour off the water. Stir to incorporate any remaining drops of water and voilà, you have guacamole that is as fresh as the day you made it. In fact, it may taste better, as the flavors will have had a chance to meld.

THE POSSIBILITIES ARE ENDLESS FOR WAYS to enjoy guacamole as a snack. Here are a few of my favorites:

- Hard-cooked egg cut in half, topped with guacamole
- Cucumber or zucchini slices topped with guacamole
- Dip for slices of grilled chicken
- Dip for crudité, crackers, or baked tortilla chips

- Dollop of guacamole atop a cup of cooked beans
- Dollop of guacamole on half of a baked potato
- Dollop of guacamole atop a piece of grilled fish
- Dollop of guacamole spread on a slice of sprouted grain bread, topped with alfalfa sprouts
- Guacamole spread on lettuce leaves, topped with shredded carrots, then rolled up burrito-style

AVOCADO CAPRESE

THIS SNACK IDEA ALSO MAKES A GREAT APPETIZER. THE AVOCADO, SLICED HORIZONTALLY TO MAKE perfect rounds, can replace the fresh mozzarella in this traditional Italian salad, or it can complement the mozzarella for a new depth of flavor. You can cut up just enough ingredients for one or two servings or multiply the recipe to feed a crowd. Any way you slice it, it's a quick and healthy way to satisfy your hunger between meals.

• Makes 2 servings •

1 avocado

2 Roma tomatoes

½ cup fresh mozzarella (can use the small balls or large round)

1 (½-ounce) bunch fresh basil leaves

2 tablespoons extra-virgin olive oil

2 tablespoons balsamic vinegar

Sea salt and freshly ground black pepper

Cut the avocado down the center lengthwise and around the pit, twist open, and remove the pit. Place each half flat-side down on the cutting surface and slice the halves in half again through the peel, so you have four quarters of avocado. Remove the peel off of each quarter. Slice each quarter into ¼-inch-thick slices.

Slice the tomatoes and mozzarella into about ¼-inch-thick rounds.

Alternate layers of tomato, mozzarella, avocado, and basil leaves on a plate. Drizzle with the oil and vinegar, then season with the salt and pepper to taste. Serve immediately.

COLD CHICKEN, ZUCCHINI, AND FETA SLIDERS

THE IDEA OF THIS SNACK IS TO USE LEFTOVER GRILLED OR BAKED CHICKEN BREASTS ALONG WITH two slices of raw zucchini (buns) to make bite-size sliders. The fillings I've offered here are my favorite flavor suggestions; you can use any fillings you like. You can also use other protein options such as chicken salad, tuna or salmon salad, egg salad, or tiny beef or turkey burgers.

• Makes 6 sliders •

3 ounces grilled or baked chicken breast, sliced into 6 pieces cut to fit the diameter of your zucchini slices (each piece should weigh about ½ ounce)

1 medium-size zucchini, cut into 12 (¼-inch-thick) rounds

3 tablespoons pizza sauce, marinara sauce, or Dijon mustard

1 Roma tomato, cut into 6 slices

6 small fresh basil or baby spinach leaves

3 (¼-inch-thick) slices of feta cheese, cut in half to make 6 pieces

Assemble the ingredients into small bite-size "sliders" by placing the chicken pieces on top of half of the zucchini slices. Add ½ tablespoon pizza sauce on top of each chicken piece. Then top each with a tomato slice, basil leaf, and slice of feta cheese. Top with the remaining slices of zucchini and place on a plate. Enjoy immediately.

QUINOA PIZZA BITES

THESE FUN LITTLE FINGER FOODS ARE A NEW WAY TO EAT QUINOA. LOADED WITH ALL THE HEALTH benefits of quinoa and the flavor profile of pizza, these bites are perfect for parties, potlucks, and after-school snacks, and even as an accompaniment to a lunch salad. The next time you cook a pot of quinoa, make extra so that you can quickly whip up a batch of these.

• Makes about 40 bites •

2 cups cooked quinoa

2 large eggs

½ cup minced yellow onion

2 teaspoons minced garlic

1 cup finely grated Parmesan cheese, or ½ cup nutritional yeast

½ cup fresh basil, chopped

1 teaspoon sweet paprika

1 teaspoon crushed dried oregano

½ teaspoon sea salt

1 cup finely chopped or crumbled cooked nitrate-free turkey or chicken Italian sausage (optional)

Warmed pizza sauce, for dipping (I use the Eden Foods organic pizza sauce that comes in a glass jar)

Preheat the oven to 350°F. Coat a baking sheet with coconut oil or line with parchment paper. Alternatively, you can use mini muffin tins; coat the muffin cups with coconut oil.

Mix together all ingredients, except the pizza sauce, in a mixing bowl.

Scoop 1 heaping tablespoon of the mixture and form it into a compact mini patty. Place it on the prepared baking sheet. If using mini muffin tins, you can pack the quinoa mixture into the oil-coated muffin cups.

Bake for 15 to 20 minutes, or until crispy on the outside.

Serve warm with pizza sauce for dipping. Store leftovers in an airtight container in the refrigerator for up to 4 days or freeze for up to 1 month.

CRUNCHY PEPITAS

PUMPKIN SEEDS, ALSO KNOWN AS PEPITAS, BRING SNACKING TO A NEW LEVEL. JUST A HANDFUL OF these crunchy seeds offers numerous health benefits, from providing protection against high blood pressure, heart disease, and cancer to promoting healthy skin and improving brain power.

After soaking and drying, pepitas are crunchy with a flavorful nutty taste all their own. Add sea salt, herbs, or spices and they're transformed into a nutritiously addictive snack; you'll see some variations here. Pepitas can also be added to trail mix, granola, muffins, and cookies and are great sprinkled on salads in place of croutons.

• Makes 2 cups •

2 cups raw pepitas

Pinch of sea salt or Himilayan pink salt

Taco Seasoning Version:

1 tablespoon taco seasoning mix (page 168 or store-bought)

Roasted Tamari Version:

1 tablespoon reduced-sodium gluten-free tamari sauce

Pumpkin Pie Version:

1 tablespoon pumpkin pie spice (page 45 or store-bought)

Soak the pepitas for 6 to 8 hours in water with a pinch of salt. Drain and blot dry using paper towels.

If you just want plain pepitas, spread them out in a single layer on baking sheets.

To make the seasoned varieties, put the pepitas in a bowl and toss with the flavorings listed.

Once the pepitas are ready, you have two options for drying them: dehydrate at very low heat to preserve the enzymes, or bake at a slightly higher temperature to dry and bring out more flavor, but lose the live enzymes.

Option 1: Preserve the enzymes, which help digestion and keep the seeds in a raw state. This is the healthiest way to dry the nuts and of course the healthiest way to eat them. You will need a dehydrator set at 110°F, or you can slightly warm your oven by leaving the oven light on. Dehydrating this way may take anywhere from 8 to 12 hours, sometimes longer. You can tell when the pepitas are dry because they will be nice and crunchy.

Option 2: Lose the enzymes and some of the nutrition but bring out the unique flavor of the roasted seeds, which is amazing. Bake for 2 hours or longer at the lowest temperature your oven will go (mine goes down to 170°F)—and no higher than 250°F, to ensure that you don't destroy the healthy oils in the seeds.

While they are baking, make sure to stir them every 15 to 20 minutes to ensure that they are drying evenly.

Once the pepitas are dry, allow them to cool to room temperature, then transfer to a glass jar with a tight-fitting lid and store in the refrigerator for up to 6 months.

SWEET 'N' SPICY MIXED NUTS

NOT ONLY ARE THEY PACKED WITH PROTEIN, THESE NUTS HAVE A UNIQUE SWEET AND SAVORY flavor and are great for snacking on at any time. Keep some in the car for emergency snack attacks!

• Makes 1 pound •

½ pound raw almonds (preferably soaked and dried)

½ pound raw cashews

2 tablespoons organic butter or virgin coconut oil

2 tablespoons unrefined whole cane sugar or coconut sugar

3 drops liquid stevia extract

¼ teaspoon cayenne pepper

¼ teaspoon sea salt or Himalayan pink salt

Preheat the oven to the lowest temperature (mine goes down to 170°F). In a large bowl, mix together the almonds and cashews.

Melt the butter in a skillet over medium-low heat. Add the sugar and stevia. Stir until the sugar is melted and blended with the butter. Add the cayenne and salt to the butter mixture. Pour the mixture over the nuts and mix well with a spoon, making sure all of the nuts get covered.

Spread the nuts evenly onto a baking sheet and roast for 45 to 60 minutes, or until the nuts are completely dry. Alternatively, place the nut mixture in a dehydrator at 145°F for 4 to 6 hours. Remove from the oven and cool to room temperature before placing in a covered container. Store in the refrigerator for up to 1 month.

CLASSIC KALE CHIPS

KALE CHIPS ARE A FUN AND TASTY WAY TO EAT THIS SUPER GREEN. WHEN BAKED OR DEHYDRATED, kale leaves take on a texture similar to that of potato chips. They've become so popular that commercial varieties are now appearing on grocery store shelves—at a premium price for a small quantity. Making your own large batch is fairly inexpensive and quite easy to do.

This recipe is for a simple version, but feel free to customize the ingredients based on your own favorites. Acceptable oils to use are extra-virgin olive oil, unrefined sesame oil, unrefined peanut oil, and virgin coconut oil. You can season them with sea salt, taco seasoning, chili powder, and other spices. For a cheesy variety, add ½ cup finely grated Parmesan cheese or nutritional yeast. You can even sprinkle on chopped nuts and seeds. The only downside to making these chips is that they'll disappear too quickly—then you have to make more!

• Makes 6 servings •

1 bunch curly kale

3 tablespoons virgin coconut oil

½ teaspoon Herbamare or sea salt

½ teaspoon garlic powder

⅓ teaspoon onion powder

Preheat the oven to 200°F. Line a large baking sheet with parchment paper.

Wash and dry the kale. Trim each kale leaf by cutting along both sides of the supporting rib with a paring knife, cutting the rib free from the leaf. Save the ribs for use in juices, broths, stir-fries, or compost.

Tear the kale leaves into chip-size pieces (they will shrink in size while baking, so don't make them too small) and place them in a large mixing bowl. Drizzle the coconut oil evenly over the kale, then gently massage the oil into the kale with your hands until the leaves are evenly coated. It's important that every piece gets coated in the oil. Sprinkle on the Herbamare, garlic powder, and onion powder and gently toss with your hands. Make sure not to overmix the ingredients, as this will cause your kale to become wilted and soggy.

TO DRY IN THE OVEN:

Evenly spread the kale chips across the prepared baking sheet. Bake until the chips begin to become slightly crispy, about 20 to 25 minutes, then use tongs to flip them over to evenly bake. Bake for another 25 to 30 minutes, or until the chips are dark green and crispy. The total baking time should last 45 to 55 minutes, but watch them closely, as they will overcook or burn quickly. Allow to cool on the baking sheet for 10 minutes, then transfer to a bowl or airtight storage container.

TO DRY IN A DEHYDRATOR:

Place the coated and seasoned kale chips on the dehydrator shelves. Set the temperature to 115°F. The drying time varies with dehydrators, anywhere from 4 to 6 hours. Transfer to a bowl or airtight storage container.

Kale chips will keep for up to 1 week when properly stored in a cool place away from direct sunlight.

ZESTY NACHO KALE KRUNCH

ONCE YOU GET THE FEEL FOR MAKING THE BASIC KALE CHIP RECIPE, YOU CAN EXPAND YOUR chip-making skills. This version involves more prep time (cashews need to be soaked for 1 hour beforehand) and baking time (anywhere from 2 to 3 hours), so it's best to plan ahead. The effort will be worth it, as the tangy cheese flavor of these chips is unbelievable. They're great for snacking but can also be crumbled to make a crunchy salad topping.

• Makes 12 servings •

3 bunches curly kale

2 tablespoons virgin coconut oil

1 cup raw cashews, soaked in water for
   1 hour, drained and rinsed

¼ cup water

1 red bell pepper, chopped

Juice of 1 lemon (about 2 tablespoons)

2 tablespoons nutritional yeast or finely
   grated Parmesan cheese

2 garlic cloves, minced

2 teaspoons chili powder

1 teaspoon onion powder

1 teaspoon ground cumin

½ teaspoon ground turmeric

½ teaspoon smoked paprika

½ teaspoon sea salt

Preheat the oven to 250°F. Line two large baking sheets with parchment paper.

Wash and dry the kale. Trim each kale leaf by cutting along both sides of the supporting rib with a paring knife, cutting the rib free from the leaf. Save the ribs for use in juices, broths, stir-fries, or compost.

Tear the kale leaves into chip-size pieces (they will shrink in size while baking, so don't make them too small) and place them in a large mixing bowl. Drizzle the coconut oil evenly over the kale, then gently massage the oil into the kale with your hands until the leaves are evenly coated. It's important that every piece gets coated in the oil.

To make the cheesy cashew coating, place the remaining ingredients into the bowl of a food processor or high-powered blender and process until very smooth and creamy, about 2 minutes.

Pour the cashew mixture over the kale, then lightly toss the kale with your hands, scrunching each leaf to ensure it gets coated as evenly as possible. Uneven layering of the coating results in a longer baking time.

TO DRY IN THE OVEN:

Evenly spread the coated kale chips across the prepared baking sheets and place them in the oven. Lower the temperature to 200°F and bake for 2 hours, flipping them every 20 to 30 minutes to evenly bake. The timing will vary based on the thickness of the coating layer and the humidity inside the oven.

When the chips are dry and crunchy, remove them from the oven and allow them to cool for at least 30 minutes. Some chips may be done before others. Remove the dry chips and return any damp chips to the oven to continue baking. Keep checking them every 10 minutes to make sure they don't burn.

TO DRY IN A DEHYDRATOR:

Place the coated and seasoned kale chips on the dehydrator shelves. Set the temperature to 115°F degrees. The drying time varies with dehydrators, anywhere from 6 to 8 hours.

When completely cool/dry, transfer to a bowl or airtight storage container. Kale chips will keep for up to 1 week when properly stored in a cool place away from direct sunlight.

SUGAR-FREE DRIED CRANBERRIES

COMMERCIAL DRIED CRANBERRIES ARE MADE WITH UNNECESSARY SUGAR, PRESERVATIVES, AND oils. Making your own dried cranberries is relatively easy, but it does take some drying time in the oven or dehydrator. Add the cranberries to homemade trail mix, sprinkle them over salads, use them in recipes, or eat them plain as a nutritious snack. To keep them from getting moldy, store them in the refrigerator for up to three months or in the freezer for up to six months.

• Makes about 1 cup •

1 cup water

1 (12-ounce) bag whole fresh cranberries

½ teaspoon liquid stevia extract or other natural sweetener equivalent to ½ cup sugar (optional)

2 tablespoons virgin coconut oil, melted

In a medium saucepan, bring the water to a boil, then turn off the heat. Add the cranberries and submerge them in the boiling water. Let the berries sit in the water until the skins pop, about 2 minutes. Do not let the cranberries boil, or they will become too mushy.

Drain the cranberries in a colander, then transfer them to a medium bowl. If using the sweetener, combine it with the melted oil in a small bowl. Add the oil or oil mixture to the cranberries, then toss to coat evenly.

TO DRY IN THE OVEN:

Preheat the oven to the lowest setting. Line a large rimmed baking sheet with parchment paper. Spread the cranberries on the prepared baking sheet and separate each individual cranberry as best you can. Place the baking sheet in the oven and let the cranberries dry, 3 to 6 hours or longer.

TO DRY IN A DEHYDRATOR:

Place the cranberries on a mesh sheet and then put them in your dehydrator until they are dry and chewy, about 16 hours.

Remove, let cool, and transfer to an airtight container. Store in the refrigerator for up to 3 months or in the freezer for up to 6 months.

Sensational Salads and Versatile Veggies

Vegetables add color to your plate and years to your life. And because they are meant to play a starring role on your plate, I've offered you an eclectic array of colorful salads and snazzy veggie recipes that can be served as side dishes or main entrées. In this section, you'll find crisp Moroccan Carrot Salad (page 192) and chewy Maple Mustard Sweet Potato Salad (page 193)—two favorites that are sure to brighten any picnic table or lunchbox. You'll also find plenty of delicious ideas for including more green leafys in your meals, such as my four Creative Kale Salads (page 199) and Thai Coconut Collard Greens (page 206). For some good old comfort food, try Skinny Stir-Fried Veggies (page 204), Roasted Tricolor Taters and Carrots (page 209), and Broccoli in Spicy Orange Sauce (page 210). All of these vegetables make a fabulous accompaniment to any grain, fish, or fowl.

CITRUS AVOCADO SALMON (OR TUNA) CUPS

THIS QUICK AND EASY SALAD MAKES THE PERFECT LUNCH OR SNACK FOOD. IT COMBINES FOUR powerhouse liver-izing foods—avocado, lemon juice, parsley, and omega-3–packed fish—to make a satisfying meal that can be enjoyed often. Pair these yummy cups with some fresh greens or a cup of warm Smoky Tomato Soup (page 216).

• Makes 2 servings •

1 large avocado

1 tablespoon freshly squeezed lemon juice

1 tablespoon chopped fresh curly parsley

5 to 6 ounces cooked or canned wild-caught salmon (or tuna)

Pinch of Herbamare or sea salt, or more to taste

Cut the avocado in half, remove the pit, and scoop the middle part of the flesh of each half of the avocado into a bowl, leaving a ¼-inch shell of avocado flesh in each half.

Add the lemon juice and parsley to the avocado in the bowl and mash everything together with a fork. Add the salmon, sprinkle with Herbamare, then stir to combine. Fill each avocado half with the salad and serve.

MOROCCAN CARROT SALAD

MOROCCAN CARROT SALADS TYPICALLY CALL FOR COOKED CARROTS, BUT I'VE OPTED FOR RAW instead. This is a wonderful alternative when you want a cool crispy salad but are not in the mood for leafy greens. The combination of cinnamon, cumin, and paprika bring out the sweet taste of the carrots, offering up a flavor that is simply stunning.

• Makes 2 servings •

- ½ pound carrots, grated (a food processor helps!)
- 2 tablespoons extra-virgin olive oil
- Juice of ½ small lemon, or more to taste
- 2 tablespoons chopped fresh cilantro or curly parsley
- 1 to 2 garlic cloves, crushed
- ¼ teaspoon ground cumin
- ½ teaspoon Spanish paprika
- ⅛ teaspoon ground cinnamon
- ½ teaspoon sea salt
- ¼ teaspoon cayenne pepper (optional)

Mix all ingredients in a large bowl. Cover and let marinate in the refrigerator for 2 hours or overnight. The salad keeps for up to 3 days in the refrigerator.

MAPLE MUSTARD SWEET POTATO SALAD

WITH ITS USE OF SWEET POTATOES AND HEALTHY OILS INSTEAD OF MAYO, THIS IS A NUTRITIOUS twist on the classic potato salad. To up the health factor, serve it over a bed of fresh organic spring mix and sprinkle with pine nuts and goat cheese or feta.

• Makes 6 servings •

- 3 pounds sweet potatoes, peeled and cut into 2-inch pieces
- 2 tablespoons virgin coconut oil, melted, plus more for the pan
- Pinch of sea salt
- ¼ cup extra-virgin olive oil
- 1 tablespoon raw organic unfiltered apple cider vinegar
- 2 tablespoons pure maple syrup
- 1 tablespoon Dijon mustard
- ⅓ cup chopped fresh curly parsley

Preheat the oven to 375°F. Coat a large baking sheet with coconut oil or line with parchment paper.
Place the sweet potatoes in a large bowl. Add the coconut oil and toss to coat.

Arrange the potatoes on the prepared baking sheet, then sprinkle with the salt. Roast the potatoes just until tender, about 20 to 25 minutes. Remove from the oven and let cool on the baking sheet.

Meanwhile, make the dressing. In a small bowl, whisk together the olive oil, vinegar, syrup, and Dijon. Set aside.

Transfer the cooled potatoes to a serving bowl. Add the chopped parsley and toss to mix. Whisk the dressing and drizzle it over the potato mixture to lightly coat, then toss gently so the potatoes don't get mashed. Serve at room temperature or chilled. Store leftovers in an airtight container in the refrigerator for up to 5 days.

AVOCADO AND BEETS WITH BALSAMIC ORANGE DRESSING

THIS DISH MAY IMPROVE YOUR MOOD, AS BEETS CONTAIN BETAINE, A COMPOUND KNOWN AS A "mood enhancer" because it enhances the brain's ability to maintain sufficient levels of the "feel good" hormones serotonin and dopamine. Beets also contain tryptophan, a compound that relaxes the mind and creates a sense of well-being, similar to chocolate.

• Makes 4 servings •

1 pound red beets (about 3 to 4 small), unpeeled

2 teaspoons balsamic vinegar (see sidebar on page 195)

Juice and zest from 1 navel orange (about 1 tablespoon zest and 2 tablespoons juice), divided

2 tablespoons extra-virgin olive oil

Sea salt and freshly ground black pepper

2 avocados

Wash the beets under cool running water, taking care not to tear the skin of the beet—this tough outer layer helps keep most of the beet's pigment inside the vegetable.

Fill the bottom of a steamer with 2 inches of water. Cut the beets into quarters, but do not peel them. When the water is steaming, place the beets in the steamer basket, cover, and steam for 15 minutes. The beets are done cooking when you can easily insert a fork or the tip of a knife into a beet. You can save the collected beet juice for adding to smoothies or just drinking as is.

Set the beets in a bowl and let sit until they are cool enough to handle. Remove the skins using a paper towel or just leave the skins on, as they are quite edible.

Cut the beet quarters into 1-inch chunks and place in a bowl. In a separate small bowl, whisk the vinegar, orange juice, and olive oil. Season with salt and pepper. Drizzle over the beets and toss. Peel and cut the avocado into chunks and layer on top of the beets. Do not toss again, as the beets will stain the avocados and the salad won't look as nice. Top with the orange zest and serve.

KNOW YOUR BALSAMIC VINEGAR

THERE ARE DIFFERENT TYPES OF BALSAMIC vinegar on grocery store shelves, so it's important to know which ones are "true" balsamic vinegar, and which ones are nothing more than a bottle of sugar. Hint: You get what you pay for, and less is more.

True balsamic vinegar, or *aceto balsamico tradizionale* as it is called in Italian, has nothing added to it—it is a reduction made purely from sweet white *trebbiano* grapes, but it is not considered a wine vinegar because the grape juice used is not fermented. The unfermented grape juice used to make balsamic is called "must" (concentrated juice).

The best balsamic vinegar comes from Modena, a city in central Italy. This true form of balsamic vinegar is aged for several years (most for 3 to 12 years, although some may be aged up to a hundred years) in a successive series of wood barrels. The result is a dark, slightly sweet, complex liquid that is quite costly due to the lengthy time needed to produce it. True *aceto* balsamic vinegar must be aged a minimum of 10 years; the better balsamic vinegars are aged 25 to 50 years. This is why "true" balsamic vinegar is very expensive—anywhere from $20 to $500 for a small bottle.

The cheap bottles of balsamic vinegar sold in the average grocery store are only aged for a few months in stainless-steel tanks, rather than wood barrels. This inexpensive form of "balsamic" is merely wine vinegar that has had brown sugar or caramelized sugar added to mimic the taste of true, aged balsamic. This is the type of balsamic used most often by cooks to make a syrupy, sweet reduction.

When shopping for balsamic, read the ingredient list to see if sugar has been added and check the label for the words *cooked grape must* or *tradizionale*, as well as the length of time the vinegar has aged.[1]

EVERYDAY RAINBOW SALAD

I EAT A VERSION OF THIS SALAD NEARLY EVERY DAY. THE VEGETABLES CAN VARY DEPENDING ON season and availability, but the goal is to make it as colorful and balanced as possible. In the note section below, I've offered some examples of possible color combinations to choose from. When the weather is hot, raw veggies make the salad light and refreshing; during the cooler months, you may want to top your raw leafy greens with some warm roasted vegetables that will make the salad more comforting and palatable.

• Makes 2 servings •

4 cups chopped raw leafy greens (lettuces, spring mix, spinach, etc.)

2 cups mixed chopped assorted colorful raw veggies (celery, cucumber, bell pepper, radish, carrot, beets, red cabbage, cauliflower, etc.)

½ cup cooked beans or lentils, or 3 ounces cooked poultry or fish

½ cup cooked whole grain (brown rice, quinoa, millet, etc.)

¼ avocado, peeled and cubed

Sprinkle of nuts or seeds of your choice (about ¼ ounce)

¼ cup salad dressing of your choice

Place the greens on the bottom of a large bowl. Top with the remaining ingredients in the order listed, toss, and enjoy!

Note:

Here are some examples of possible color combinations for your everyday salad. Select one or more items from each color category and try to rotate different items to maximize variety and nutrients. For example, if you buy a bag of carrots and use them in your salads one week, go for orange bell peppers or squash the next week.

Green: *arugula, asparagus, avocado, basil, broccoli, Brussels sprouts, cabbage, celery, chard, cilantro, cucumber, green beans, green bell peppers, green onion, kale, lettuces, mint, mustard greens, parsley, sugar snap peas, spinach, spring mix, zucchini*

Yellow/Orange: *carrot, golden beet, orange squashes (acorn, butternut, pumpkin, kabocha, etc.), rutabaga, sweet corn, sweet potato, yellow or orange bell pepper, yellow squash, yellow tomato*

Red: *radish, red beet, red bell pepper, rhubarb, tomato*

Purple/Blue: *eggplant, purple cabbage, purple potato, red onion*

White: *cauliflower, garlic, ginger, jicama, mushrooms, onions, parsnips, potatoes, turnips*

Brown: *beans, cooked whole grains, lentils, nuts, seeds*

MEXICAN CAESAR SALAD WITH CILANTRO PEPITA DRESSING

TRADITIONAL CAESAR SALADS CONSIST OF MAINLY ROMAINE, CHEESE, CROUTONS, AND DRESSING. This southwestern version adds more veggies and replaces the croutons with pepitas. The cheese is in the flavorful dressing!

• Makes 2 servings of salad, 1 cup of dressing •

SALAD

4 cups chopped romaine lettuce

10 Roma tomatoes, cut in half

2 carrots, diced or shredded

¼ small red onion, thinly sliced

1 cup thinly sliced purple cabbage

1 avocado, pitted, peeled, and sliced

2 tablespoons pepitas (see page 185)

DRESSING

½ cup coconut milk

¼ cup water

1 teaspoon freshly squeezed lime juice

¼ cup Parmesan cheese

1 garlic clove

¼ cup pepitas (see page 185)

¼ cup chopped fresh cilantro leaves

½ teaspoon raw organic unfiltered apple cider vinegar

1 tablespoon extra-virgin olive oil

⅛ teaspoon sea salt

To make the salad, toss all ingredients except the avocado and pepitas in a bowl. Divide the salad between 2 serving plates, then top each with half of the sliced avocado and 1 tablespoon pepitas.

To make the dressing, place all ingredients in a blender and run until well blended. If the dressing is too thick, thin it out with a small amount of water until the desired consistency is reached. Drizzle on top of the salad. Store the remainder of the dressing in the refrigerator for up to 3 days.

DANDELION GREENS SALAD WITH SWEET CITRUS DRESSING

O N THEIR OWN, DANDELION GREENS ARE QUITE BITTER, SO ADDING A BIT OF SWEET CITRUS TO the dressing and letting the greens sit for a bit removes some of their bite. Dandelion greens contain nearly all the vitamins (except vitamin D) and are a rich source of protein, calcium, iron, antioxidants, and other minerals that not only heal and cleanse the liver but also fight against cancer and reduce inflammation. This is more than just a salad—it's life-force energy in a bowl!

• Makes 4 servings •

Zest and juice of 1 lime

Zest and juice of 1 orange plus 2 large oranges, divided

2 teaspoons raw honey or coconut nectar

1 teaspoon sea salt

3 tablespoons extra-virgin olive oil

1 bunch dandelion greens, stems trimmed, chopped into bite-size pieces

¼ cup packed fresh mint leaves

2 radishes, finely chopped

¼ cup raw walnut halves

Zest the lime and one of the oranges into a large salad bowl. Cut the lime and the orange in half and squeeze the juice into the bowl. Add the honey, salt, and olive oil and whisk together.

Add the dandelion greens to the bowl with the dressing. Toss and let sit for 10 minutes.

Peel the remaining 2 oranges and separate the segments. Top the greens with the orange segments, mint leaves, radishes, and walnuts and toss. Transfer to plates and serve immediately.

RAISIN, PINE NUT, AND GOAT CHEESE KALE SALAD

ACINATO KALE ALSO GOES BY THE NAME DINOSAUR, *CAVOLO NERO*, TUSCAN, OR BLACK KALE. THIS type of kale has long, spear-shaped blue-green leaves with a pebbled, or scaly, appearance that resembles dinosaur skin. The raisins in this salad add a nice touch of sweetness to complement the kale's deep earthy and nutty flavor.

• Makes 2 to 3 servings for large lunch or dinner salads,
or 4 servings for small side salads •

1 bunch Lacinato kale, stems and ribs removed,
leaves chopped into small pieces

¼ cup extra-virgin olive oil

2 tablespoons freshly squeezed lemon juice
(about the juice of 1 lemon)

2 garlic cloves, pressed

¼ teaspoon sea salt

¼ cup raisins

¼ cup crumbled goat cheese

20 raw pine nuts (about 2 grams)

Place the chopped kale in a large serving bowl. In a small bowl, whisk together the olive oil, lemon juice, pressed garlic, and salt. Pour over the kale and use your hands to massage the dressing into the kale for 2 to 5 minutes. Make sure all of the kale is evenly coated with the dressing. Add the raisins and goat cheese and toss well. The salad may be served immediately or stored in the refrigerator for up to 3 days before serving. To keep the pine nuts from getting soggy, wait to sprinkle them over the top of the salad just before serving.

VARIATIONS

- Swap sugar-free dried cranberries (page 189) for the raisins.
- Change out the pine nuts for any other favorite raw nut.
- Replace the goat cheese with feta, Parmesan, or another favorite cheese.
- Add sliced hard-cooked egg, cooked chicken, chickpeas, or whole grains such as brown rice or quinoa to balance the salad into a complete meal.

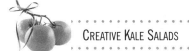
KALE IS KNOWN AS THE "QUEEN OF Greens," owing to its extremely high levels of beta-carotene, vitamin C, vitamin K, and the all-important alkalizing mineral calcium. It also packs a number of phytonutrients, including sulforaphane, a compound whose potent anticancer properties are particularly enhanced when the vegetable is chopped or minced.

Despite its many health virtues, raw kale can be a tough sell for those who are new to incorporating the dark green leaves into their meals. Unlike the soft, easy-to-chew texture of raw spinach or arugula, raw kale can be hard to chew, unless you know the secret to making it soft and loveable—*massage*. Massaging raw kale with healthy oil, sea salt, and lemon juice transforms the taste and chewability of its leaves. The citric acid from the lemon juice combined with the salt and oil helps to break down the cell walls in the kale, which softens its leaves and changes its taste from bitter to sweet. Massaging kale gives it the "wilted" appearance of being lightly cooked, yet it still retains a crunchy texture.

To make a basic massaged kale salad, start with one bunch of washed kale. Trim each kale leaf by cutting along both sides of the supporting rib with a paring knife, cutting the rib free from the leaf. Save the ribs for use in juices, broths, stir-fries, or compost. Tear or chop the leaves into small bite-size pieces. The smaller the better, to make massaging and chewing easier.

Add 2 tablespoons healthy unrefined oil (such as extra-virgin olive oil) or half of an avocado, 1 tablespoon freshly squeezed lemon juice, and ¼ teaspoon of sea salt or Himalayan pink salt. Using both hands, "massage" the oil, lemon juice, and salt into the kale, squeezing it as you go along, until the kale begins to "wilt" and get soft, about two to five minutes. The longer you massage, the softer and sweeter the kale becomes. Add other dressings or salad toppings as desired.

Unlike other salads that wilt several hours after being tossed in dressing, massaged kale's sturdy leaves hold up for several days in the refrigerator without losing their crunchy texture.

ZESTY SOUTHWESTERN KALE SALAD

AVOCADO, LIME JUICE, CILANTRO, AND MEXICAN SEASONINGS GIVE THIS SALAD A ZESTY southwestern kick. If you don't have any Mexican seasoning on hand, you can use a 1:1 ratio of cumin and chili powder in its place. Queso fresco, a traditional Latin American cheese, is a soft, crumbly, and mild-tasting white cheese commonly used in Mexican recipes. It's delicious in tacos and enchiladas, it complements black beans beautifully, and it's a wonderful addition to salads.

• Makes 2 to 3 servings for large lunch or dinner salads,
or 4 servings for small side salads •

1 bunch Lacinato kale, stems and ribs removed, leaves chopped into small pieces

2 tablespoons freshly squeezed lime juice

2 teaspoons taco seasoning mix (page 168) or Spice Hunter Mexican Seasoning (see Resources, page 281)

¼ teaspoon sea salt

1 large avocado, pitted and peeled

1 cup cooked black beans

1 medium tomato, diced

½ yellow or red bell pepper, diced

¼ cup chopped red onion

½ cup chopped fresh cilantro

½ cup seeded and chopped roasted Hatch green chiles (page 75), or ½ cup of your favorite salsa

¼ cup crumbled queso fresco or other favorite cheese (optional)

2 tablespoons Crunchy Pepitas (page 185)

Place the chopped kale in a large serving bowl and drizzle the lime juice over it. Sprinkle with taco seasoning and salt, then add the avocado. Massage the kale with your hands while mashing the avocado for 2 to 5 minutes, making sure to mix all ingredients evenly. Add the beans, tomato, bell pepper, onion, cilantro, green chiles, and cheese, if using. Toss to combine. Sprinkle with the pepitas just before serving.

SESAME ASIAN KALE SALAD

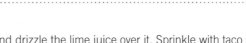

TOASTED SESAME OIL AND SESAME SEEDS INFUSE THE KALE WITH A FLAVORFUL ASIAN FLAIR. TRY adding the toasted nori sheet for added flavor, vitamins, minerals, iodine, and protein.

• Makes 2 to 3 servings for large lunch or dinner salads,
or 4 servings for small side salads •

- 1 bunch curly kale, stems and ribs removed, leaves chopped into small pieces
- 1 tablespoon freshly squeezed lime juice
- 1 tablespoon unrefined toasted sesame oil
- 2 teaspoons reduced-sodium gluten-free tamari sauce
- ¼ teaspoon ground ginger
- 1 avocado, divided
- 2 medium carrots, shredded or finely chopped
- 2 radishes, thinly sliced
- ½ red, yellow, or orange bell pepper, thinly sliced
- 2 green onions, chopped (green part only)
- 1 sheet toasted nori seaweed, crumbled (optional)
- 2 teaspoons toasted sesame seeds

Place the chopped kale in a large serving bowl and drizzle the lime juice, sesame oil, and tamari over it. Sprinkle with the ground ginger. Cut the avocado in half; add one half to the salad bowl to use for massaging the salad, then dice the other half and set aside.

Massage the kale with your hands while mashing the avocado for 2 to 5 minutes, making sure to mix all ingredients evenly. Add the carrot, radish, bell pepper, green onion, and nori, if using, and toss. Just before serving, top the salad with the diced avocado and sesame seeds.

GREEK-STYLE KALE SALAD

THE ROMAINE LETTUCE IS REPLACED BY KALE IN THIS MEDITERRANEAN FAVORITE.

• Makes 2 to 3 servings for large lunch or dinner salads,
or 4 servings for small side salads •

- 1 bunch Lacinato kale, stems and ribs removed, leaves chopped into small pieces
- ¼ cup extra-virgin olive oil
- 2 tablespoons freshly squeezed lemon juice (about the juice of 1 lemon)
- 2 garlic cloves, pressed
- 2 tablespoons red wine vinegar
- ¼ teaspoon liquid stevia extract, or 1 tablespoon raw honey
- ¼ teaspoon sea salt
- 1 medium cucumber, sliced
- 2 Roma tomatoes, quartered lengthwise
- 16 Kalamata olives, pitted and cut in half lengthwise
- ¼ small red onion, sliced into very thin strips
- 1 cup coarsely chopped fresh curly parsley leaves
- ½ cup (2 ounces) crumbled feta cheese
- 20 raw pine nuts (about 2 grams; optional)

Place the chopped kale in a large serving bowl. In a small bowl, whisk together the olive oil, lemon juice, garlic, vinegar, stevia, and salt. Pour over the kale and use your hands to massage the dressing into the kale for 2 to 5 minutes. Make sure all of the kale is evenly coated with the dressing. Add the cucumber, tomatoes, olives, onion, parsley, and feta and toss well. If using, sprinkle the pine nuts over the top of the salad just before serving.

GINGER ASIAN SLAW

THIS COLORFUL CABBAGE SALAD IS CHOCK-FULL OF NUTRIENTS, INCLUDING VITAMIN C, AND INDOLES, powerful cancer-fighting and liver-cleansing compounds. When cabbage is sliced or chopped, additional anticancer compounds called glucosinolates are formed and activated, making all types of cabbage true superfoods. Red cabbage also contains anthocyanins, the same purple pigment that gives blueberries their strong antioxidant properties. Toss in a few more veggies and a tasty toasted sesame dressing, and you have a winning salad that can be enjoyed alongside your favorite fish, meat, or vegetarian entrée. This slaw goes great with Apricot Sweet and Sour Meatballs (page 233).

• Makes 6 servings •

DRESSING

1 garlic clove, minced

1 teaspoon grated fresh ginger

1 tablespoon reduced-sodium gluten-free tamari sauce or soy sauce

1 tablespoon brown rice vinegar

1 tablespoon raw honey

1 tablespoon unrefined toasted sesame oil

Juice of 1 lime

Pinch of cayenne pepper

¼ cup unrefined peanut oil or extra-virgin olive oil

Pinch of sea salt and freshly ground pepper (optional)

SLAW

3 cups thinly sliced napa cabbage

2 cups thinly sliced purple cabbage

1 cup shredded carrot

1 red bell pepper, diced

1 cup chopped sugar snap peas

3 green onions, chopped (white and green parts)

½ cup chopped fresh cilantro leaves

¼ cup chopped fresh mint leaves

½ cup raw slivered almonds

1 tablespoon toasted sesame seeds

Prepare the dressing by combining all ingredients except the peanut oil and salt/pepper in a medium bowl. While whisking everything together, slowly stream in the peanut oil. Taste and add salt and pepper, if needed. Set aside.

In a large bowl, combine the cabbages, carrot, bell pepper, snap peas, green onions, cilantro, and mint. Add the dressing and toss to coat the vegetables in the dressing. Sprinkle with the almonds and sesame seeds. Serve immediately or chill up to a day ahead of time. This slaw keeps in the refrigerator for up to 3 days.

SKINNY STIR-FRIED VEGGIES

THIS STIR-FRY GETS ITS DEPTH OF FLAVORS FROM JUST A FEW SIMPLE INGREDIENTS—FRESH GINGER, garlic, tamari sauce, and toasted sesame oil. Because the cooking process is fast, it's a good idea to have all the ingredients chopped, measured, and ready to go before you start cooking. The veggies in this stir-fry are my faves, but they can be adapted to just about any vegetable you have in your fridge.

• Makes 4 servings •

1 tablespoon reduced-sodium soy sauce or gluten-free tamari sauce

1 tablespoon unrefined toasted sesame oil

2 teaspoons arrowroot

½ cup water (can also use vegetable or chicken broth)

2 tablespoons virgin coconut oil

2 cups fresh broccoli florets

2 large carrots, sliced into thin coins

1 small red onion, quartered and thinly sliced

8 asparagus spears, ends trimmed, cut on the diagonal into 2-inch-long pieces

1 red bell pepper, cut into 1-inch chunks

1 tablespoon grated fresh ginger

4 garlic cloves, minced

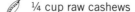 ¼ cup raw cashews

Whisk together the soy sauce, sesame oil, arrowroot, and water in a small bowl. Set aside.

Heat the coconut oil in a large, dry skillet or wok over medium-high heat. When it is hot, add the broccoli and carrots. Stir-fry for about 3 minutes, then add the onion, asparagus, bell pepper, ginger, and garlic and stir-fry for another 2 to 3 minutes.

Reduce the heat to medium low, then add the cashews and soy sauce mixture. Cook, stirring, for 2 minutes, or until the sauce has thickened. Serve immediately.

BASIC BRAISED GREENS

Braising is a simple, quick, and delicious way to prepare any variety of greens. Some of my favorites are beet greens, kale, mustard greens, napa cabbage, and spinach. Braising is a cooking technique that means foods are cooked in both fat and liquid. Many traditional braising recipes call for bacon fat, which gives great flavor, but I've found that coconut oil, garlic, and a little smoked paprika do the same trick. Other healthy fats that can be used are butter, duck fat, and sesame oil, which all lend their own unique flavors. For the liquid, water is the simplest. Richer flavors can be infused by using your favorite broth, lemon juice, apple cider, cooking wine, or coconut milk.

For every bunch of greens (about ½ pound), you can use 2 tablespoons fat and ¼ cup liquid in a large skillet, give or take a little depending on the tenderness or toughness of the greens. Simply heat the fat in the skillet over medium heat, add the chopped greens, drizzle the liquid over them, and stir. If all of the liquid evaporates before the greens are fully cooked, add a little bit more. Tender greens like spinach will cook very quickly, in about two minutes, whereas tougher greens like kale or cabbage can take anywhere from ten to fifteen minutes. Most greens take about five to seven minutes and should still be bright green when they are served. Overcooking greens turns their color dark and their texture mushy, so watch the greens closely while braising—it may take less time than you think!

• Makes 2 servings •

---

2 tablespoons virgin coconut oil
½ pound greens of your choice (kale, beet
    greens, mustard greens, etc.)

2 garlic cloves, minced
½ teaspoon smoked paprika
¼ cup water or broth

Heat the oil in a large skillet over medium-high heat. Add the greens and garlic, stirring to coat with oil. Sprinkle the paprika over the greens and drizzle in the water. Stir until the greens are tender but still bright green. Serve immediately.

THAI COCONUT COLLARD GREENS

I N THIS RECIPE, I'VE ENHANCED THE SIMPLE BRAISE OF THE GREENS BY USING COCONUT MILK AND the signature spices of Thai food. The result is a slightly sweet, creamy vegetable dish that pairs well with grains, beans, fish, or poultry.

• Makes 2 servings •

2 tablespoons virgin coconut oil

½ cup diced red onion

½ red bell pepper, diced

1 large bunch collard greens, leaves sliced evenly into ½-inch strips, stems cut into ¼-inch pieces

2 teaspoons Thai spice mix (store-bought or recipe follows; combine all spices in a small bowl)

2 garlic cloves, minced

1 tablespoon minced fresh ginger

¾ cup coconut milk

2 tablespoons chopped fresh basil

THAI SPICE MIX

¼ teaspoon sea salt

¼ teaspoon ground coriander

¼ teaspoon ground cumin

¼ teaspoon ground cloves

¼ teaspoon ground cinnamon

¼ teaspoon ground cardamom

¼ teaspoon freshly ground black pepper

⅛ teaspoon chili powder

⅛ teaspoon ground turmeric

Heat the oil in a large skillet over medium-high heat. Add the onion, bell pepper, collard stems, and Thai spice and sauté until the onions are soft and translucent, about 3 minutes. Add the garlic, ginger, and sliced collard leaves and stir well to coat everything in the oil. Add the coconut milk and basil, stir, cover, and cook for 10 to 15 minutes, or until the greens are very tender. Serve immediately.

> **NOTE:**
>
> *As with all greens, it is important not to overcook collard greens. When overcooked, collard greens will give off the familiar but unpleasant smell of sulfur associated with overcooking other cruciferous vegetables such as broccoli and Brussels sprouts. To help collard greens cook more quickly, make sure the leaves are sliced evenly into ½-inch slices and the stems cut into ¼-inch pieces. Let them sit on the cutting board for at least 5 minutes before cooking to bring out their health-promoting qualities.*

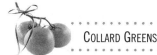

COLLARD GREENS

MOST OFTEN THOUGHT OF AS A SALTY dish of the American South, collard greens are gaining new respect as a superfood. Part of the cabbage family, or cruciferous vegetables, they're loaded with disease-fighting beta-carotene, vitamin C, calcium, and fiber. Steaming or braising collards increases their cholesterol-lowering properties, and they outshine other cruciferous vegetables like broccoli, Brussels sprouts, cabbage, and kale in this regard.

Collard greens are a superb weight loss food, as they are an excellent liver-izing vegetable. They contain compounds that uniquely support the liver's ability to break down fat and toxins, and they play a dual role in stopping the formation of cancer cells. You'll want to include collard greens in your meals on a regular basis if you want to receive these fantastic health benefits. Finding new and delicious ways to enjoy this powerful vegetable, such as Thai Coconut Collard Greens, is a great way to start!

PIÑON-TOPPED LEMONY KALE

THIS RECIPE IS A ZESTY VERSION OF BRAISED KALE. THE ADDITION OF LEMON JUICE, LEMON ZEST, and piñons (pine nuts) brightens up the flavor and superstardom of kale. Pine nuts are a rich source of pinolenic acid, a unique fatty acid that triggers the body to release hormones that suppress appetite, making them an excellent weight loss aid. The peel of a lemon contains five to ten times more vitamins and health benefits than its juice. This recipe is a perfect pairing for Coconut Oil Garlic-Roasted Chicken (page 234), Chickpea Garden Patties (page 243), and any grilled fish.

• Makes 2 servings •

---

2 tablespoons organic butter or virgin coconut oil

1 small red onion, chopped

2 garlic cloves, minced

1 pound Lacinato kale, stems and ribs removed, leaves coarsely chopped

Zest and juice of 1 lemon

1 tablespoon raw pine nuts

Heat the butter in a large skillet over medium heat. Add the onion and sauté for 3 to 4 minutes, or until soft and translucent. Add the garlic and kale, lemon zest and lemon juice, and cook, stirring often, about 10 minutes, or until the kale is tender and wilted, adding small amounts of water to the pan, if needed. Remove from the heat, sprinkle with pine nuts, and serve.

CARROT, BRUSSELS SPROUT, AND PURPLE CABBAGE SAUTÉ

THE SWEETNESS OF THE CARROTS BALANCES THE EARTHY TONES OF THE CRUCIFEROUS VEGETABLES in this buttery sauté. Pile these veggies on a bed of cooked grains or add some chicken or beef to the sauté for a simple weeknight meal.

• Makes 4 servings •

3 tablespoons organic butter, divided

1 large shallot, chopped

1 pound carrots, cut on the diagonal into ½-inch-thick pieces

1 pound Brussels sprouts, halved lengthwise

3 garlic cloves, minced

½ teaspoon sea salt

¼ teaspoon freshly ground black pepper

⅓ cup water or vegetable or chicken broth (pages 59 or 56, or store-bought)

½ pound purple cabbage, cored and thinly sliced

1½ tablespoons raw organic unfiltered apple cider vinegar

Heat 2 tablespoons of the butter in a large skillet over medium heat, stirring occasionally, until softened, 1 to 2 minutes. Add the shallot, carrots, Brussels sprouts, garlic, salt, and pepper and cook, stirring occasionally, until the vegetables begin to brown, 3 to 4 minutes.

Increase the heat to medium high, add the water and purple cabbage, cover, and cook until the vegetables are tender, 5 to 8 minutes. Stir in the vinegar and the remaining tablespoon of butter. Remove from the heat and serve.

PURPLE POTATOES PREVENT CANCER AND HELP LOWER BLOOD PRESSURE

PURPLE POTATOES ARE NEARLY IDENTICAL to russet potatoes when it comes to calories, carbs, fiber, and protein per serving. But they are significantly different when it comes to antioxidant content; purple potatoes contain four times as much antioxidants as russets.

Like all purple/blue plant foods, purple potatoes contain a class of phytonutrients called anthocyanins, which give them their distinctive color and their health-protective properties. The anthocyanins in purple potatoes are a type called flavonoids— substances with powerful anti-aging, anti-cancer, and heart-protective effects. Flavonoids also stimulate the immune system and protect against age-related memory loss.

A study conducted by Joe Vinson, a chemistry professor at the University of Scranton in Pennsylvania, among overweight participants suffering from hypertension reported that consuming six to eight small purple potatoes, with skins (baked, not fried), at both lunch and dinner for one month reduced blood pressure by an average of 4 percent. None of the subjects gained weight.[2]

While these studies didn't exist 7,000 years ago, the ancients must have known there was more to this vegetable than its striking hue. In fact, purple spuds, considered a sacred food, were reserved for Incan kings in their native Peru.

ROASTED TRICOLOR TATERS AND CARROTS

THREE COLORS OF POTATOES, ROASTED AND SEASONED, BRING A LOT OF VISUAL IMPACT TO THIS healthy side dish (see note on page 208 on purple potatoes). They're a great addition to just about any meal. Eat them with eggs for breakfast, toss them into your salad at lunch, or serve them with a turkey burger for dinner.

• Makes 4 servings •

½ pound Yukon gold potatoes

½ pound red-skinned new potatoes

½ pound purple-skinned potatoes

3 large carrots

2 tablespoons virgin coconut oil, melted

1 tablespoon dried basil or Herbes de Provence

Sea salt

Preheat the oven to 375°F. Wash the potatoes and carrots and pat dry to remove excess moisture. Line a large baking sheet with parchment paper.

Quarter the potatoes and place them in a large bowl. Cut the carrots in half lengthwise down the center, then slice each of the carrot halves diagonally in 1½-inch-thick slices and add them to the bowl with the potatoes. Drizzle the coconut oil into the bowl, then sprinkle with the herbs and season with salt. Toss to coat the potatoes and carrots evenly.

Spread the vegetables onto the prepared baking sheet in one layer. Roast in the oven for 30 minutes, or until tender. Remove from the oven and serve. Store leftovers in an airtight container in the refrigerator for up to 4 days or freeze for up to 3 months.

BROCCOLI IN SPICY ORANGE SAUCE

I T'S MORE FUN TO EAT BROCCOLI WHEN IT'S ALL DRESSED UP IN A FRAGRANT CITRUS SAUCE. ENJOY this veggie dish with just about anything—it even pairs well with scrambled eggs for breakfast. Make a big batch and freeze it for meals throughout the month.

• Makes 6 servings •

1 tablespoon arrowroot

3 tablespoons water

Zest and juice of 1 large orange (about ⅓ cup juice)

3 tablespoons reduced-sodium soy sauce or gluten-free tamari sauce

2 tablespoons virgin coconut oil

2 garlic cloves, minced

2 pounds broccoli, florets and stems (trim florets into 1½-inch-long pieces; cut stems crosswise into ⅓-inch-thick pieces)

12 green onions, chopped (white and green parts)

½ teaspoon ground ginger

¼ teaspoon red pepper flakes

2 tablespoons unrefined toasted sesame oil

In a small bowl, mix the arrowroot with the water until dissolved. Add the orange zest, orange juice, and soy sauce. Stir and set aside.

Heat the coconut oil over medium heat in a large skillet or wok. Sauté the garlic for 30 seconds. Add the broccoli, green onions, ginger, pepper flakes, and sesame oil. Stir-fry for 2 minutes, or until the broccoli is slightly tender. Add the orange juice mixture and stir for 2 more minutes, or until the sauce is thickened. Serve immediately.

MAPLE-ROASTED BRUSSELS SPROUTS WITH PECANS

FORGET ANY PRECONCEIVED NOTION YOU MAY HAVE HAD ABOUT THESE BITTER, SMALL, LEAFY GREEN buds. The roasted, partially caramelized vegetables are just slightly sweet, thanks to the coconut oil, maple syrup, and pecans.

• Makes 6 servings •

1½ pounds Brussels sprouts

¼ cup virgin coconut oil

2 tablespoons pure maple syrup

Sea salt and freshly ground black pepper

½ cup raw pecans, coarsely chopped

Preheat the oven to 375°F.

Remove any yellow or brown outer leaves from the Brussels sprouts, cut off the stems, and quarter.

In a large bowl, toss the Brussels sprouts with the coconut oil and maple syrup and season with salt and pepper. Spread the sprouts on a large baking sheet. Roast for 15 minutes, then stir the sprouts with a spatula to even out the browning. Roast for 15 minutes more, or until fork-tender, then remove from the oven. Sprinkle with chopped pecans and serve. Store leftovers in an airtight container for up to 2 days or freeze for up to 1 month.

JUST VEGGIE CREOLE

THIS DISH IS A VEGGIE VERSION OF A CLASSIC CAJUN SEAFOOD RECIPE. IN ADDITION TO THE CAJUN holy trinity (onions, bell peppers, and celery), I've included a few more star players—carrots, parsnips, green beans, and okra. These are my favorites, but feel free to substitute any vegetables you have on hand. This hearty dish can be served as a side vegetable to chicken or fish, or it can be a meal in itself when served over cooked brown rice, quinoa, or millet. Leftovers taste even better the next day, after all of the vegetables and spices have released their flavors.

• Makes 6 servings •

2 tablespoons virgin coconut oil

1 medium yellow or white onion, finely chopped

1 large red or green bell pepper (or half of each), chopped

2 celery stalks with leaves, chopped

2 large carrots, sliced

4 garlic cloves, minced

1 (14½-ounce) can diced tomatoes, with juice

1 (15-ounce) can tomato sauce

2 cups water

1 cup fresh or frozen green beans

1 parsnip, diced

16 ounces fresh or frozen okra (thaw if using frozen), cut into ½-inch chunks (2 cups)

1 lemon wedge

2 teaspoons chili powder

½ teaspoon sea salt or Himalayan pink salt

¼ teaspoon freshly ground black pepper

½ teaspoon dried basil

½ teaspoon dried thyme

2 bay leaves

⅛ teaspoon cayenne pepper

¼ cup chopped fresh curly parsley

Heat the oil in a large stockpot over medium heat. Add the onion, bell peppers, celery, and carrots and sauté until the onions are translucent and the peppers are soft, about 5 minutes. Add the garlic and cook for 1 minute more.

Add the remaining ingredients except the parsley and stir together to mix well. Allow the mixture to come to a boil, then reduce the heat to low and cover. Simmer for 40 minutes, or until the carrots are tender, stirring occasionally.

Remove the lemon wedge and bay leaves before serving. Garnish with the parsley. Store leftovers in an airtight container in the refrigerator for up to 4 days or freeze for up to 4 months.

A SURPRISING NUTRITIONAL SUPERSTAR, okra is an excellent liver-izing vegetable that also contains a high amount of epicatechin and catechin—two antioxidants also found in cocoa and green tea—which provide strong protection against heart disease and cancer. While some people don't like its somewhat "slimy" quality, its gelatinous juice contains a superior fiber that has been shown in studies to slow the absorption of blood sugar, lower cholesterol, and rid the body of toxins.

PECAN-TOPPED GREEN BEANS

GREEN BEANS ARE A GREAT SOURCE OF FOLATE, FIBER, AND VITAMIN K, IN ADDITION TO A WIDE array of antioxidants with anti-inflammatory and antidiabetic properties. This favorite bean dish makes a great addition to whole grains, steamed vegetables, and winter squashes.

• Makes 6 servings •

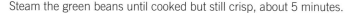

1 pound green beans, trimmed

1 tablespoon virgin coconut oil

3 garlic cloves, minced

½ cup chopped red pearl onions

½ red bell pepper, cut into 2-inch pieces

1 cup chopped raw pecans

Steam the green beans until cooked but still crisp, about 5 minutes.

Heat the coconut oil in a large skillet over medium heat. Add the garlic, onions, and bell pepper and cook until the onions are soft, about 2 minutes. Add the green beans and stir.

Place the green bean mixture into a serving bowl and sprinkle the pecans over the top. Serve hot. Store leftovers in an airtight container for up to 2 days or freeze for up to 1 month.

12

Soups, Stews, Grains, and Legumes

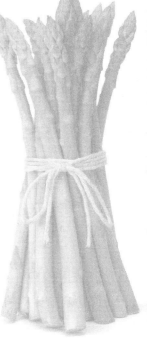

The recipes you'll find in this section are as varied as they are versatile. They can be a simple meal addition, a filling afternoon snack, or an entire lunch or light evening meal. Some can even be eaten for breakfast! You'll find everything from the quick and surprisingly delicious Creamy Zucchini Cashew Soup (page 217) to my family's favorite earthy comfort food—Mexican Ground Beef and Potato Stew (page 223), which we eat wrapped in warm tortillas.

In keeping with my veggie-centric theme, you'll find the soups, stews, and side dishes in this section don't skimp on color, flavor, variety, or nutrition. I've included several types of legumes, nuts, grains, and herbs in an assortment of different ethnic styles, while keeping the kitchen time and skill level within your realm. If you're a fan of chili and Mexican mole sauce, you'll want to try the Pumpkin Chickpea

Chili (page 221), which, despite its seasonal main ingredient, can be made any time of year with canned pumpkin. And speaking of seasonal recipes, if you need a gluten-free alternative to the boxed stovetop stuffing mix, I've got you covered with my Cranberry Quinoa Stovetop Stuffing (page 224), which can actually be made anytime you've got a hankering for those seasonal flavors.

Since many of the recipes call for broth, it's important to understand the value of making your own broth and keeping some on hand to use in everyday recipes; you'll find instructions for doing so in chapter 4. With a nutritious broth, you can make a variety of great-tasting, healthy meals in one pot.

SMOKY TOMATO SOUP

THIS WARM, COMFORTING SOUP IS QUICK AND EASY TO MAKE FOR A NICE LUNCH OR DINNER accompaniment, or it can even be eaten for breakfast with some scrambled eggs. Since the soup is all about the robust flavor of tomatoes, use high-quality organic jarred or canned tomatoes for best results.

• Makes 4 servings •

2 (14½-ounce) cans fire-roasted tomatoes, with juice

3 cups chicken or vegetable broth (pages 56 or 59, or store-bought)

1 tablespoon virgin coconut oil or organic butter

1 medium yellow onion, diced

1 large carrot, diced

2 to 3 garlic cloves, minced

½ teaspoon smoked paprika

2 tablespoons arrowroot

2 tablespoons cold water

Sea salt and freshly ground black pepper

2 tablespoons chopped fresh curly parsley

Place the tomatoes with their juice and the broth in a blender. Set aside.

Heat the coconut oil in a stockpot over medium heat. Add the onions and carrot and cook, stirring frequently, until the onions are translucent, about 3 minutes. Add the garlic and paprika and cook another minute. Remove from the heat and transfer the onion mixture to the blender with the tomatoes and broth. Blend on high until smooth and well combined.

Return the blended mixture back to the pot and simmer over medium-low heat for 20 minutes. Dissolve the arrowroot in the water, then add to the simmering mixture and stir until the soup thickens. Remove from the heat, season with salt and pepper to taste, sprinkle in the chopped parsley, stir, and serve.

STORING AND FREEZING SOUPS AND STEWS

THERE'S NOTHING QUITE LIKE A BOWL OF homemade soup—but sometimes you just don't have time to make a batch. Most of the recipes in this chapter lend themselves well to refrigerating for a short period or freezing for longer. You may want to make a double batch and save half for the week and freeze the other half. For easy grab-'n'-go lunches, freeze portions in single-serving containers. Thaw frozen containers of soup in the refrigerator the night before, then grab one on your way out the door in the morning or have it for dinner when you come home.

I suggest storing leftovers in glass containers. The same procedure and tips for freezing and thawing broth on page 61 can be used for soups and stews.

CREAMY ZUCCHINI CASHEW SOUP

YOU HAVE TO TRY THIS SOUP TO APPRECIATE ITS SURPRISING YUMMINESS—IT'S SO CREAMY, YOU'D never guess it is completely dairy-free. With a little preplanning—the cashews need to be soaked for at least an hour ahead of time to soften them, and the zucchini needs to be lightly steamed—it's a snap to make in your blender. It makes a nice accompaniment to one of the kale salads on pages 199–202.

• Makes 2 servings •

½ cup raw cashews

3 to 4 medium zucchini, cut into chunks and lightly steamed (save the warm steaming water to use for the soup)

2 teaspoons dried herb seasoning, such as Italian seasoning, or 2 tablespoons chopped fresh herbs, such as basil or dill (optional)

¼ teaspoon Herbamare or sea salt, or more to taste

Put the cashews in a bowl and add enough water to cover them completely. Allow them to soak in the water for at least 1 hour. After the cashews have soaked, drain off the water, rinse, and place them in a blender. If needed, the cashews can be soaked a day ahead of time, then drained, rinsed, and placed in a container in the refrigerator until ready to use.

Add the steamed zucchini and seasonings to the blender and blend until smooth, adding small amounts of the warm steaming water as needed for the desired consistency. Serve immediately or save to be eaten later. It can be gently reheated in a saucepan over low heat. Do not boil. Store leftovers in an airtight container in the refrigerator for up to 2 days. This soup does not freeze well.

EASY WAKAME MISO SOUP

MISO SOUP IS THE JAPANESE VERSION OF OUR CHICKEN SOUP—A COMBINATION SOUL FOOD AND comfort food. This basic soup takes only minutes to prepare and is loaded with alkalizing and liver-izing nutrients. Wakame contains high amounts of calcium and magnesium, omega-3 fatty acids, and a unique phytochemical called fucoxanthin that has been shown to burn belly fat, reduce fatty liver, lower blood pressure, and improve blood sugar levels. Combined with miso's protein, probiotics, and immune-boosting properties, this soup can improve your health dramatically if you include a cup of it regularly with your meals.

• Makes 1 serving •

2 cups plus 2 to 3 tablespoons water, divided

1 tablespoon white or yellow miso paste

2 tablespoons dried wakame flakes

1 green onion, thinly sliced (white and green parts)

Bring 2 cups of the water to a boil, then remove from the heat. In a small bowl, mix the miso paste with the remaining 2 to 3 tablespoons of water to make a thin paste. Add this mixture to the boiled water. Stir in the wakame and green onion. Let sit for a few moments, stir, and serve hot. Store leftovers in an airtight container in the refrigerator for up to 2 days. Reheat gently and do not boil (see note). This soup does not freeze well.

> **NOTE:**
>
> *To preserve its nutritional properties, miso should not be boiled. Mix it with a few tablespoons of room temperature water to make a paste, then add the paste to hot water or soup after it has been removed from direct heat.*

HEARTY VEGETABLE MISO SOUP

THIS IS AN AMPED-UP AND MORE FILLING VERSION OF EASY WAKAME MISO SOUP (PAGE 218). Fresh vegetables are always best, but a frozen mixed-vegetable medley of broccoli, cauliflower, and carrots also works great for this recipe.

• Makes 2 servings •

1 tablespoon virgin coconut oil

1 tablespoon finely chopped yellow onion

1 garlic clove, minced

1 small carrot, thinly sliced on the diagonal

1 small celery stalk, thinly sliced on the diagonal

½ teaspoon finely grated fresh ginger (optional)

2 cups plus 2 to 3 tablespoons water, divided

1 cup mixed fresh vegetables (broccoli florets, cauliflower, shredded cabbage, green beans, snow peas, etc.)

2 tablespoons dried wakame flakes

1 tablespoon white or yellow miso paste

1 green onion, thinly sliced (white and green parts; optional)

½ teaspoon unrefined toasted sesame oil (optional)

Heat the coconut oil in a stockpot over medium heat. Add the onion, garlic, carrot, celery, and ginger, if using, and sauté for 5 minutes, or until fragrant. Add 2 cups of the water and simmer on low for 20 minutes, or until the carrots and celery are tender. Add the vegetables and wakame. Stir and simmer until tender but not overcooked; the vegetables should remain crisp. Remove from the heat.

In a small bowl, mix the miso paste with the remaining 2 to 3 tablespoons of water to make a thin paste. Add this mixture to the simmered mixture. Stir in the green onion and sesame oil, if using. Let sit for a few moments, stir, and serve hot. Store leftovers in an airtight container in the refrigerator for up to 2 days. Reheat gently and do not boil (see note on page 218). This soup does not freeze well.

ROASTED GARLIC, CAULIFLOWER, AND FRESH PARSLEY SOUP

THE COMBINATION OF GARLIC, CAULIFLOWER, AND PARSLEY MAKES THIS A SOUP-ER ALKALIZING, liver-izing, and scrumptious meal. For a heartier soup, feel free to add additional ingredients such as cooked chicken, grains, or beans after the soup has been puréed.

• Makes 4 to 6 servings •

4 roasted garlic heads (see page 76)

1 tablespoon virgin coconut oil

3 shallots, chopped

6 cups vegetable or chicken broth (pages 59 or 56, or store-bought)

1 large head cauliflower, chopped (about 5 cups)

¾ teaspoon sea salt or Himalayan pink salt

¼ teaspoon freshly ground black pepper

½ cup chopped fresh curly parsley

Roast the garlic according to the method on page 76. Allow it to cool slightly, then squeeze out the garlic from each clove. Set aside.

Heat the coconut oil in a stockpot over medium heat. Add the shallots and sauté until tender and beginning to brown, about 6 minutes. Add the broth, cauliflower, roasted garlic, salt, and pepper. Bring to a boil, then reduce the heat to low, cover, and simmer for 15 to 20 minutes, or until the cauliflower is soft enough to pierce with a fork but not mushy.

Transfer the soup to a blender or food processor and purée until smooth and creamy. Return to the pot, sprinkle in the parsley, stir, and serve. Store leftovers in an airtight container in the refrigerator for up to 2 days or freeze for up to 1 month.

PUMPKIN CHICKPEA CHILI

THE COMBINATION OF SPICES, PUMPKIN, AND CHICKPEAS GIVES THIS CHILI A FLAVOR THAT IS reminiscent of Mexican mole sauce. Pumpkin and chickpeas both pack an amazing array of antioxidant phytonutrients, with health benefits ranging from lowering the risk of heart disease to prevention of breast, lung, and colon cancer.

The ground turkey can be replaced with ground chicken, bison, or grass-fed beef. To make this a vegetarian chili, omit the ground turkey and add another 2 cups of chickpeas.

• Makes 10 (1-cup) servings •

2 tablespoons virgin coconut oil

1 pound ground turkey

2 celery stalks, diced

1 large carrot, diced

1 medium yellow onion, finely chopped

6 garlic cloves, chopped

1 teaspoon sea salt, divided

1 (15-ounce) can crushed tomatoes, with juice

1 (6-ounce) can tomato paste

2 cups pumpkin purée (page 70), or
    1 (15-ounce) can

3 cups water

1 small sweet potato, peeled and diced

2 tablespoons plus 1 teaspoon chili powder

1 tablespoon ground cumin

1 tablespoon unsweetened cocoa powder

2 teaspoons pumpkin pie spice (page 45 or
    store-bought)

2 cups cooked chickpeas, or 1 (15-ounce) can,
    drained and rinsed

2 roasted Hatch green chiles (page 75), seeded
    and diced (optional)

Diced avocado and chopped fresh cilantro or
    curly parsley, for garnish (optional)

Heat the coconut oil in a large stockpot over medium heat. Add the ground turkey, celery, carrot, onion, garlic, and ½ teaspoon salt. Break up the turkey into small crumbles and cook, stirring frequently, until the onions are translucent and the turkey is no longer pink.

Add the tomatoes with juice, tomato paste, pumpkin, and water. Stir and then add the sweet potato, chili powder, cumin, cocoa powder, pumpkin pie spice, and remaining ½ teaspoon salt. Stir, reduce the heat to low, and simmer for 45 minutes, or until the sweet potatoes are cooked through and tender. Add the chickpeas and green chiles, if using, and simmer for 15 minutes more. Adjust the seasonings if needed and serve.

Garnish each bowl with diced avocado and fresh cilantro, if desired. Store leftovers in an airtight container in the refrigerator for up to 4 days or freeze for up to 4 months.

YELLOW LENTIL DAL

*D*AL IS AN EAST INDIAN WORD FOR ALL TYPES OF DRIED LEGUMES, BUT THE TERM IS MORE commonly used to describe a simple lentil stew made with nourishing vegetables and spices. Any type of lentil can be used in this recipe, but if using green or black beluga lentils instead of red, yellow, or brown, you'll need to increase the cooking time by ten to fifteen minutes. Serve with cooked brown rice, quinoa, or sprouted grain pita bread and a fresh green salad.

• Makes 6 servings •

2 tablespoons virgin coconut oil

1 medium yellow onion, finely diced

3 teaspoons whole cumin seeds

¼ teaspoon ground cardamom

2 teaspoons red pepper flakes

4 garlic cloves, minced

2 tablespoons minced fresh ginger

2 cups yellow lentils, soaked and rinsed

4 cups organic vegetable broth (page 59 or store-bought)

1½ cups chopped tomatoes, with juice

½ cup chopped fresh cilantro or curly parsley

1 tablespoon freshly grated turmeric, or 1 teaspoon ground turmeric

1 teaspoon sea salt or Himalayan pink salt

Heat the oil in a large pot over medium heat. Add the onions and cook until translucent, about 5 minutes. Add the cumin seeds, cardamom, pepper flakes, garlic, and ginger and cook, stirring often, until fragrant, about 2 minutes more.

Add the lentils, broth, tomatoes with juice, cilantro, turmeric, and salt and bring to a boil. Reduce the heat to medium low, cover, and simmer for 15 to 25 minutes, or until the lentils are soft and the liquid is absorbed. Ladle into bowls and serve. Store leftovers in an airtight container in the refrigerator for up to 3 days or freeze for up to 1 month.

MEXICAN GROUND BEEF AND POTATO STEW

THIS SIMPLE STEW HAS BEEN A STAPLE COMFORT FOOD IN MY FAMILY FOR GENERATIONS. THE original recipe called for just ground beef, potatoes, tomato sauce, water, and spices. I've since updated it for my veggie-centric palate, but I have kept the simplicity and flavors intact. The key ingredient is the potatoes, which infuse it with high amounts of heart-healthy potassium while thickening it to a chili-like texture. For a vegetarian version, see the variations. Serve with warm whole grain or corn tortillas and a tossed green salad.

• Makes 6 (1½-cup) servings •

1 tablespoon virgin coconut oil

1 large yellow onion, finely chopped

4 garlic cloves, minced

1 pound organic grass-fed ground beef
(if grass-fed beef is not available, use
90–95 percent lean)

1 (8-ounce) can tomato sauce

2 to 3 cups water or chicken broth (page 56
or store-bought)

5 large organic Yukon gold potatoes,
unpeeled, cut into ½-inch chunks

1 large carrot, sliced into ¼-inch-thick rounds

1 cup frozen organic corn kernels

1 cup fresh or frozen green beans

1 tablespoon ground cumin

2 bay leaves

1 teaspoon sea salt or Himalayan pink salt, or
more to taste

½ teaspoon freshly ground black pepper

Heat the oil over medium heat in a stockpot and sauté the onion and garlic for 2 to 3 minutes. Add the ground beef and brown until it is evenly cooked and shows no signs of pink.

Add the tomato sauce, water, potatoes, carrots, corn, green beans, cumin, and bay leaves. Stir to combine. Add more water if needed to cover the vegetables, bring to a boil, then lower the heat to medium and cook until the potatoes are done and the stew has thickened, about 20 to 25 minutes. Add more water during cooking, if necessary, but allow the stew to thicken as it cooks. Remove the bay leaves. Season with the salt and pepper.

Remove from the heat, ladle into bowls, and serve hot. The family tradition is to spoon a portion of the stew onto a tortilla, roll it up, and eat it burrito-style.

Store leftovers in an airtight container in the refrigerator for up to 4 days or freeze for up to 4 months.

VARIATIONS

- Ground turkey or ground chicken can replace the ground beef.
- For a vegetarian version, omit the ground beef, use vegetable stock or water, and add 2 cups cooked chickpeas after the stew has been removed from the heat. Wait 10 minutes before serving to allow the chickpeas to warm through.

CRANBERRY QUINOA STOVETOP STUFFING

LOOK NO FURTHER FOR A FLAVORFUL GLUTEN-FREE ALTERNATIVE TO TRADITIONAL STUFFING MIX. (And if you use coconut oil, it's vegan, too!) The dried cranberries lend a nice tartness in contrast with the savory flavors of the vegetables.

• Makes 8 servings •

2 tablespoons virgin coconut oil or organic butter

1 red onion, chopped

2 garlic cloves, minced

1 large carrot, diced

2 celery stalks, diced

1 cup quinoa, soaked and rinsed

2 cups vegetable or chicken broth (pages 59 or 56, or store-bought)

¾ teaspoon sea salt

¼ teaspoon freshly ground black pepper

1 tablespoon chopped fresh rosemary

1 tablespoon chopped fresh curly parsley

¼ cup raw pine nuts

½ cup sugar-free or naturally sweetened dried cranberries (see sidebar; for homemade, see page 189)

Heat the oil over medium heat in a large pot. Add the onion, garlic, carrot, and celery and sauté until the onion is translucent (about 10 minutes).

When the vegetables have been cooked, add the quinoa, broth, salt, pepper, and rosemary. Turn the heat up to medium high, bring the mixture to a boil, cover, and reduce the heat to a low simmer. After 15 to 20 minutes, the quinoa should have absorbed all the liquid. Transfer the mixture to a large bowl and toss in the parsley, pine nuts, and cranberries. Serve hot.

ALTERNATIVE SLOW COOKER METHOD:

Place all ingredients except parsley, pine nuts, and cranberries in a slow cooker and cook on low for 4 to 6 hours. Toss in the parsley, pine nuts, and cranberries just before serving. Store leftovers in an airtight container in the refrigerator for up to 3 days or freeze for up to 1 month.

DRIED CRANBERRY CONUNDRUM

IT IS INCREDIBLY DIFFICULT TO FIND sugar-free or naturally sweetened dried cranberries—even in natural food markets. And when you do find them, they still tend be less than healthy. So, like any respectable processed-free foodie, I've taken to making my own. However, if I'm in a pinch I buy them from Cherry Bay Orchards, the only company I have found that offers unsweetened, un-oiled, and unpreserved dried cranberries. See Resources (page 280) for more info. They do come with a pretty hefty price tag, so you may want to try your hand at making them yourself (see page 189).

LEMON TURMERIC QUINOA

LEMON AND TURMERIC, TWO POWERFUL LIVER CLEANSERS, GIVE A REFRESHING AND TANGY FLAVOR to the quinoa. To make this a complete meal, add a sprinkle of pine nuts and 2 cups of a steamed vegetable medley.

• Makes 4 servings •

1 tablespoon virgin coconut oil

1 small onion, chopped

2 garlic cloves, minced

1 teaspoon ground cumin

1 cup quinoa, soaked and rinsed

½ teaspoon ground turmeric

½ teaspoon Herbamare or sea salt

2 cups water

Juice of 1 lemon (about 2 tablespoons)

½ cup grape tomatoes, halved

½ cup chopped fresh curly parsley

¼ cup thinly sliced purple cabbage, for garnish (optional)

Thinly sliced peel from 1 lemon, for garnish (optional)

Heat the oil over medium-high heat in a large skillet. Add the onion, garlic, and cumin and cook until the garlic is soft, but not burned, about 1 minute. Add the quinoa and turmeric and stir to combine with the onion mixture. Add the Herbamare and water and stir again. Allow the water to come to a boil, then reduce the heat to low, cover, and cook for about 15 minutes, or until all the water is absorbed. When done, the quinoa appears soft and translucent, with the germ ring visible along the outer edge of the grain. Turn off the heat. Add the lemon juice, tomatoes, and parsley and stir to combine. Garnish with the cabbage and lemon peel, if desired.

MILLET PILAF WITH BRAISED CARROTS AND FENNEL

COOKED MILLET IS A VERSATILE GRAIN WITH A LIGHT FLUFFY TEXTURE AND A MILD CORN FLAVOR. It makes a wonderful pilaf but can also be cooked with any type of milk to make a creamy breakfast porridge. It boasts a long list of health benefits, most notably reducing the risk of type 2 diabetes and breast cancer. This tiny little gluten-free grain is also a good source of protein, anti-oxidants, and the alkaline-forming mineral magnesium, which helps to lower high blood pressure and reduce the risk of heart attack.

Millet pilaf can be made with any cooked veggies—steamed, braised, or roasted. Here I use a combination of braised fennel, carrot, and onion to sweetly accent the flavor of millet. This pilaf can serve as a meal on its own or as a colorful side dish to any entrée. Try it with Coconut Oil Garlic-Roasted Chicken (page 234) or Unwrapped Cabbage Rolls (page 237).

• Makes 4 servings •

MILLET

1 cup millet, soaked and rinsed

2 cups water or broth (page 56 or store-bought)

¼ teaspoon sea salt (optional)

1 tablespoon virgin coconut oil or organic butter

BRAISED CARROTS AND FENNEL

1 tablespoon virgin coconut oil or organic butter

1 yellow onion, diced

2 large carrots, chopped

1 large fennel bulb, finely chopped (set aside a tablespoon of the fronds for garnish; save the stalks and the remaining fronds to use in salads)

1 garlic clove, minced

¾ cup chicken or vegetable broth (pages 59 or 56, or store-bought)

Heat a large, dry saucepan over medium heat. Add the millet and toast for 4 to 5 minutes, or until it turns a rich golden brown and the grains become fragrant.

Add the water and salt, if using, stir the mixture, then increase the heat to high and bring to a boil.

Reduce the heat to low, add the oil, stir, cover, and simmer until the grains absorb most of the water, about 15 minutes.

Remove the pan from the heat and allow it to sit, covered, for about 10 minutes to let the millet fully absorb the liquid. Remove the cover and fluff it with a fork. Transfer the millet to a large bowl.

While the millet is cooking, braise the vegetables.

Heat the oil in a large skillet over medium heat. Add the onion, carrots, and fennel. Cook for 5 to 7 minutes, or until the vegetables are soft. Reduce the heat to medium and add the garlic and broth. Cover and cook for 10 more minutes, or until the vegetables are done.

Add the vegetables to the cooked millet in the bowl, toss to combine, then sprinkle on the reserved fennel fronds. Serve warm. Pilaf may be stored in the refrigerator for up to 3 days or frozen for up to 1 month.

ANCIENT GRAINS TABBOULEH

THE WHEAT IN THIS CLASSIC MIDDLE EASTERN SIDE DISH IS REPLACED WITH A TRIO OF NATURALLY gluten-free ancient grains—amaranth, millet, and quinoa. These three tiny grains, which are actually seeds, have a nutty flavor and a pleasing texture when cooked together.

The main benefit of ancient grains is that they are higher in protein, vitamins, minerals, and phytonutrients than modern wheat. They are also naturally gluten-free, making them a good choice for everyone.

I chose red quinoa for this recipe because its dark color creates a nice contrast with the other brightly colored ingredients, but the white or black varieties will work as well.

• Makes 6 servings •

⅓ cup amaranth, soaked and rinsed

⅓ cup millet, soaked and rinsed

⅓ cup red quinoa, soaked and rinsed

2¼ cups water

1 cucumber, seeded and diced

2 Roma tomatoes, seeded and chopped

1 red bell pepper, diced

2 radishes, diced

1 small red onion, diced

1 bunch curly parsley, chopped

10 fresh mint leaves, chopped

3 garlic cloves, minced

Zest and juice of 2 lemons

¼ cup extra-virgin olive oil

½ teaspoon dried oregano

Herbamare or sea salt and freshly
    ground black pepper

Place the grains in a 3-quart saucepan. Add the water, stir, and bring the mixture to a boil.

Cover, reduce the heat, and simmer for 15 to 20 minutes, or until the grains have absorbed all the water.

Remove the pan from the heat and allow it to sit, covered, for about 10 minutes to let the grains fully absorb the water. Remove the cover and fluff them with a fork. Transfer the grains to a large bowl and allow them to cool.

While the grains are cooking, prep the rest of the ingredients.

When the grains are cool, add the remaining ingredients to the bowl and toss to combine. The tabbouleh can be enjoyed immediately; however, the flavors become more pronounced when the salad is left to chill for a few hours or overnight, covered, in the refrigerator. Tabbouleh may be kept in the refrigerator for up to 3 days.

SESAME BROWN RICE

Brown rice is a staple in my home, but I rarely eat it as a plain grain. By cooking it in broth and flavorful toasted sesame oil, the experience of eating brown rice is completely transformed. Brown rice also offers a number of unique health benefits, especially in the areas of weight loss and heart health. It absorbs waste and flushes fat out of the liver and also lowers LDL (bad) cholesterol.

• Makes 4 servings •

1 cup brown basmati rice

1½ cups water or chicken or vegetable broth (pages 59 or 56, or store-bought)

1 tablespoon reduced-sodium gluten-free tamari sauce or soy sauce

1 tablespoon unrefined toasted sesame oil

2 teaspoons sesame seeds, for garnish

1 tablespoon chopped green onions (green part only), for garnish

In a medium saucepan, bring the rice and water to a boil for 5 minutes. Add the tamari sauce and toasted sesame oil. Reduce the heat to low, cover, and simmer for 40 to 50 minutes, or until the liquid is absorbed.

While the rice is cooking, toast the sesame seeds. Place the seeds in a dry skillet over low heat, shaking frequently to prevent burning, until fragrant and barely colored, about 5 minutes.

When the rice is done, fluff it with a fork and sprinkle the sesame seeds and green onions over the top. Serve immediately. Store leftovers in an airtight container in the refrigerator for up to 5 days or freeze for up to 3 months.

SLOW-COOKED BOSTON BAKED BEANS

THESE SLOWLY COOKED BEANS ARE PACKED WITH FLAVOR, FIBER, AND CANCER-FIGHTING antioxidants. They're meant to be cooked in a slow cooker but can also be baked in the oven. To make this a vegan dish, you can leave out the turkey bacon and increase the smoked paprika by 1 teaspoon.

• Makes 12 servings •

1 pound (2 to 2¼ cups) dried white beans (such as navy, Great Northern, or cannellini), or 5½ cups canned white beans, drained and rinsed

2 cups hot water

⅓ cup unsulphured blackstrap molasses

⅓ cup organic unrefined whole cane sugar

2 tablespoons Dijon mustard

2 tablespoons yellow mustard

⅛ teaspoon ground cloves

1 teaspoon smoked paprika

¾ teaspoon ground turmeric

1 (6-ounce) can tomato paste

½ pound nitrate-free turkey bacon, cut into ½-inch to 1-inch pieces

1½ cups yellow diced onion (about 1 medium)

3 garlic cloves, minced

Sea salt (optional)

If using dried beans, soak them in a large pot of water overnight or for at least 8 hours. Drain and rinse.

Combine the hot water, molasses, and sugar in a mixing bowl. Stir to dissolve the sugar and mix thoroughly. Add the Dijon, yellow mustard, cloves, paprika, turmeric, and tomato paste. Stir again to combine.

Line the bottom of a slow cooker (or Dutch oven if you're baking in the oven) with half of the turkey bacon. Layer over half of the drained beans. Add all of the onions and garlic in one layer, then top with another layer of beans and the remaining turkey bacon. Pour the molasses mixture over the beans.

Place the cover on the slow cooker (or Dutch oven) and cook on the low setting (or in a 250°F oven) for 8 hours, or until the beans are tender. (If you are using canned beans, the cooking time is reduced to 5 hours.) Check the water level a few hours in and add more water if necessary. Season to taste with salt, if desired.

NOTE:
Your beans may take more or less time to cook, depending on your slow cooker and the freshness of the beans (fresher beans take less time to cook than older beans).

13

Meaty and Meatless Mains

From the crowd-pleasing Apricot Sweet and Sour Meatballs (page 233) to the vegetarian favorite Chickpea Garden Patties (page 243), there's something for everyone in this section. You'll find an assortment of made-over classics and some inventive creations, including casseroles, tacos, and rice dishes. For special occasions, there's the red, white, and green Festive Spinach Lasagna (page 240) and Three Sisters Casserole (page 246). For quick weeknight meals, whip up some Seared Southwest Mahimahi Fish Tacos (page 242) or Veggie Egg Fried Rice (page 245). Many of the veggie dishes can be made meaty by adding chicken or beef, and vice versa—the meat can be swapped out for beans in some of the meaty dishes. Whatever your protein preference, I know you'll enjoy these kitchen-tested favorites. So put on your apron and get cooking!

ASPARAGUS AND SUN-DRIED TOMATO–STUFFED CHICKEN

I N THE SAME WAY A JAVELIN IS USED AS A WEAPON, THE SPEAR-SHAPED FORM OF ASPARAGUS IS symbolic of its powerful weaponry against toxins, free radicals, cancer, and aging. It is a particularly rich source of glutathione, a liver-detoxifying compound that destroys carcinogens and free radicals. Wrapping a chicken breast around asparagus spears is a fun way to beat cancer! The dish pairs well with Roasted Tricolor Taters and Carrots (page 209).

• Makes 4 servings •

½ cup sun-dried tomatoes

4 (4- to 5-ounce) organic chicken breasts, boneless and skinless

Melted virgin coconut oil, for coating the chicken

4 garlic cloves, minced

12 asparagus spears, trimmed

1 teaspoon Herbamare or sea salt

½ teaspoon freshly ground black pepper

1 teaspoon dried basil

Chicken broth (page 56 or store-bought) or water, for filling the baking dish

Preheat the oven to 350°F.

Place the sun-dried tomatoes in a small bowl; cover with hot water. Allow to sit for 5 minutes. Drain well and pat dry. Cut into thin strips.

Pound the chicken breasts with a meat mallet to flatten. Brush both sides of the chicken breast with coconut oil. Spread a quarter of the minced garlic down the center of each breast, then top each with 3 trimmed asparagus spears and a quarter of the sun-dried tomatoes. Bring in the sides of the chicken and tie in one or two places with kitchen string. Season with Herbamare, pepper, and dried basil.

Add ¼ inch of broth to a 2-quart casserole dish; cover with a lid or aluminum foil and bake for 20 minutes. Remove the cover and cook for 20 minutes more, or until the chicken is cooked through. Serve. Store leftovers in an airtight container in the refrigerator for up to 3 days or freeze for up to 3 months.

APRICOT SWEET AND SOUR MEATBALLS

APRICOTS, FULL OF BETA-CAROTENE, POTASSIUM, AND FIBER, ARE THE SECRET INGREDIENT IN this recipe, which is always a hit with kids and grown-ups alike. These meatballs make great party appetizers but are also a meal in their own right. The versatile sweet and sour sauce can also be used to flavor vegetables, grains, chicken, and tempeh without spiking your blood sugar.

• Makes 8 servings •

MEATBALLS

1½ pounds ground turkey or grass-fed ground beef

1 teaspoon garlic powder

1 teaspoon dried basil

1 teaspoon dried parsley

1 teaspoon dried oregano

1 teaspoon sea salt

¼ teaspoon freshly ground black pepper

2 green onions, chopped (green parts only)

1 egg

½ cup oat bran

SAUCE

¼ cup brown rice vinegar

¾ cup 100 percent fruit apricot jam (page 164 or store-bought)

1 cup sugar-free ketchup (page 158 or store-bought)

1 teaspoon dried oregano

4 tablespoons unrefined peanut oil, divided

¼ cup diced yellow onion

Preheat the oven to 350°F.

Combine all the meatball ingredients in a large bowl and mix together. Form the mixture into balls no greater than 1 level tablespoon in size. Place the meatballs on a parchment-lined baking sheet. Bake for 20 minutes. Remove from the oven.

While the meatballs are baking, make the sauce. In a large bowl, whisk together the vinegar, apricot jam, ketchup, oregano, and 3 tablespoons of the peanut oil. Set aside.

Heat a stockpot over medium and pour in a small amount of water and the remaining tablespoon of peanut oil. Add the onion and sauté until it is translucent. Add the jam mixture and cook until bubbling, then lower the heat and simmer until thick, stirring occasionally, about 5 minutes. Add the baked meatballs to the sauce and stir to coat.

Serve hot. They go well with Sesame Brown Rice (page 229) and Ginger Asian Slaw (page 203) or steamed carrots and broccoli. Store leftovers in an airtight container in the refrigerator for up to 3 days or freeze for up to 4 months.

COCONUT OIL
GARLIC-ROASTED CHICKEN

THE PAN WATER KEEPS THIS CHICKEN MOIST WHILE ROASTING, AND THE COCONUT OIL MAKES THE skin brown and crispy. Once it's done, you can pull the chicken off the bones to use in tacos, sandwiches, wraps, salads, soups, or main entrées. Roast two chickens at a time, then freeze the leftovers so you've always got ready-to-eat chicken on hand.

• Makes 6 servings •

1 (5- to 6-pound) whole organic chicken

Sea salt and freshly ground black pepper

1 large lemon, sliced in half

1 garlic head (about 10 cloves), peeled and cloves cut in half

¼ cup virgin coconut oil, melted

½ teaspoon sweet paprika

Preheat the oven to 425°F. Prepare a roasting pan with a rack by filling the pan halfway with water and setting the rack in place.

Remove the giblets from the chicken (they can be frozen and used later to make broth, see page 56), wash the chicken in hot tap water, and pat dry with paper towels. Liberally season the cavity with sea salt and pepper. Squeeze the juice of each lemon half into the cavity, then stuff the squeezed lemon halves and the garlic clove halves into the cavity.

Brush the melted coconut oil all over the chicken and season with salt, pepper, and paprika. Place the chicken on the roasting rack.

Place in the oven for 10 minutes at 425°F. Reduce the heat to 350°F and roast for 1 hour more, or until the juices run clear when the chicken is pricked between the leg and thigh. Store leftovers in an airtight container in the refrigerator for up to 3 days or freeze for up to 4 months.

> **NOTE:**
> *Save the juices and coconut oil that collect in the pan water. This makes a great "broth" to use for cooking grains, soups, or vegetable sautés. After you've pulled all the meat off the chicken bones, use the carcass to make a highly nutritious bone broth (page 56).*

THAI BASIL CHICKEN IN CREAMY COCONUT SAUCE

This recipe is always a hit when I teach it in cooking classes. It's a way to show people how to incorporate coconut milk and a variety of health-promoting spices in a tasty dish that's quick and easy to prepare. To avoid having to buy bottles of each individual spice, I encourage you to buy spices from the bulk area at your local natural food market. You may want to make up a larger batch of the spice mix to have on hand so you can make this recipe often. The spices in this recipe are mild, but the heat can easily be turned up a notch by adding a pinch of cayenne.

• Makes 4 servings •

1 pound organic boneless, skinless chicken breast or thighs, cut into 1-inch pieces

4 teaspoons Thai spice mix (store-bought or recipe follows; combine all spices in a small bowl)

2 tablespoons virgin coconut oil, divided

1 cup chopped red onion

5 garlic cloves, minced

1 (14-ounce) can coconut milk

1 teaspoon reduced-sodium soy sauce or gluten-free tamari sauce

1 tablespoon minced fresh ginger

1 tablespoon arrowroot

1 to 2 tablespoons water

2 cups julienned or grated carrots

2 cups snow peas

3 tablespoons chopped fresh basil

THAI SPICE MIX

½ teaspoon sea salt

½ teaspoon ground coriander

½ teaspoon ground cumin

½ teaspoon ground cloves

½ teaspoon ground cinnamon

½ teaspoon ground cardamom

½ teaspoon freshly ground black pepper

¼ teaspoon chili powder

¼ teaspoon ground turmeric

Place the chicken pieces in a mixing bowl and sprinkle the spice mix over all the pieces. Toss to coat well and let sit at room temperature while you prep the rest of your ingredients. You may also leave the seasoned chicken in the refrigerator, covered, for several hours before you are ready to make the recipe.

Heat 1 tablespoon coconut oil in a large skillet over medium heat. Add the onions and cook for 3 minutes. Add the garlic and cook for 1 minute more. Remove the onions and garlic from the skillet and put in a medium bowl. Set aside. Use the same skillet for the next step.

Add the remaining 1 tablespoon coconut oil to the skillet and heat over medium. Add the chicken pieces, spreading them out in the pan so that they are not crowded. Brown for a few minutes on each side. When the chicken pieces are cooked through and no pink remains, transfer them to the bowl with the onions and garlic.

Return the skillet to the burner over medium heat, then add the coconut milk, soy sauce, and ginger to the skillet.

In a small bowl, dissolve the arrowroot in the water by stirring it until it is a milky-white consistency. Add the arrowroot mixture to the coconut milk and stir to mix it in.

Cook over medium heat and stir until thick and bubbly. Add the carrots and snow peas and cook for 5 minutes. Add the chicken mixture, onions, and garlic back to the skillet. Then add the fresh basil. Cook for 2 minutes more to cook through. Serve with cooked brown rice, if desired. Store leftovers in an airtight container in the refrigerator for up to 3 days or freeze for up to 4 months.

PASTA E FAGIOLI

I'VE MODIFIED THE CLASSIC *FAGIOLI* (ITALIAN FOR "BEAN") SOUP INTO A MEAL THAT MORE RESEMBLES a pasta skillet dish. You can modify it even further to make it a vegetarian dish by using twice the amount of beans and removing the turkey. Serve with a large portion of leafy green salad or steamed vegetables.

• Makes 8 servings •

½ pound brown rice penne

1½ pounds organic ground turkey or nitrate-free organic turkey sausage

1 large yellow onion, chopped

4 large garlic cloves, minced

½ teaspoon sea salt

¼ teaspoon freshly ground black pepper

1½ teaspoons dried oregano

1½ teaspoons dried thyme

1½ teaspoons dried basil

½ teaspoon sweet paprika

1 teaspoon freshly grated lemon zest

1 (28-ounce) can diced tomatoes, with juice

1 (6-ounce) can tomato paste

1½ cups cooked cannellini beans, or 1 (15-ounce) can, drained and rinsed

½ cup shaved or grated Parmesan cheese, divided

¼ cup chopped fresh curly parsley

Cook the pasta according to package directions. Drain, rinse, and set aside.

Heat a heavy saucepan over medium heat. Add the turkey, onion, garlic, salt, pepper, oregano, thyme, basil, paprika, and lemon zest. Break up the turkey with a spatula and cook until the meat is cooked through, about 5 to 7 minutes. Add the diced tomatoes with their juice and the tomato paste. Simmer for 5 minutes.

Add the beans, cooked penne, ¼ cup Parmesan cheese, and chopped parsley. Stir to combine and heat through, about 5 minutes. Remove from the heat, sprinkle the remaining ¼ cup Parmesan on top, and serve. Store leftovers in an airtight container in the refrigerator for up to 5 days or freeze for up to 2 months.

NOTE:

You can replace the dried herbs and lemon zest with 1½ tablespoons Spice Hunter Pasta Seasoning Blend (see Resources, page 281).

UNWRAPPED CABBAGE ROLLS

THIS SKILLET DISH PROVIDES ALL OF THE INGREDIENTS AND HEALTH BENEFITS OF CABBAGE ROLLS, without the time-consuming labor. Cabbage in general—but napa cabbage in particular—has high levels of a compound that has unique cancer-preventive properties with respect to bladder cancer, colon cancer, and prostate cancer. Like collard greens, you'll want to slice cabbage into ¼-inch pieces and let it sit on the cutting board for five minutes or more before cooking to enhance its health-promoting benefits.

The cancer-fighting benefits of cabbage are lost when cabbage is cooked too long; therefore, it is best to cook it for no longer than five minutes.

Serve this tasty skillet meal with cooked grains or Rosemary-Topped Flourless Cornbread (page 137) and a small raw salad for a great-tasting meal.

• Makes 5 servings •

1½ pounds grass-fed ground beef or ground turkey

1 medium yellow onion, chopped

2 garlic cloves, crushed

1 (28-ounce) can diced tomatoes, with juice

1 cup (8 ounces) tomato sauce

2 tablespoons freshly squeezed lemon juice

½ teaspoon freshly ground black pepper

½ teaspoon ground nutmeg

½ teaspoon ground cinnamon

1 teaspoon sea salt

1 small head green cabbage or ½ head napa cabbage, coarsely chopped

Begin browning the ground beef in a heavy skillet over medium heat. Add the onion and garlic. Cover the pan and let the mixture cook for 3 to 4 minutes, or until the meat is no longer pink.

Stir in the tomatoes with juice, tomato sauce, lemon juice, pepper, nutmeg, cinnamon, and salt. Bring to a simmer.

Stir the cabbage into the beef mixture a little at a time—it will come close to overflowing the skillet. Stir the mixture carefully so it cooks evenly. Cover and let simmer for 5 minutes, then serve. Store leftovers in an airtight container in the refrigerator for up to 3 days or freeze for up to 3 months.

SWEET POTATO AND GROUND TURKEY SHEPHERD'S PIE

SWEET POTATOES AND FRESH GINGER PUT A TASTY TWIST ON THE TRADITIONAL MASHED POTATO—topped shepherd's pie. Sweet potatoes lend a hefty dose of potassium, a nutrient that regulates heartbeat and reduces cholesterol, while ginger reduces inflammation in the body and fires up the digestive juices for better absorption of essential nutrients. For a meatless version, you can use crumbled tempeh (see the variations).

• Makes 6 servings •

FILLING

2 tablespoons virgin coconut oil

1 medium yellow onion, chopped

1 celery stalk, chopped

2 large carrots, chopped

1 pound lean ground turkey

3 garlic cloves, minced

½ tablespoon minced fresh ginger

½ tablespoon curry powder

¼ cup brown rice flour

1 cup chicken broth (page 56 or store-bought)

10 ounces frozen mixed vegetables (green beans, peas, corn, etc.)

½ cup chopped fresh curly parsley, divided

Sea salt and black pepper

TOPPING

2½ pounds sweet potatoes (about 4 medium), baked, or 2½ cups canned sweet potato purée

¼ cup coconut milk or Greek-style yogurt

¼ cup chicken broth (page 56 or store-bought)

Sea salt and freshly ground black pepper

Preheat the oven to 375°F.

To make the filling, heat the oil in a large skillet over medium heat. Add the onion, celery, and carrots and cook until slightly softened, 6 to 7 minutes. Add the ground turkey and cook, breaking up the turkey with a spoon, until it is no longer pink. Add the garlic, ginger, and curry powder and cook for 1 to 2 minutes, or until fragrant.

Sprinkle the brown rice flour over the meat mixture, stir, and cook another 1 to 2 minutes. Add the chicken broth, frozen vegetables, and ¼ cup parsley. Stir and simmer another couple of minutes until thickened. Season the filling with salt and pepper. Spoon 1 cup of the meat mixture into each of six individual oven-safe dishes or ramekins, or spoon the entire mixture into a 3-quart casserole dish.

To make the topping, cut the prebaked sweet potatoes in half and scoop the flesh from the skins into a large bowl. If using canned purée, scoop it into a large bowl. Add the coconut milk and broth. Mash the mixture together with your hands or a potato masher. Season the mixture with salt and pepper.

Spread ½ cup of the sweet potato topping evenly over the filling in each individual dish, or if using a larger casserole dish, spread the topping over the entire dish, spreading it all the way to the edges. Alternatively, you can pipe the topping on with a pastry bag. Bake uncovered, 20 to 25 minutes, or until the filling is warm and the top is lightly browned. Remove from the oven and garnish with the remaining chopped parsley. Let cool for 10 minutes before serving.

Store leftovers in an airtight container in the refrigerator for up to 5 days or freeze for up to 2 months.

VARIATIONS

- Replace the ground turkey and chicken broth with the same amounts of organic grass-fed ground beef and organic beef broth.
- For a meatless version, replace the ground turkey and chicken broth with 1 pound tempeh (crumbled or pulsed in a food processor to the consistency of ground beef), equivalent amounts of vegetable broth, and 3 tablespoons gluten-free tamari sauce.

FESTIVE SPINACH LASAGNA

THIS LASAGNA GETS ITS FESTIVE COLORS FROM THE RED MARINARA SAUCE AND THE GREEN spinach. The cheese and pasta make it a heavy meal; therefore, it's a recipe I only make for the holidays or special occasions when company is coming. For a vegetarian option, it can be made without the ground meat. I serve it with a large green salad to help balance the heavy cheese and starch in the meal.

• Makes 12 servings •

8 ounces whole grain lasagna noodles (preferably brown rice or whole spelt noodles)

1 pound ground turkey or grass-fed ground beef (optional)

Sea salt and freshly ground black pepper

2 pounds fresh spinach, trimmed of thick stems

2 cups raw pine nuts

3 garlic cloves, finely chopped

⅔ cup plus 2 tablespoons extra-virgin olive oil, divided

½ cup grated Parmesan cheese

1 (32-ounce) container ricotta cheese (4 cups)

2 large eggs

6 to 8 cups fresh marinara sauce (page 160 or store-bought)

1 cup shredded organic mozzarella cheese

Preheat the oven to 350°F. Cook the lasagna noodles according to package directions. If using, season the ground turkey with salt and pepper and brown it in a large skillet over medium heat. Cook until the meat is no longer pink, about 10 to 12 minutes. Drain off the fat and set aside.

Make a spinach pesto by adding the spinach, pine nuts, and 3 garlic cloves to the bowl of a food processor. Pour in 2 tablespoons extra-virgin olive oil and pulse until everything is chopped up. With the food processor running, stream in the remaining ⅔ cup extra-virgin olive oil and add the Parmesan cheese. Transfer the pesto to a mixing bowl and season with salt and pepper. Stir in the ricotta cheese and egg, mix well, and set aside.

Assemble the lasagna by ladling a small amount of the marinara sauce into the bottom of a 13 x 9-inch baking dish. Top the sauce with 3 lasagna noodles and cover those with half of the meat (if using) and half of the spinach pesto mixture. Top the spinach pesto with 3 more lasagna noodles, then ladle half of the remaining sauce on top of that. Cover that layer with 3 more noodles and top them off with the remaining meat and spinach pesto.

Place the last 3 noodles over that layer and spoon the remaining sauce over the top. Sprinkle the mozzarella cheese on top and cover the pan with aluminum foil. Bake the lasagna for 30 minutes, then remove the cover and bake for 10 to 15 minutes more, or until the cheese is bubbly and melted. Serve hot. Store leftovers in an airtight container in the refrigerator for up to 5 days or freeze for up to 2 months.

HERB-CRUSTED SALMON ON GREENS

CHOPPED FRESH HERBS INFUSE MORE THAN JUST COLOR AND FLAVOR IN THIS QUICK AND EASY dish. Dill, basil, and parsley provide calcium and antioxidants with antibacterial and cancer-fighting properties. Serving this fish over fresh greens makes a light yet satisfying meal for lunch or dinner.

• Makes 2 servings •

DRESSING
2 tablespoons freshly squeezed lime juice

1 teaspoon minced fresh ginger

2 teaspoons Dijon mustard

1 tablespoon unrefined toasted sesame oil

Sea salt and freshly ground black pepper

SALMON AND GREENS
2 (6-ounce) wild-caught salmon fillets
   (about 1-inch thick, skin removed)

1 tablespoon virgin coconut oil, melted,
   plus more for brushing the salmon

2½ tablespoons fresh dill, divided

2½ tablespoons fresh basil, divided

2½ tablespoons fresh curly parsley, divided

4 cups mixed baby greens

To make the dressing, whisk together the lime juice, ginger, and mustard in a small bowl. Slowly whisk in the sesame oil. Season with salt and pepper. Set aside.

Brush the salmon lightly on both sides with coconut oil, then sprinkle ½ tablespoon each of dill, basil, and parsley onto each side of the salmon filets. Press the herbs to adhere.

Heat 1 tablespoon coconut oil in a large skillet over medium heat. Add the salmon to the skillet, herb-side down, and sauté for 4 minutes. Gently turn each fillet over and sauté until the salmon is just opaque in the center, about 5 minutes.

Toss the greens in a bowl with the remaining herbs and some dressing. Divide between 2 plates. Top with the warm salmon and remaining dressing. Serve immediately. Store any leftover salmon in an airtight container in the refrigerator for up to 2 days or freeze for up to 2 months. Fresh salad greens tossed with dressing should be consumed immediately. They do not store well, as the greens become wilted and soggy.

SEARED SOUTHWEST MAHIMAHI FISH TACOS

SOME YEARS AGO, WHILE LIVING IN SAN DIEGO, I FELL IN LOVE WITH FISH TACOS. NOT THE deep-fried battered version—the real fish tacos that most likely originated in Mexico. When I moved back to Arizona, I decided to start making them myself. My take on this popular delicacy consists of a pan-seared white fish served in a corn tortilla and topped with finely shredded green or red cabbage, chopped cilantro, a sprinkle of white cheese, avocado slices, and a most vital spritz of lime. When you buy the ingredients to make these, you'll have plenty of extra veggies to make a crisp slaw to accompany your tacos.

My favorite fish for tacos is mahimahi, but salmon, cod, and halibut are great substitutes.

The secret to searing the fish without having it stick to the pan is to make sure it is completely dry before cooking, and the oil should be hot but not smoking.

• Makes 6 tacos •

⅛ teaspoon cayenne pepper

1 teaspoon ground cumin

1 tablespoon chili powder

Pinch of sea salt and freshly ground black pepper

6 corn tortillas (page 139 or store-bought)

1 pound Mahimahi or other white fish fillets

2 tablespoons virgin coconut oil

1 cup shredded green or red cabbage

1 cup shredded jack cheese

1 avocado, pitted, peeled, and cut into 12 slices

½ cup chopped fresh cilantro

2 limes, quartered

Combine the cayenne, cumin, chili powder, salt, and pepper in a small bowl. Set aside.

Warm the tortillas in a dry skillet or on a griddle, then wrap in a clean kitchen towel to keep warm.

Pat the Mahimahi fillets dry with paper towels and season both sides with the spice mixture.

Heat the coconut oil in a skillet over medium-high heat. When the oil is hot, carefully place the fish in the skillet. Cook the fish for 3 to 5 minutes per side, depending on the thickness of the fillets (the fish will whiten around the bottom and outside as it cooks).

Remove the fish from the skillet and divide into 6 equal portions.

Assemble the tacos by topping each tortilla with a portion of the fish, shredded cabbage, shredded cheese, avocado slices, cilantro, and a generous squeeze of fresh lime juice. Store any leftover fish in an airtight container in the refrigerator for up to 3 days or freeze for up to 2 months.

CHICKPEA GARDEN PATTIES

ALSO CALLED GARBANZO BEANS, CHICKPEAS RANK HIGH ON THE LIST OF WEIGHT LOSS SUPERFOODS due to their high amount of resistant starch, a special type of fiber that helps your body burn more fat. These veggie patties are definitely satisfying and filling. Enjoy them with steamed vegetables or your favorite leafy green salad.

• Makes 6 patties •

1 cup cooked chickpeas

1 cup cooked brown rice or quinoa

½ cup mixed frozen organic vegetables (peas, carrots, green beans, corn, etc.)

½ cup diced yellow onion

2 garlic cloves, minced

½ cup brown rice flour or any whole grain flour (preferably sprouted)

1½ teaspoons ground cumin

1 teaspoon Herbamare or sea salt

1 large egg (or use a chia seed egg replacement, page 133)

2 tablespoons virgin coconut oil

Add all ingredients except the coconut oil to the bowl of a food processor. Pulse until well blended but not puréed (you should still be able to see chunks of vegetables in the mixture). Transfer the mixture to a large bowl.

Form the mixture into 6 patties. Heat the coconut oil in a large skillet over medium heat. Cook the patties for 5 to 7 minutes on each side, or until lightly browned and crispy on the outside, turning carefully so they don't break apart.

Place the cooked patties on a plate lined with paper towels to absorb excess oil. The patties will be soft and moist on the inside and slightly crispy on the outside. Serve with a fresh green salad or as a complement to cooked veggies. You may also eat a patty like a burger on a sprouted grain bun. Store leftover patties in an airtight container in the refrigerator for up to 3 days or freeze for up to 3 months.

CHILI CON TEMPEH

FINELY CHOPPED TEMPEH SUBSTITUTES FOR GROUND BEEF IN THIS DARING VERSION OF A WELL-loved classic, though unsuspecting dinner guests may not be able to tell the difference! Masa harina, a traditional thickener, adds a distinguishing southwestern flavor to the chili. Serve with a tossed green salad.

• Makes 8 servings •

4 tablespoons virgin coconut oil, divided

1 medium yellow onion, chopped

2 carrots, cut into ½-inch pieces

8 garlic cloves, minced, divided

3 celery stalks, chopped

1 red or yellow bell pepper, cut into ½-inch pieces

2 small jalapeño peppers, seeded and minced

1 (14½-ounce) can diced tomatoes, with juice (can also use fire-roasted diced tomatoes)

1 (6-ounce) can tomato paste

2 cups water

2 teaspoons ground cumin

2 teaspoons dried oregano

3 tablespoons chili powder, divided

2 (8-ounce) packages tempeh

1½ cups cooked pinto or black beans

2 tablespoons masa harina (corn flour; optional)

¼ cup cold water (optional)

Heat 2 tablespoons of coconut oil in a large stockpot over medium heat. Add the onion, carrots, and half of the minced garlic. Cook over medium heat until the onions are translucent, about 5 minutes.

Add the celery, bell pepper, and jalapeños and continue to cook for about 5 minutes more.

Once the vegetables are softened, add the diced tomatoes with juice, tomato paste, water, cumin, oregano, and 2 tablespoons chili powder to the veggies. Bring the mixture to a boil, then lower the heat to simmer for 15 minutes.

While the veggie mixture is simmering, break up the tempeh and put it in the bowl of a food processor. Add the remaining minced garlic and 1 tablespoon chili powder. Pulse the mixture until the tempeh appears crumbled.

Heat the remaining 2 tablespoons coconut oil over medium heat in a skillet. Add the crumbled tempeh and cook for 5 minutes, or until the tempeh is golden brown.

Add the tempeh and beans to the simmering veggie mixture. If using masa harina, combine it with the water to form a thin, watery paste and then add it to the chili. Stir to combine well. Simmer, uncovered, for 15 minutes more, stirring occasionally. Remove from the heat and serve. Store leftovers in an airtight container in the refrigerator for up to 4 days or freeze for up to 4 months.

VEGGIE EGG FRIED RICE

ALTHOUGH OFTEN EATEN AS A SIDE DISH, FRIED RICE CAN COMFORTABLY SERVE AS A COMPLETE meal on its own if you balance the rice with loads of vegetables and throw in a little bit of protein. The rice needs to be cooked and then chilled in the refrigerator, so it's best to prepare the rice at least a day ahead of time before making this recipe (see note on page 246).

• Makes 4 servings •

4 large eggs

½ teaspoon sea salt

2 tablespoons virgin coconut oil, divided

1 bunch asparagus, trimmed and cut into 1-inch pieces

4 carrots, cut on a slight angle to form thinly sliced ovals

1 red bell pepper, thinly sliced into 1-inch pieces

4 green onions, thinly sliced (white and green parts)

4 garlic cloves, minced

1 tablespoon minced fresh ginger, or 1 teaspoon ground ginger

1 cup snow peas

4 teaspoons reduced-sodium gluten-free tamari sauce or soy sauce

2½ cups cooked long-grain brown rice, chilled

2 teaspoons unrefined toasted sesame oil

1 tablespoon toasted sesame seeds, for garnish (optional)

In a small bowl, lightly beat the eggs and salt.

Add 1 tablespoon of the coconut oil to a large skillet and heat over medium heat. Pour in the eggs and cook, stirring gently, until just set, about 2 minutes. Transfer the eggs to a plate and chop into small pieces.

Using the same skillet, add a small amount of water and the remaining 1 tablespoon coconut oil and heat over medium-high heat; add the asparagus and carrots and cook, stirring, for 2 minutes. Add the bell pepper, green onions, garlic, ginger, snow peas, and tamari sauce and cook, stirring, until the vegetables are just tender, about 2 minutes.

Stir in the rice and eggs until well mixed. Continue to cook, stirring, until the rice is heated through and the liquid is absorbed, about 1 to 2 minutes. Remove from the heat, drizzle in the sesame oil, and stir. Divide evenly between 4 plates, sprinkle with toasted sesame seeds, if desired, and serve.

The consensus among professionals in Asian cookery is that fried rice should be made with long-grain rice, and more importantly, the rice needs to be cold—like refrigerator cold. Freshly cooked rice is too soft and moist and will turn sticky when it hits the hot oil, making "fried mush" instead of fried rice. Refrigerating the rice overnight firms up the grains and gets rid of the excess moisture. It also allows the rice grains to separate easily instead of sticking together when stir-fried. If you can't wait a day, at least let the rice cool for a few hours in an airy spot before making fried rice.

THREE SISTERS CASSEROLE

A Native American expression, "the three sisters" refers to the practice of growing beans, corn, and squash together because they nourish and protect each other from garden pests when planted next to each other. Native Americans consider these three foods— (known as the "sustainers of life")—to be special gifts from the earth. When eaten together, they provide a complete vegetarian protein and are packed with blood sugar–stabilizing fiber and cancer-fighting phytonutrients.

This filling main dish is a colorful sight to behold. Serve it alongside a crisp green salad.

• Makes 6 servings •

THREE SISTERS FILLING

3 tablespoons virgin coconut oil, divided, plus more for the pan

1 cup chopped yellow onion

1 red bell pepper, chopped

2 cups peeled and cubed butternut squash (1-inch cubes)

1 (15-ounce) can diced tomatoes, with juice, or 2 cups seeded and diced fresh tomatoes

½ cup seeded and diced roasted green chiles (page 75)

2 garlic cloves, minced

1 teaspoon ground coriander

1 teaspoon ground cumin

½ cup water

½ teaspoon sea salt

2 cups cooked red kidney beans

1 cup fresh or frozen organic corn kernels

POLENTA TOPPING	2 tablespoons chili powder
1½ cups course-grind whole grain organic cornmeal	¼ teaspoon sea salt
	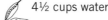 4½ cups water

Preheat the oven to 375°F. Coat an 11 x 8-inch baking dish with coconut oil.

To make the polenta topping, whisk together the cornmeal, chili powder, salt, and water in a double boiler, or place in a large metal bowl over barely simmering water. Cook for 40 minutes, or until the polenta is thick and stiff, stirring 3 or 4 times. Remove from the heat.

To make the filling, heat 2 tablespoons oil in a large saucepan over medium heat. Add the onion and cook for 7 minutes, or until softened, stirring often. Add the bell pepper and cook 5 minutes more, stirring often.

Stir in the squash, tomatoes, chiles, garlic, coriander, and cumin. Cook for 5 minutes, stirring occasionally. Stir in the water and salt. Bring the mixture to a boil. Reduce the heat to medium low and simmer, partially covered, 10 to 15 minutes, or until the squash is tender. Stir in the beans and corn and cook for 5 minutes, or until slightly thickened, stirring occasionally.

Spread 2 cups polenta over the bottom of the prepared dish. Spoon the squash mixture over the polenta. Smooth the remaining polenta (about 2½ cups) over the top.

Score the casserole into 6 squares with a knife. Brush the top with the remaining 1 tablespoon oil. Bake for 30 minutes, or until heated through and the top is lightly browned. Serve warm. Store leftovers in an airtight container in the refrigerator for up to 5 days or freeze for up to 2 months.

CHICKPEA TIKKA MASALA WITH CINNAMON BROWN RICE

THE CLASSIC RECIPE FOR TIKKA MASALA IS TRADITIONALLY HEAVY ON THE CHICKEN, WITH A LONG list of hard-to-find spices. This version is a lighter weeknight vegetarian meal using easy-to-find spices and coconut milk instead of heavy cream, along with the addition of kale, turmeric, and ginger for their anti-inflammatory benefits. Served over a bed of cinnamon brown rice, this dish hits the spot on chilly winter evenings.

• Makes 6 servings •

CHICKPEA TIKKA MASALA

2 tablespoons virgin coconut oil

1 yellow onion, chopped

4 garlic cloves, minced

1 (1-inch) piece fresh ginger, peeled and coarsely chopped

1 tablespoon garam masala

1 tablespoon chili powder

½ teaspoon ground turmeric, or 1½ teaspoons freshly grated turmeric

½ teaspoon sea salt

1 (28-ounce) can diced tomatoes, with juice

1 tablespoon tomato paste

1 (15-ounce) can coconut milk

2 teaspoons unrefined raw whole cane sugar or coconut sugar

1 cup sliced carrots (¼-inch-thick rounds)

1 cup chopped Lacinato kale leaves

3½ cups cooked chickpeas

½ cup chopped fresh cilantro

CINNAMON BROWN RICE

2 cups jasmine brown rice

4½ cups water

1½ teaspoons ground cinnamon

⅛ teaspoon ground cloves

½ teaspoon ground cardamom

½ teaspoon sea salt

To make the tikka masala, heat the oil in a large stockpot over medium heat. Add the onion and sauté until soft, stirring often, about 5 minutes. Add the garlic and ginger and stir for 1 minute. Mix in the garam masala, chili powder, turmeric, and salt; stir until fragrant, a minute or so.

Add the tomatoes with their juice, tomato paste, coconut milk, and sugar. Bring to a simmer.

Add the carrots, kale, and chickpeas. Cover and simmer over medium-low heat until the vegetables are tender, stirring occasionally, about 20 minutes. Turn off the heat, add the cilantro, and stir. To serve, place about ½ cup of the cinnamon brown rice on a serving plate, then top with 1 heaping cup of the tikka masala. Store leftovers in an airtight container in the refrigerator for up to 4 days or freeze for up to 2 months.

To make the rice, add the rice, water, spices, and salt to a medium saucepan.

Bring to a boil, then reduce the heat to medium low.

Cover and simmer until the liquid is absorbed and the rice is tender, about 45 minutes.

To make in a rice cooker, place all ingredients in the rice cooker, stir, and cook on the setting for brown rice. Store leftovers in an airtight container in the refrigerator for up to 4 days or freeze for up to 6 months.

SALSA VERDE SPINACH AND SWEET POTATO ENCHILADAS

USING SPROUTED CORN TORTILLAS FOR THIS RECIPE UPS THE ALKALIZING FACTOR WITHOUT ALTERING the yum factor. Baked sweet potatoes are preferred for this recipe, but canned organic sweet potato purée works just as well.

• Makes 10 enchiladas •

2½ cups salsa verde (page 156)

1½ pounds sweet potatoes, baked, or 2 (15-ounce) cans organic sweet potato purée (see Resources, page 277)

1 tablespoon virgin coconut oil, plus more for the pan and brushing the tortillas

2 shallots, chopped

4 garlic cloves, minced

1 pound fresh baby spinach

2 tablespoons taco seasoning mix (page 168)

10 corn tortillas (page 139 or store-bought)

½ cup crumbled goat cheese

Preheat the oven to 350°F. Lightly coat a large baking sheet with coconut oil. Set aside.

Cover the bottom of a 13 x 9-inch baking dish with a thin layer of the salsa verde. Set aside.

Cut open the baked sweet potatoes and scoop the flesh into a large bowl (discard the skins). Mash with your hands or a spoon, just enough to break it up. There can still be some lumps left. Set aside.

Heat 1 tablespoon oil in a skillet over medium heat. Add the shallot and garlic; cook for a few minutes until fragrant but not brown. Stir in the spinach and taco seasoning and cook until the spinach is just lightly wilted, about 2 to 3 minutes. Remove from the heat and add to the bowl of mashed sweet potato. Mix well.

Lightly brush each side of the tortillas with coconut oil and place them on the baking sheet. Place in the oven for 4 minutes, or until soft and warm.

Remove from the oven and spoon about ⅓ cup of the sweet potato mixture onto the center of the tortilla. Roll up and place seam-side down in the baking dish. Repeat with the remaining tortillas.

When all the enchiladas are in the baking dish, pour the remaining salsa generously over the top and sprinkle with the goat cheese.

Bake for 15 to 20 minutes, or until the sauce is bubbling and the cheese is melted. Store leftovers in an airtight container in the refrigerator for up to 4 days or freeze for up to 2 months.

14

Sweet Indulgences

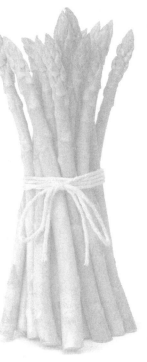

wholeheartedly believe that you can follow a processed-free lifestyle and still indulge your sweet tooth every once in a while. It's one of the reasons so many *Science of Skinny* followers have found the processed-free lifestyle doable for the long term. The recipes in this section prove that "nutritious" and "dessert" can coexist! I've offered up some of my best tried-and-true recipes, including Grain-Free Nutty Peanut Butter Cookies (page 252) and Guiltless Grain-Free Brownies (page 254)—two specialties that have won over hundreds of die-hard cookie and brownie lovers. For the amateur chocolatier, you'll enjoy making your own Simply Skinny Chocolate Bars (page 262) and Joyful Chocolate Almond Bars (page 264). For the holidays, favorites like Simply Perfect Pumpkin Pie (page 260) and Whole Grain Gingerbread Cookies (page 255) will please the whole crowd. I've included something for everyone here—

some recipes are grain-free, some are gluten-free, and all are dairy-free with the exception of my Honey Lemon Cream Cheese Frosting (page 265). Some of them are quick and easy to put together, and some will take a little time and patience. All of these recipes use natural sweeteners. You can refer back to the chart on page 47 for a comprehensive description of the most popular alternative sweeteners. Finally, I'm not suggesting that the goodies included in this section should be a part of your daily nutrition plan, but when company comes or you just need a little indulgence, these are the recipes that will nourish your body as well as your soul.

GRAIN-FREE NUTTY PEANUT BUTTER COOKIES

DIE-HARD PEANUT BUTTER COOKIE LOVERS DON'T MISS THE FLOUR IN THESE YUMMY MORSELS. I use chunky peanut butter in this recipe because I like the crunchiness of the peanuts in the cookies, but the creamy style can be used as well.

• Makes 24 (2-inch) cookies •

1 cup chunky natural peanut butter (see note)

¾ cup organic unrefined whole cane sugar or coconut sugar

1 teaspoon baking soda

1 large egg

½ teaspoon pure vanilla extract, or ¼ teaspoon vanilla powder

Preheat the oven to 350°F. Line a baking sheet with parchment paper.

Using an electric mixer, cream together the peanut butter, sugar, and baking soda in a bowl until well combined. Add the egg and vanilla and mix for about 1 minute, or until well combined. The "dough" may be slightly crumbly, but you can pack it easily into a large ball with your hands.

Measure tablespoon-size pieces of dough and form them into small balls. Place the balls 1 inch apart on the lined baking sheet. Press each ball with the prongs of a fork to flatten them and create a crisscross pattern.

Bake for 12 minutes, or until lightly browned. Cool on the baking sheet for 5 minutes, then transfer to wire racks to cool completely. Store in an airtight container for up to 1 week or place in a freezer-safe container for up to 1 month.

> **NOTE:**
>
> *Most jars of natural peanut butter have a layer of oil at the top of the jar. Before measuring the peanut butter for this recipe, be sure to stir the oil into the peanut butter so that it is well combined. If the peanut butter is more dry and crumbly, you can add a tablespoon of coconut oil to the dough to get the right consistency.*

GRAIN-FREE ALMOND SPICE COOKIES

YOU WON'T BELIEVE THESE COOKIES ARE GRAIN-FREE! THEY'RE PERFECT FOR THE KIDS' LUNCHBOXES or as a nice snack with some afternoon tea. This recipe works best with a stand mixer, but you can also mix it the old-fashioned way, by hand.

• Makes 24 (2-inch) cookies •

1 cup natural almond butter (page 72 or store-bought; see note)

½ cup almond meal (page 71 or store-bought), plus more as needed

¾ cup organic unrefined whole cane sugar or coconut sugar

1 teaspoon baking soda

1 large egg

1 teaspoon almond extract

¼ teaspoon ground cinnamon

¼ teaspoon ground cardamom

¼ teaspoon ground ginger

24 raw almonds

Preheat the oven to 350°F. Line a baking sheet with parchment paper.

Using an electric mixer, cream together the almond butter, almond meal, sugar, and baking soda in a bowl. Add the egg, almond extract, cinnamon, cardamom, and ginger, mixing until incorporated. If the dough is too thin and oily, you can bulk it up by adding more almond meal, a tablespoon at a time, mixing well after each addition. The "dough" may be slightly crumbly, but you can pack it easily into a large ball with your hands.

Measure tablespoon-size pieces of dough and form them into small balls. Place the balls 1 inch apart on the lined baking sheet. Lightly press a whole almond into each ball, but don't press down too hard that you flatten them. If you flatten the cookies, they will spread too much and become flat during baking. Leave them as round balls and they will turn out just right!

Bake for 10 to 12 minutes, or until lightly browned. Cool on the baking sheet for 5 minutes, then transfer to wire racks to cool completely. Store in an airtight container for up to 1 week or place in a freezer-safe container for up to 1 month.

> **NOTE:**
>
> *Most jars of natural almond butter have a layer of oil at the top of the jar. Do not stir it in, as too much oil can affect the texture of this recipe. Instead, pour as much of the oil as possible into a separate container before measuring out the almond butter. You can add the oil back to the jar afterward.*

GUILTLESS GRAIN-FREE BROWNIES

B E PREPARED FOR A SURPRISE INGREDIENT HERE: PURÉED BLACK BEANS REPLACE THE FLOUR IN these chocolaty brownies. They make a high-fiber, low-sugar treat that truly tastes great!

• Makes 1 (8-inch) square pan •

4 large eggs

2 tablespoons virgin coconut oil, melted, plus more for the pan

¼ cup unsweetened cocoa powder

½ cup coconut sugar

1 teaspoon aluminum-free baking powder

1 teaspoon pure vanilla extract, or ½ teaspoon vanilla powder

1½ cups cooked black beans, or 1 (15-ounce) can, drained and rinsed

1 cup chopped raw walnuts

Preheat the oven to 350°F. Coat an 8-inch square baking dish with coconut oil or butter.

Place the eggs, coconut oil, cocoa powder, sugar, baking powder, and vanilla into the bowl of a food processor. Process until the mixture is well combined, about 1 minute. Add the black beans and process until the mixture is smooth and creamy, about 1 to 2 minutes. Remove the blade from the food processor, then fold the walnuts into the batter.

Pour the batter into the prepared baking dish and smooth the top with a spatula. Bake for 30 minutes, or until a toothpick inserted in the center comes out clean. Allow to cool completely, then cut into equal-size squares. Store in an airtight container for up to 1 week or place in a freezer-safe container for up to 1 month.

WHOLE GRAIN GINGERBREAD COOKIES

WHY WAIT UNTIL THE HOLIDAYS TO MAKE GINGERBREAD COOKIES? I USE A HEART-SHAPED COOKIE cutter and serve these chewy sprouted grain favorites year-round.

• Makes 24 (1½-inch) cookies •

¼ cup virgin coconut oil, melted

¼ cup (½ stick) organic butter, at room temperature

½ cup organic unrefined whole cane sugar or coconut sugar

½ cup unsulphured blackstrap molasses

1 large egg

3 cups sprouted spelt flour

½ teaspoon baking soda

½ teaspoon sea salt

1 teaspoon ground ginger

½ teaspoon ground cinnamon

½ teaspoon ground cloves

In a large mixing bowl, combine the coconut oil and butter. Add the sugar, molasses, and egg. Mix well to combine.

In a separate mixing bowl, combine the flour, baking soda, salt, ginger, cinnamon, and cloves. Add this mixture to the oil/sugar mixture. Mix well to combine until it forms a dough. Wrap the cookie dough in waxed paper and chill in the refrigerator for at least 1 hour.

After the dough has chilled, preheat the oven to 325°F. Line a baking sheet with parchment paper.

Place the dough between 2 large sheets of clean waxed paper. Use a rolling pin to roll out the dough to ⅓-inch thickness between the 2 pieces of waxed paper. Cut out shapes using a cookie cutter and place them on the prepared baking sheet.

Gather the leftover dough from the cutouts and roll again between the waxed paper so you can cut out more cookies. Repeat until you have used up all the dough. Once all of the cookies are on the baking sheet, place the baking sheet in the freezer for about 12 minutes to chill the cookies before placing them in the oven.

Bake for 12 to 15 minutes. Cool on the baking sheet for 10 minutes, then transfer to wire racks to cool completely. Store in an airtight container for up to 1 week or place in a freezer-safe container for up to 1 month.

SKINNY MACAROONS

THESE SIMPLE MACAROONS ARE GLUTEN-FREE, GRAIN-FREE, LACTOSE-FREE, SULFITE-FREE, AND refined-sugar-free—and deliciously flavor-full! Naturally sweetened with a small amount of nutritious coconut nectar, they also provide a nice dose of immune-boosting medium-chain triglycerides from coconut for quick, fast-burning energy.

• Makes 36 (1-inch) macaroons •

4 large egg whites

½ cup coconut nectar or raw honey, divided

1 teaspoon pure vanilla extract

3 cups unsweetened shredded coconut, plus more as needed

Preheat the oven to 350°F. Line a baking sheet with parchment paper.

Place the egg whites in a mixing bowl and beat with an electric mixer until stiff peaks form (the meringue should be very stiff and foamy).

Turn off the mixer, add half of the coconut nectar and all of the vanilla, then beat again with the mixer to thoroughly combine. Turn off the mixer and add the remaining coconut nectar, then beat again with the mixer until the mixture is thick and stiff again.

Fold in the shredded coconut by hand with a spatula. Be gentle, so as not to deflate the egg whites. The mixture should be firm. If necessary, add a bit more shredded coconut to thicken up the mixture.

Scoop and press the mixture into a tablespoon-size cookie scoop or round-shaped measuring spoon (the idea is to compact the mixture) to make small, half-dome-shaped macaroons. Space them 1 inch apart on the baking sheet.

Bake for 10 minutes, or until the tops are golden brown. Cool on the baking sheet for 5 minutes, then transfer to wire racks to cool completely. Store in an airtight container for up to 1 week or place in a freezer-safe container for up to 6 months.

VARIATIONS

- For larger macaroons, keep the recipe as is but measure out larger portions for each macaroon and bake for a longer period of time depending on size.
- For almond-flavored macaroons, replace the vanilla extract with almond extract. And, if desired, wrap the coconut mixture around a whole almond before baking.
- Place the cooled macaroons in the freezer for 10 minutes, then dip or drizzle the chilled macaroons with melted homemade chocolate (see recipe 262) and place the macaroons in the refrigerator to allow the chocolate to harden.

DECADENT DAIRY-FREE ICE CREAM

COCONUT MILK, WITH ITS HEALTHY MEDIUM-CHAIN FATS AND CREAMY TEXTURE, MAKES A PERFECT nondairy ice cream that is just as satisfying as milk-based versions, and much healthier! The addition of arrowroot powder helps prevent ice crystals from forming in the ice cream and keeps it soft and scoopable after being stored in the freezer. This recipe is for vanilla ice cream, but it can serve as the base to make many different flavors and varieties of coconut milk ice cream. Use the stevia for a completely sugar-free version.

• Makes 1 quart •

1 tablespoon arrowroot

2 (14-ounce) cans coconut milk, divided

½ cup natural sweetener of choice (see note), or ½ teaspoon liquid stevia extract

1 vanilla bean, or ½ teaspoon vanilla powder

In a small bowl, stir the arrowroot with 2 tablespoons of the coconut milk until thoroughly dissolved. Set aside.

Add the remaining coconut milk, sweetener, and vanilla to a saucepan. (If using a vanilla bean, cut a slit lengthwise in the bean and then add it to the milk mixture in the pan.) Heat the mixture over medium-low heat just until bubbles form at the edges of the pan, stirring to dissolve the sweetener. Do not boil. Remove the pan from the heat.

If you used a vanilla bean, remove it from the pan and scrape out the seeds into the mixture. The more seeds you get, the more vanilla flavor. Discard the vanilla bean pod.

Transfer the mixture to a mixing bowl, cover, and place it in the refrigerator until cold, about 2 hours. When cold, remove it from the fridge and whisk in the arrowroot mixture. Pour the mixture into an ice cream maker and freeze according to the manufacturer's instructions. Store leftovers in an airtight container in the freezer for up to 2 weeks.

VARIATIONS

- To make chocolate ice cream, add ¾ cup unsweetened cocoa powder to the mixture at the same time you add the sweetener and increase the sweetener to ¾ cup (¾ teaspoon stevia).

- To make fresh mint ice cream, add 1 cup coarsely chopped fresh mint leaves to the pan with the coconut milk, sweetener, and vanilla. Allow the mixture to steep in the pan, covered, for 20 minutes once you remove it from the heat. Strain the mixture into a mixing bowl to remove the mint leaves (and vanilla bean, if using) before adding the arrowroot and chilling in the refrigerator.

NOTES:

- You can experiment with different sweeteners in this recipe, like organic unrefined whole cane sugar, coconut crystals, pure maple syrup, coconut nectar, or raw honey. They each give a different flavor. Coconut crystals or nectar provide a caramel flavor, while the raw honey gives the ice cream an almost marshmallow flavor. If you are using stevia, you may want to try a vanilla crème–flavored variety for a more pronounced vanilla flavor.
- Starting from this simple base recipe, you can mix in other ingredients to create your own flavor combos. Extracts and flavoring oils (citrus, mint, lavender, almond, etc.) can be added into the mixture, as well as fresh or frozen fruits. Add solid extras—such as nuts, cacao nibs, chopped or shaved dark chocolate, etc.—after the ice cream has reached the consistency of soft-serve.

CHOCO-CADO MOUSSE

Y OU WON'T BELIEVE THAT THIS DELECTABLE MOUSSE IS MADE FROM AVOCADOS. YOU WON'T taste the avocado, but you'll benefit from its high fiber content and blood sugar–stabilizing compounds. For a sugar-free version, 1 teaspoon of liquid stevia extract can be used in place of the coconut nectar or honey. I highly recommend using a flavored stevia extract, such as chocolate raspberry or vanilla crème. The rose water is optional, but it adds a beautiful depth and flavor to the mousse.

• Makes 8 servings •

4 medium avocados

1 cup coconut nectar or raw honey

1 tablespoon pure vanilla extract

1 cup unsweetened cocoa powder

1 teaspoon organic rose water (page 166 or store-bought; optional)

24 fresh raspberries or other favorite berries, for garnish

1 bunch fresh mint leaves, for garnish

Cut open each avocado and scoop the creamy flesh into the bowl of a food processor. Discard the pits and peels. Add the coconut nectar, vanilla, cocoa powder, and rose water, if using. Process the mixture until fully blended, about 1 to 2 minutes, stopping to scrape down the sides of the bowl if necessary. The mixture should be smooth with no visible chunks of avocado.

The mousse can be served immediately; however, it is recommended to let it chill in the refrigerator for at least 1 hour to allow the flavors to meld and the mousse to firm up. When ready to serve, spoon into 8 custard cups and garnish with fresh berries and mint leaves. This mousse can be stored in the refrigerator for up to 3 days.

SIMPLY PERFECT PUMPKIN PIE

With just a few simple ingredient upgrades, this holiday favorite is transformed into a healthy dessert. You can use any type of crust: whole grain, sprouted grain, or no grain (see options below). You can even go crustless by baking just the filling in a well-oiled pie dish.

• Makes 8 servings •

¾ cup unrefined organic whole cane sugar or coconut sugar

1½ teaspoons ground cinnamon

¾ teaspoon ground ginger

¼ teaspoon ground cloves

½ teaspoon sea salt

2 large eggs

2 cups pumpkin purée (page 70), or 1 (15-ounce) can organic pumpkin purée

¾ cup coconut milk

1 unbaked 9-inch pie crust (see recipes on page 261)

Preheat the oven to 425°F. Mix the sugar, cinnamon, ginger, cloves, and salt in a small bowl. In a large bowl, beat the eggs. Stir in the pumpkin and then add the sugar-spice mixture. Gradually stir in the coconut milk and mix until well blended.

Pour into the unbaked pie shell. Bake for 15 minutes, then reduce the oven temperature to 350°F and bake for an additional 40 to 50 minutes, or until a knife inserted into the center comes out clean. Cool on a wire rack for 2 hours. Serve immediately or refrigerate for up to 1 week. Freeze in a freezer-safe container for up to 1 month.

PIE CRUST OPTIONS:

Store-bought pie crust: If you're not into making your own pie crusts, or if you're in a pinch for time, you can buy a premade 9-inch frozen crust made by a company called Wholly Wholesome. They sell organic whole wheat and whole spelt pie crusts that have a fairly clean ingredient list (they use a negligible amount of organic sugar). You'll find them in the frozen section of natural food markets.

Homemade pie crust: See the recipes on page 261 for whole grain pie crust and grain-free pie crust.

HOMEMADE WHOLE GRAIN OR SPROUTED GRAIN PIE CRUST

HERE'S A SIMPLE RECIPE FOR MAKING YOUR OWN 9-INCH PIE CRUST. YOU CAN USE WHITE WHOLE wheat flour, traditional whole wheat flour, whole spelt flour, or the sprouted versions of these flours. To make two crusts, double all ingredients and divide dough in half.

• Makes 1 (9-inch) pie crust •

1 cup whole grain or sprouted grain flour

½ teaspoon sea salt

⅓ cup virgin coconut oil or organic butter, chilled

2 tablespoons cold water, plus more as needed

1 teaspoon raw organic unfiltered apple cider vinegar

Combine the flour and salt in a medium bowl; cut in the oil with a pastry cutter or two knives until the mixture is crumbly. Sprinkle with the water and vinegar and blend until the mixture holds together. Add an additional tablespoon of cold water if needed.

Shape the dough into a ball and place on a lightly floured surface. Roll out the dough to ⅛ inch thickness. Coat a 9-inch pie dish with butter or coconut oil. Line the pie dish with the crust. Turn the edges under and crimp as desired. Fill with pie filling and bake according to the recipe.

GLUTEN-FREE, GRAIN-FREE COCONUT FLOUR PIE CRUST

THIS CRUST WILL BE FLAKY AND BUTTERY, BUT DIFFERENT FROM A REGULAR FLOUR CRUST. THE taste and texture is reminiscent of shortbread and is surprisingly tasty.

• Makes 1 (9-inch) pie crust •

¼ cup organic butter, at room temperature

2 tablespoons virgin coconut oil, at room
    temperature, or coconut milk

1 cup coconut flour

3 large eggs

Pinch of sea salt

 1 tablespoon water

Place all ingredients into a mixing bowl and blend well with an electric mixer until it forms a ball of dough. Coat a 9-inch pie dish with coconut oil or butter. Place the ball of dough into the pie dish, and press down to spread and shape the crust evenly across the bottom and up the sides. Crimp the edges as desired. Fill with pie filling and bake according to the recipe.

SIMPLY SKINNY CHOCOLATE BARS

THE ADVANTAGE OF MAKING YOUR OWN CHOCOLATE IS THAT YOU CAN CONTROL THE TYPE AND amount of sweetener and leave out undesirable additives that often show up even in organic dark chocolate bars. Not only is it healthier, homemade chocolate is fun, quick, and easy. All you need are a few simple ingredients you probably already have in your kitchen. Start with this simple basic recipe, then experiment with adding other ingredients such as chopped nuts, goji berries, sea salt, mint extract, chili powder, etc. The possibilities are endless!

• Makes 16 (1-ounce) servings •

½ cup virgin coconut oil

¼ cup coconut nectar, or 1 teaspoon liquid
    stevia extract

1 teaspoon pure vanilla extract, or ½ teaspoon
    vanilla powder

1 cup raw cacao powder or unsweetened
    cocoa powder

Warm the coconut oil in a small saucepan over low heat until melted and warm to the touch. Transfer the coconut oil to a small mixing bowl and whisk in the coconut nectar and vanilla. Add the cacao powder and whisk again until smooth and thick.

Pour into a small (about 6 x 3-inch) rectangular or square container with sides, such as a Pyrex dish or other type of storage container, or use truffle-size candy molds. Place the container in the freezer until the chocolate is completely hardened.

Once the chocolate has hardened, cut it into bars, chop or break it into chunks, or chop it into small pieces to use for chocolate chips. Store in the refrigerator or freezer for up to 1 month.

To use the chocolate as a coating for dates, bananas, cookies, etc., use it before hardening.

CHOCOLATE-COVERED FROZEN BANANA BITES

THESE SNACK-SIZE, SUGAR-FREE, HEALTHY BONBONS ARE THE PERFECT BITE WHEN THAT CRAVING for "a little something sweet" hits. Bananas frozen at their peak of ripeness are as creamy and sweet as ice cream. When sliced and dipped in chocolate, they're absolutely divine!

• Makes about 30 (½-inch) pieces •

2 large ripe bananas, peeled and sliced into
   ½-inch pieces
¼ cup virgin coconut oil
1 teaspoon pure vanilla extract

1 teaspoon liquid stevia extract
¼ cup raw cacao powder or unsweetened
   cocoa powder
½ cup raw chopped walnuts

Line a baking sheet with waxed paper. Skewer each piece of banana with a toothpick and place on the baking sheet. Freeze until hard, about 1 hour.

While the banana pieces are freezing, warm the coconut oil in a small saucepan over low heat until melted and warm to the touch. Transfer the coconut oil to a small mixing bowl and whisk in the vanilla and stevia. Add the cacao powder and whisk again until smooth and thick. Set aside.

Once the banana pieces are frozen, spread the chopped walnuts on a plate. Use the toothpicks to dip each banana piece in the chocolate mixture. Coat completely and then quickly roll the chocolate-covered banana bite in the chopped walnuts to coat. Place the banana bite back onto the lined baking sheet. Repeat with the remaining pieces of banana. Place the banana bites back in the freezer to allow the chocolate to harden, about 5 minutes. When the chocolate has hardened, enjoy!

Store the banana bites in a tightly sealed freezer-safe container for up to 3 months. Eat the bites directly from the freezer; once they thaw, the chocolate melts and the bananas become mushy.

JOYFUL CHOCOLATE ALMOND BARS

WITH JUST A FOOD PROCESSOR AND A FEW SIMPLE INGREDIENTS, YOU CAN CREATE AN AMAZING and nutritious rival to the processed Almond Joy candy bar. If you don't feel like a nut, you can leave the almonds out!

• Makes 12 pieces •

1 cup unsweetened shredded coconut

¼ cup plus 3 tablespoons virgin coconut oil, melted, divided

2 tablespoons coconut nectar or raw honey

2 teaspoons pure vanilla extract, divided

Small pinch of sea salt (just a few grains)

24 raw almonds

2 teaspoons liquid stevia extract

½ cup raw cacao powder or unsweetened cocoa powder

Place the shredded coconut, 3 tablespoons of the coconut oil, coconut nectar, 1 teaspoon of the vanilla, and salt into the bowl of a food processor. Process until it forms a thick paste, about 2 minutes. Squeeze a small amount of the coconut mixture in the palm of your hand to see if it sticks and holds together. If it's still too loose, process the mixture again for another 2 minutes.

Line a tray or plate with waxed paper. Divide the mixture into 12 tablespoon-size balls and place them on the tray. Press each coconut ball down to flatten, and then use your fingers to shape and compact them into ovals. Top each oval with two almonds, pressing down slightly to create an indentation.

Place the coconut bars in the freezer for 10 to 20 minutes, or until hard.

While the coconut ovals are freezing, warm the remaining ¼ cup coconut oil in a small saucepan over low heat until it is warm to the touch. Transfer the warm coconut oil to a small mixing bowl and whisk in the stevia and remaining teaspoon of vanilla. Add the cacao powder and whisk again to combine until the chocolate is smooth and thick.

Once the coconut bars are hard, use a toothpick as a skewer to dip each bar into the chocolate mixture to completely coat with chocolate. Return it to the waxed paper and remove the toothpick.

Place the bars in the refrigerator for a few minutes to let the chocolate completely harden. Store in an airtight container in the refrigerator for up to 3 months. Eat the bars directly from the refrigerator; if they are left out for too long the chocolate starts to melt.

HONEY LEMON CREAM CHEESE FROSTING OR FILLING

THIS RECIPE GIVES YOU A HEALTHIER ALTERNATIVE TO THE CONVENTIONAL FROSTINGS MADE FROM powdered sugar and shortening. It can be used to frost cakes and cupcakes, but is versatile enough to be a filling for muffins (see page 133) or stuffed dates, a spread for toast or crackers, or a dip for apple slices, celery, and jicama.

• Makes ¾ cup •

¾ cup organic Neufchâtel cream cheese, at room temperature

2 tablespoons raw honey

1 tablespoon freshly grated lemon zest

¼ teaspoon pure vanilla extract

Place all ingredients in a large bowl and stir with a rubber spatula until well blended. Store in an airtight container in the refrigerator for up to 2 weeks.

GRAIN-FREE, NO-BAKE
CHOCOLATE ORANGE CAKE

MAKE THIS CAKE FOR SPECIAL OCCASIONS SUCH AS BIRTHDAYS AND OTHER CELEBRATIONS. THIS IS A nutrient-rich, decadent treat made entirely from raw ingredients, with a consistency remarkably like a real chocolate cake. There's no baking involved, but you will need a good food processor or high-powered blender. This cake can be decorated with just fresh fruit, if desired, but for a more cake-like experience, you can make the cashew frosting. It's delicious either way. If you've never had a raw cake, prepare to be amazed!

• Makes 1 (8-inch) layered cake or 2 (8-inch) single cakes •

CAKE

14 Medjool dates, pitted

3 cups almond meal (page 71 or store-bought)

Peel from 2 oranges or 4 tangerines (the entire peel, not just the zest), finely chopped using a mini food chopper or high-powered blender

½ cup raw cacao powder

1 tablespoon virgin coconut oil

½ cup raw honey

1 teaspoon pure vanilla extract

½ teaspoon sea salt

½ cup unsweetened shredded coconut, plus more as needed

FROSTING

1 cup raw cashews, soaked for 1 hour, then drained, rinsed, and patted dry

¼ cup water

¼ cup coconut cream concentrate

2 tablespoons raw honey

1 teaspoon pure vanilla extract

1 teaspoon almond extract

½ teaspoon sea salt

TOPPING DECORATIONS

1 cup assorted fresh berries (blueberries, raspberries, and sliced kiwis or strawberries work best)

A few fresh mint leaves

 15 to 20 raw cashew halves or other nuts

To make the cake, place the dates in a food processor or blender and pulse until they form a sticky paste. Add the almond meal and orange peel and pulse again to combine thoroughly. Add the rest of the cake ingredients and process until it forms a big ball of firm "dough." If the mixture is not firm enough, add more shredded coconut.

Place the ball of dough onto a flat plate. At this point you can decide what presentation you want to make (desired shape, frosting, fruit toppings). Using your hands, press the dough into your desired shape. For example, shape the dough into a cake shape. Decorate it with just fresh fruit or make the frosting recipe, frost it, and then decorate with fruit and nuts.

You could also split the dough in half and press each half into a cake shape, add some fruit or frosting to the top of the bottom half, then put the other half on top for a layer-cake effect.

Once shaped, refrigerate until chilled.

To make the frosting, place all of the frosting ingredients into a food processor or high-powered blender and process on high until it becomes thick, smooth, and creamy like a frosting. If it's too thick, add water by the tablespoon until you get the right consistency.

Spread the frosting evenly over the cake(s). Decorate with fruit, mint leaves, and nuts as desired. The cake may be served immediately, but it is best when refrigerated for at least 2 hours to allow both the cake and the frosting to chill and harden up a bit. The cake itself and the frosting will keep in the refrigerator for up to 1 week, so if you are making the cake ahead of time, you may want to wait before topping it with fresh fruit. Store in an airtight cake keeper or other large covered container, or wrap carefully with plastic wrap after the cake has chilled and hardened for 2 hours, to prevent the wrap from sticking to the frosting.

NOTE:

To make a smaller quantity of dough for just one layer, you can reduce the number of dates in the recipe by half, without changing the amounts of the other ingredients. You can also shape the dough into small individual "cupcakes."

Metric Conversions

The recipes in this book have not been tested with metric measurements, so some variations might occur.

Remember that the weight of dry ingredients varies according to the volume or density factor: 1 cup of flour weighs far less than 1 cup of sugar, and 1 tablespoon doesn't necessarily hold 3 teaspoons.

General Formula for Metric Conversion

Ounces to grams	Multiply ounces by 28.35
Grams to ounces	Multiply grams by 0.035
Pounds to grams	Multiply pounds by 453.5
Pounds to kilograms	Multiply pounds by 0.45
Cups to liters	Multiply cups by 0.24
Fahrenheit to Celsius	Subtract 32 from Fahrenheit temperature, multiply by 5, divide by 9
Celsius to Fahrenheit	Multiply Celsius temperature by 9, divide by 5, add 32

Volume (Liquid) Measurements

1 teaspoon = ⅙ fluid ounce = 5 milliliters
1 tablespoon = ½ fluid ounce = 15 milliliters
2 tablespoons = 1 fluid ounce = 30 milliliters
¼ cup = 2 fluid ounces = 60 milliliters
⅓ cup = 2⅔ fluid ounces = 79 milliliters
½ cup = 4 fluid ounces = 118 milliliters
1 cup or ½ pint = 8 fluid ounces = 250 milliliters
2 cups or 1 pint = 16 fluid ounces = 500 milliliters
4 cups or 1 quart = 32 fluid ounces = 1,000 milliliters
1 gallon = 4 liters

Linear Measure

½ inch = 1⅓ cm
1 inch = 2½ cm
6 inches = 15 cm
8 inches = 20 cm
10 inches = 25 cm
12 inches = 30 cm
20 inches = 50 cm

Volume (Dry) Measurements

¼ teaspoon = 1 milliliter	½ cup = 118 milliliters
½ teaspoon = 2 milliliters	⅔ cup = 158 milliliters
¾ teaspoon = 4 milliliters	¾ cup = 177 milliliters
1 teaspoon = 5 milliliters	1 cup = 225 milliliters
1 tablespoon = 15 milliliters	4 cups or 1 quart = 1 liter
¼ cup = 59 milliliters	½ gallon = 2 liters
⅓ cup = 79 milliliters	1 gallon = 4 liters

Weight (Mass) Measurements

1 ounce = 30 grams
2 ounces = 55 grams
3 ounces = 85 grams
4 ounces = ¼ pound = 125 grams
8 ounces = ½ pound = 240 grams
12 ounces = ¾ pound = 375 grams
16 ounces = 1 pound = 454 grams

Oven Temperature Equivalents Fahrenheit (F) and Celsius (C)

100°F = 38°C
200°F = 95°C
250°F = 120°C
300°F = 150°C
350°F = 180°C
400°F = 205°C
450°F = 230°C

Acknowledgments

Writing this cookbook, including its previous iterations, has been over ten years in the making. It started as a simple collection of recipes designed to help people enjoy tasty meals without white flour and white sugar. With each iteration, it has evolved into something much greater than I could have imagined. At times it felt like an arduous chore, and I often wondered if I could actually ever finish it. In my head, I knew exactly what I wanted to put into the book, but getting it out of me and onto the page proved to be more challenging than I ever realized. To make matters more difficult, my recipe collection kept growing, and it took great restraint and discernment to stay focused on my original selections. In the end, this cookbook is exactly what I have always intended it to be—a resource for processed-free living that you can come back to over and over again.

At each step in its development, many special people have freely contributed their time and talent in numerous ways to support my work. First, it is nearly impossible to find words to express my deep love and appreciation for Michael, my partner and husband extraordinaire. Your dreams for me have always surpassed my own. It was from your loving prompting that *Dee's Mighty Cookbook* was born, and from your continued love and unwavering support that *The Science of Skinny* and this companion cookbook are possible. You wore many hats in the development of this book—from graciously tasting nearly every recipe and offering your unbiased comments, to coordinating and styling the food for the photo sessions. You are a remarkable man who I am unbelievably blessed and grateful to have as my life partner. Thank you for being the man of my life.

The following people round out my culinary and literary gratitude list:

My mother, Carol, for your love, strength, and encouragement to live my dreams. I kept you close in my heart during my marathon writing sessions.

My sister Rene, my lifelong friend and cooking partner. Thank you for your recipe suggestions and for always believing in me. Your love is a cherished gift.

Silvio Rone, for your keen eye, artistic suggestions, and exceptionally gifted photography. Your warm sense of humor made our culinary photo sessions an effortless joy. Thank you for your kindness, generosity, and longstanding friendship.

Nancy Dirstine, our valued Processed-Free America board member and treasured friend. Thank you for lending your time, your home, your dishes, and your creative eye for our culinary photo sessions. We are deeply grateful for your amazing support and dedication to our mission.

Kristine Heidrich, my recipe-creation partner, fitness coach, mirror, and role model. Thank you for sharing your kitchen with me. It is always a pleasure to cook for you and with you. Your love and support inspire me to live fully.

Tanner Goodsell, my biggest fan, supporter and contributor of recipes and encouraging words to our online community. Your selfless dedication and passion for healthy cooking is über appreciated and incredibly inspiring. I know you *will be* a fabulous natural chef someday.

Lavonia Nowell, who singlehandedly set all of east Texas on fire for *The Science of Skinny* and Processed-Free Living. You are my loudest cheerleader and my cherished friend. Words cannot convey my gratitude for your deep faith and devotion to my work.

Bob Cash, who holds the distinct talent of being both a fabulous cook and an extraordinary editor. Thank you for inspiring me to write about cooking.

Jerry Bolfrass, whose culinary expertise, enthusiasm, and charisma infused our early test kitchen with high energy and fierce love for cooking. Thank you for your contributions in making many of my recipes exciting and tasty. I value and treasure your loyalty and friendship.

An enormous thank you to my editor, Renée Sedliar, at Da Capo Lifelong Books for your encouragement, support, guidance, and belief in me and my work. This author has never been so grateful and humbled by your amazing understanding and kindness. Thank you for filling in the holes, moving my words into place, and boosting my spirits more than you'll ever know.

Much appreciation goes to the talented editorial, design, publicity, and marketing teams at Da Capo Lifelong Books. Thank you for bringing this project to life.

I offer my heartfelt gratitude to my literary agent, Andrea Somberg, who believed in *The Science of Skinny* from the very beginning.

Also, my deepest appreciation goes to WNPR Connecticut talk show host Faith Middleton for her wonderful repeated airplay of *The Science of Skinny* interview. You have truly made an impact in spreading the processed-free message.

Thank you also to my wonderful clients, students, processed-free support group leaders and members, and online friends and followers. Your kind words and positive *Science of Skinny* experiences are inspiring and a testament to the healing power of whole natural foods. Thank you for attending my lectures, cooking workshops, and online classes—many of you have been with me since the early days when *Dee's Mighty Muffins* and *Dee's Mighty Cookbook* first appeared in our local natural food markets over ten years ago. I would not be where I am today without your continued admiration and support.

Resources

Recommended Foods and Products Guide

This section contains information to help you find products and foods that are healthy and free of processed ingredients. Some are available in natural food markets or mainstream grocery stores, and some are only available through online retailers.

To the best of my knowledge, I am recommending products and companies whose health goals are closely aligned with mine at the time of this writing. However, please understand that companies reserve the right to change their goals or ingredients without notifying customers. Such changes may render the product out of alignment with a processed-free lifestyle; therefore, it is always important to read ingredient lists and to do your own checking on any product that you buy.

I have no connection to any of the companies or products listed. They are all recommended without compensation from the company. However, many of the items I recommend are available through the Processed-Free America Amazon affiliate link.

What this means is that if you shop through our Amazon affiliate store, a very small percentage of your entire order goes back to Processed-Free America, and it doesn't cost you any more than what you would normally pay when shopping on Amazon. The small commission we receive helps to fund the nutrition programs we offer to children, and it's a nice way to say "thanks" for the wealth of information that we freely share on our website.

If you are going to purchase any of the recommended items through Amazon, please consider buying them through our Amazon affiliate store at www.processedfreeamerica.org /store.

Wild-Caught Fish

Vital Choice Wild Seafood and Organics:
www.vitalchoice.com

Vital Choice offers home delivery of the world's finest wild seafood and organic fare: premium frozen, canned, and pouched fish products, including many no-salt-added and kosher options.

WILD PLANET FOODS:

www.wildplanetfoods.com

Wild Planet offers sustainably caught wild tuna, salmon, and sardines in cans and single-serve pouches. Available in natural food markets, Costco, and online.

Organic Grass-Fed Meats and Pastured Poultry

The following websites offer a good selection of meats and poultry. Some also carry organic grass-fed butter and raw cheeses:

GRASSLAND BEEF:

www.grasslandbeef.com

GRASS-FED TRADITIONS:

www.grassfedtraditions.com

AMERICAN GRASS-FED BEEF:

www.americangrassfedbeef.com

TROPICAL TRADITIONS:

www.tropicaltraditions.com

Organic Deli Meat

APPLEGATE FARMS:

www.applegatefarms.com

Applegate Farms does not use grass-fed meats or pastured poultry, but if you are going to eat deli meats, this is the brand you want. Products are available in natural food markets and the company's online store.

Organic Grass-Fed Milk, Butter, Raw Cheeses, and Other Dairy Products

ORGANIC VALLEY:

www.organicvalley.coop

Organic Valley is the only national brand to produce organic milk from cows that are 100 percent grass-fed. This specialty milk, called Grassmilk, is minimally pasteurized and not homogenized, and still has the cream on top. Organic Valley produces two varieties of organic raw Cheddar cheese made from Grassmilk.

The company also produces a variety of other organic dairy foods from cows that are grass-fed (but not 100 percent). Organic Valley dairy products are sold in natural food markets, supermarkets, and food cooperatives nationwide. Check the website for store locations.

KALONA SUPER NATURAL DAIRY PRODUCTS:

www.kalonasupernatural.com

Kalona offers organic dairy products that come from small, sustainable farms raising grass-fed cows. The milk is minimally pasteurized and not homogenized. Products include milk, yogurt, sour cream, cottage cheese, and butter. Check the website for store locations. Kalona Super Natural butter is also available at www.tropicaltraditions.com.

COONRIDGE ORGANIC GOAT CHEESE:

www.coonridge.com

This amazing company based in Pie Town, New Mexico, offers sixteen varieties of gourmet organic herbed goat cheeses. The goats are never fed any grains, and they freely roam for long distances to feed on wild high-desert plants. They also offer a raw goat milk feta with fresh garlic oil that is out of this world! Available through their online store.

KERRYGOLD BUTTER:

www.kerrygoldusa.com

Kerrygold relies on a cooperative of small Irish dairy farmers with centuries of natural traditions to turn the sweet, rich, grass-fed cow's milk into delicious cheese and butter. The milk is not homogenized and is minimally pasteurized. Kerrygold butter and cheese are sold in natural food markets and mainstream grocery stores nationwide.

REDWOOD HILL FARM GOAT MILK PRODUCTS:

www.redwoodhill.com

This family-owned goat dairy farm and creamery offers artisan goat milk cheese, yogurt, and kefir. Redwood Hill Farm products are sold in natural food markets and supermarkets nationwide, and also through their online store. Check the website for store locations.

GREEN VALLEY ORGANICS LACTOSE-FREE YOGURT, KEFIR, AND SOUR CREAM:

www.greenvalleylactosefree.com

Green Valley Organics is dedicated to producing the purest, best-tasting milk for their lactose-free dairy products. No chemicals are used, and the nutritional components of the milk are not altered in any way. Green Valley Organics products are sold in natural food markets. Check the website for store locations.

Organic Grass-Fed Whey Protein Concentrate

The highest-quality whey protein powder consists only of whey protein concentrate, is derived from the milk of organic grass-fed cows, and is free of chemicals, GMOs, soy lecithin, sugar, and artificial sweeteners. Additionally, it is cold processed (as opposed to heat processed) without the use of acid. This method preserves the whey's protein structures in their biologically active forms. The following whey protein concentrate powders meet this criteria:

RAW ORGANIC WHEY:

www.raworganicwhey.com

Available at www.processedfreeamerica.org/store.

ONE WORLD WHEY:

www.sgn80.com/one-world-whey

Available at www.processedfreeamerica.org/store.

Sprouted Breads and Bread Products

FOOD FOR LIFE BAKING COMPANY:

www.foodforlife.com

Food for Life is the maker of Ezekiel 4:9 breads, tortillas, English muffins, buns, pocket breads, pasta, and cereals. Available nationwide in natural food markets and some mainstream grocery stores.

Sprouted Whole Grains and Sprouted Flours for Cooking and Baking

TO YOUR HEALTH SPROUTED FLOUR COMPANY:

www.organicsproutedflour.net

This is your one-stop online shop for organic sprouted grains and organic sprouted flours, as well as organic unsprouted grains and flours.

ONE DEGREE ORGANIC FOODS:

www.onedegreeorganics.com

One Degree offers organic sprouted wheat flour and organic sprouted spelt flour in five-pound bags.

WILD ROOTS FOODS:

www.wildrootsfoods.com

Wild Roots Foods sells sprouted brown rice in a sealed four-pound package. Available at select Walmart, Sam's Club, and Costco stores. Check the website for store locations.

TRU ROOTS:

www.truroots.com

Tru Roots sells a variety of sprouted grains, beans, and legumes individually and in blends. Available in natural food markets.

Whole Grains, Whole Grain Flour, Whole Grain Pasta, Non-GMO Masa Harina

BOB'S RED MILL:
www.bobsredmill.com
Bob's Red Mill offers a large line of natural, certified-organic, non-GMO cornmeal, masa harina, gluten-free grains, flours, dried beans, and baking mixes.

EDEN FOODS:
www.edenfoods.com
Eden Foods has a unique offering of uncommon whole grains and pastas such as kamut, spelt, buckwheat, and quinoa in a variety of shapes and sizes.

WILDERNESS FAMILY NATURALS:
www.wildernessfamilynaturals.com
Wilderness Family Naturals has a selection of exotic rice and organic ancient grains such as teff, amaranth, and quinoa.

ANCIENT HARVEST QUINOA:
www.quinoa.net
Ancient Harvest offers a line of quinoa products including flakes, flour, and pasta.

PURCELL MOUNTAIN FARMS:
www.purcellmountainfarms.com
Purcell Mountain Farms offers non-GMO masa harina and a variety of organic grains, beans, exotic rice, and chiles.

TINKYADA PASTA JOY:
www.tinkyada.com
Tinkyada offers a wide variety of brown rice pasta in many different shapes and sizes.

VITASPELT:
www.natureslegacyforlife.com

VitaSpelt offers organic whole grain spelt kernels, spelt flour, and spelt pastas.

Coconut Flour

These brands are available in natural food markets and www.processedfreeamerica.org/store.

COCONUT SECRET:
www.coconutsecret.com
NUTIVA:
www.nutiva.com
BOB'S RED MILL:
www.bobsredmill.com

Almond Meal (Unblanched Almond Flour)

These brands are available in natural food markets and www.processedfreeamerica.org/store.

NOW FOODS NATURAL UNBLANCHED ALMOND FLOUR:
www.nowfoods.com
HONEYVILLE FARMS NATURAL ALMOND FLOUR (UNBLANCHED):
www.shop.honeyville.com/
TRADER JOE'S Almond Meal:
www.traderjoes.com

Canned and Jarred Items (Beans, Tomatoes, Pumpkin)

EDEN FOODS:
www.edenfoods.com
Eden Foods provides a large selection of organic cooked beans, lentils, and other bean favorites, all in BPA-free cans. The company also produces many other healthy organic products such as jarred tomatoes, tomato-based sauces, whole grains and pastas, unrefined oils, sea vegetables, condiments, dried herbs, spices, and more. Available in most natural food markets.

FARMER'S MARKET:

www.farmersmarketfoods.com

Farmer's Market brand provides canned organic pumpkin purée, organic sweet potato purée, and organic butternut squash in BPA-free cans and tetrapaks. Available in most natural food markets.

Unrefined Culinary Oils

The following oils are available in natural food markets, through the company's online store, and at www.processedfreeamerica.org/store.

Organic Virgin Coconut Oil

TROPICAL TRADITIONS:

www.tropicaltraditions.com

Also, at www.processedfreeamerica.org there are links to Tropical Traditions coconut oil and other products. If you order by clicking on any of those links and have never ordered from Tropical Traditions in the past, you will receive a free book on virgin coconut oil, and I will receive a discount coupon for referring you. It's a win-win for all of us!

Organic Extra-Virgin Olive Oil

BRAGG:

www.bragg.com

EDEN FOODS:

www.edenfoods.com

Unrefined Sesame Oil, Unrefined Toasted Sesame Oil:

EDEN FOODS:

www.edenfoods.com

SPECTRUM ORGANICS:

www.spectrumorganics.com

Unrefined Peanut Oil

SPECTRUM ORGANICS:

www.spectrumorganics.com

Non-hydrogenated Organic Palm Oil Shortening

SPECTRUM ORGANICS:

www.spectrumorganics.com

TROPICAL TRADITIONS:

www.tropicaltraditions.com

Vinegars

The following vinegars are available in natural food markets, through the company's online store, and at www.processedfreeamerica.org/store.

Apple Cider Vinegar, Raw Organic Unfiltered

BRAGG:

www.bragg.com

EDEN FOODS:

www.edenfoods.com

Balsamic Vinegar

FINI MODENA Balsamic Vinegar of Modena (Aceto Balsamico di Modena)**:**

www.acetaiafini.it

VILLA MANODORI Organic Aceto Balsamico di Modena**:**

www.demedici.com

Brown Rice Vinegar

EDEN FOODS:

www.edenfoods.com

Coconut Vinegar

TROPICAL TRADITIONS:

www.tropicaltraditions.com

Coconut Secret:
www.coconutsecret.com

Red Wine Vinegar, Raw Unpasteurized
Eden Foods:
www.edenfoods.com

Dressings and Condiments

The following dressings and condiments are available in natural food markets, through the company's online store, and at www.processed freeamerica.org/store.

Liquid Aminos
Bragg Liquid Aminos:
www.bragg.com
Coconut Secret Coconut Aminos:
www.coconutsecret.com

Mayonnaise
Wilderness Family Naturals:
www.wildernessfamilynaturals.com
Wilderness Family Naturals offers the best mayonnaise available anywhere, along with a unique selection of items not found in the chain natural food markets. Along with natural food items, you'll find kitchen tools and appliances, books, and beauty products.

Mirin (Rice Cooking Wine)
Eden Foods:
www.edenfoods.com

Salad Dressing
Bragg:
www.bragg.com
Wilderness Family Naturals:
www.wildernessfamilynaturals.com

Tahini
Joyva:
www.joyva.com
Arrowhead Mills:
www.arrowheadmills.com

Tamari Sauce, Gluten-Free, Reduced Sodium
San-J:
www.san-j.com

Jams/Fruit Preserves
Bionaturae:
www.bionaturae.com
St. Dalfour:
www.stdalfour.us

Grass-Fed Gelatin

The best gelatin is produced from the highest-quality grass-fed cows using methods that virtually eliminate the formation of monosodium glutamate (MSG). The following two brands meet this criteria. Both are available at www .processedfreeamerica.org/store.
Bernard Jensen:
www.bernardjensen.com
Great Lakes:
www.greatlakesgelatin.com

Agar-Agar, Sea Vegetables, and Miso

Sea vegetables are typically found in Asian markets or natural food markets. The following brands can also be found at www.processedfree america.org/store.

Agar-Agar Powder
Telephone Brand:
www.amazon.com

NOW Foods:
www.nowfoods.com

Agar-Agar Flakes
Eden Foods:
www.edenfoods.com

Sea Vegetables
Marine Coast Sea Vegetables:
www.seaveg.com
Eden Foods:
www.edenfoods.com

Miso
Eden Foods Shiro Miso, Reclosable Pouch:
www.edenfoods.com
Marukome All-Natural Miso, Reduced Sodium:
www.marukomeusa.com

Organic Fruit Juices
Lakewood Organic:
www.lakewoodjuices.com
Available in natural food markets and at www
.processedfreeamerica.org/store.

Sweeteners
The following sweeteners are available in natural food markets, through the company's online store, and at www.processedfreeamerica.org/store.

Stevia
SweetLeaf Stevia Concentrate Dark Liquid, Stevia Clear Sweet Drops, and Stevia Powders:
http://www.sweetleaf.com

Organic Barley Malt Syrup
Eden Foods:
www.edenfoods.com

Blackstrap Molasses, Unsulphured Organic
Wholesome Sweeteners:
www.wholesomesweeteners.com

Brown Rice Syrup
Lundberg Family Farms:
www.lundberg.com

Coconut Nectar
Coconut Secret:
www.coconutsecret.com

Coconut Crystals, Coconut Sugar
Coconut Secret:
www.coconutsecret.com
Navitas Naturals:
www.navitasnaturals.com
Madhava:
www.madhavasweeteners.com

Date Sugar
NOW Foods:
www.nowfoods.com
Bob's Red Mill:
www.bobsredmill.com

Organic Whole Cane Sugar, Unrefined and Unbleached
Rapunzel:
www.internaturalfoods.com/brands (also available at www.tropicaltraditions.com)

Sucanat
Wholesome Sweeteners:
www.wholesomesweeteners.com

Raw Honey

Wholesome Sweeteners:
www.wholesomesweeteners.com
Y.S. Organic Bee Farm:
www.ysorganic.com
Really Raw Honey:
www.reallyrawhoney.com

Pure Maple Syrup, Maple Sugar

Coombs Family Farms:
www.coombsfamilyfarms.com

Cacao/Chocolate/Carob

The following products are made from pure ingredients without soy lecithin or refined sugars. Available in natural food markets and through the company's online stores.

Raw Cacao Nibs/Raw Cacao Powder

Navitas:
www.navitasnaturals.com
Sunfood Super Foods:
www.sunfood.com
Wilderness Family Naturals:
www.wildernessfamilynaturals.com

Unsweetened Baking Chocolate Bar, 100 percent Cacao

Sunspire:
www.sunspire.com

Organic Chocolate Chips (soy-free, vegan, and gluten-free)

Equal Exchange Organic Bittersweet Chocolate Chips (70 percent Cacao) and Organic Semi-Sweet Chocolate Chips (55 percent Cacao):
www.equalexchange.coop (also available at www.tropicaltraditions.com)

Organic Chocolate Bars

Equal Exchange Organic Panama Extra Dark Chocolate Bar 80 percent Cacao:
www.equalexchange.coop/products/chocolate
Righteously Raw Chocolate Bars:
www.righteouslyrawchocolate.com

Carob Powder

Bob's Red Mill:
www.bobsredmill.com
Chatfield's:
www.chatfieldsbrand.com

Raw Nuts and Seeds

Living Nutz:
www.livingnutz.com

Cranberries, Dried Unsweetened

Cherry Bay Orchards:
www.cherrybayorchards.com
My only known source of unsweetened dried cranberries without oil. Available from their online store and at www.processedfreeamerica.org/store.

Herbal Coffee

Dandy Blend:
www.dandyblend.com
This tasty instant herbal coffee substitute is caffeine-free, gluten-free, and non-GMO. Made from a blend of the extracts of dandelion root, beetroot, chicory, barley, and rye, it has a rich, full-bodied flavor with the smoothness and texture of real coffee. Available from their online store and at www.processedfreeamerica.org/store.
Teeccino:
www.teeccino.com

This herbal coffee is a delicious blend of herbs, grains, fruits, and nuts that are roasted and ground to brew and taste just like coffee. The Teeccino line offers a variety of roast types and unique flavors. Teeccino is distributed to natural food and specialty grocery stores nationwide, is available through their online store, and at www.processedfreeamerica.org/store.

Coconut Milk

The following are brands that are truly 100 percent coconut milk with no preservatives. Available in natural food markets and at www.processedfreeamerica.org/store.

Natural Value (comes in BPA-free cans): www.naturalvalue.com

Aroy-D (comes in a BPA-Free aseptic carton): www.importfood.com/naturalcoconutmilk.html

Golden Star: www.goldenstartrading.com

Coconut Cream Concentrate (Coconut Butter)

These are the best coconut cream concentrates you'll find anywhere. Tropical Traditions has better pricing per ounce. Artisana is available in natural food markets. Both are available at www.processedfreeamerica.org/store.

Tropical Traditions Coconut Cream Concentrate: www.tropicaltraditions.com

Artisana Coconut Butter: www.artisana.com

Coconut Water

Harmless Harvest 100% Raw and Organic Coconut Water:

www.harmlesscoconut.com Available at natural food markets nationwide. Check the website for locations.

Coco Libre Pure Organic Coconut Water: www.cocolibreorganic.com

Spices, Seasonings, Extracts, and Flavors

Herbamare: www.herbamare.us

Sea Salt

Eden Foods: www.edenfoods.com

Real Salt: www.realsalt.com

Himalayan Pink Salt

Trader Joe's: www.traderjoes.com

Himalania: www.himalania.com (also available at www.tropicaltraditions.com)

Spices

Simply Organic Spices: www.simplyorganic.com

Frontier Natural Products Co-op: www.frontiercoop.com

Spice Hunter: www.spicehunter.com

Vanilla Extracts, Flavors, and Powders

The Vanilla Company: www.vanilla.com

Sun Food Superfoods: www.sunfood.com

Rose Water

Organic Bulgarian Rose Water:

www.bulgarianrosewater.com (also available at www.processedfreeamerica.org/store)

Alkalizing and Liver-izing Supplements

The following are recommended supplements for helping you balance your body pH and support your body's main detoxifying and fat-burning organ. All products are available at www.processedfreeamerica.org/store.

Amazing Grass Green SuperFood Powder:

www.amazinggrass.com

Amazing Grass is a blend of dehydrated alkalizing and detoxifying greens, fruits, and supportive herbs combined into a delicious-tasting powder that mixes well with water, nondairy milk, juice, smoothies, or your favorite beverage.

Oregon's Wild Harvest Milk Thistle & Dandelion Root:

www.oregonswildharvest.com

Many clinical studies have demonstrated that milk thistle provides potent antioxidant protection against free radicals and other liver toxins. Dandelion has been used traditionally to stimulate the liver to produce more bile and assists in breaking down fats.

pHion Diagnosis pH Test Strips:

www.phionbalance.com

These are the best pH testing strips available. Use them to see if your body is overly acidic or in an optimal pH state.

Kitchen Equipment and Supplies

The Bluapple:

www.thebluapple.com

An absorbent pouch housed in a small blue apple-shaped plastic container that can be placed in your crisper drawers, on the shelves in your refrigerator, or anywhere you keep fruits and vegetables. The Bluapple absorbs ethylene gas and extends the useful storage life of your produce up to three times longer than normal. This really works! Available in the produce department of grocery stores and online at www.processedfreeamerica.org/store.

Coconut Meat Knife Tool:

www.thecoconuttool.com

Makes removing the meat out of a mature coconut very easy. Available online at www.processedfreeamerica.org/store.

Nut-Milk Strainer Bag:

www.processedfreeamerica.org/store, www.purejoyplanet.com

This drawstring bag is made of nylon that can be used over and over again to make your own nut milk, juice, or sprouts. Also, if you don't have a juicer, you can use a blender and strain the pulp through a nut-milk strainer bag. There are a variety of nut-milk strainer bags available through our Amazon affiliate store.

Harvest Essentials:

www.harvestessentials.com

Harvest Essentials carries a wide selection of everything you need to make food preparation easy and enjoyable, including rice cookers, grain mills, food processors, yogurt makers, blenders, juicers, dehydrators, nut-milk strainer bags, sprouters, and more.

Vitamix (high-powered blender/ food processor):

www.vitamix.com

Buy a Vitamix once and have it for life. It is the best-performing and most reliable blender/food processing appliance for creating recipes from whole-food ingredients. If you're considering making the investment, you can get free shipping ($25 savings) by using my affiliate code: 06–007608. Order online or call 1-800-848-2649.

BREVILLE JUICERS:

www.brevilleusa.com

The Breville Juicer Fountain Series offers a large selection of juicers with a variety of features and price ranges. From the economically priced Juice Fountain Compact to the top-of-the-line Juice Fountain Duo (a juicer and high-powered blender in one), Breville juicers are high-quality appliances that are easy to clean and make juicing a fun and enjoyable health practice.

Helpful Websites

PROCESSED-FREE AMERICA:

www.processedfreeamerica.org

To help others make the transition to a processed-free lifestyle, my husband Michael and I founded Processed-Free America—a nonprofit organization dedicated to providing nutrition education and support services to both young and old. Through online and in-person classes, volunteer-led support groups, one-on-one nutrition and weight loss counseling, books, and videos, our processed-free message is reaching thousands around the country and overseas.

We carry out our mission in several ways:

+ Through the free information provided on our website: We have a large archive of podcasts, articles, videos, and recipes on the site. New material is added weekly.
+ Through our free monthly e-newsletter: Each month we provide new cutting-edge information on health and nutrition topics to keep you informed and inspired. The newsletter is also our way of letting you know about upcoming classes and events. Sign up on the website to receive the e-newsletter.
+ Through our free message-board forum: Members of our online community ask questions, post comments and recipes, and get online support from others.
+ Through free volunteer-led support groups: The Processed-Free Support Groups are "peer-to-peer" gatherings of like-minded people who meet in person to support each other in their processed-free journey. Processed-Free Support Groups have formed in cities across the United States and Canada. Groups that are currently meeting are listed on our website. If there is not a group in your area, you can start one!
+ Through nutrition classes for both children and adults: Classes are offered throughout the year in varying formats (in person, teleclasses, webinars). Some classes require a fee, some are free of charge. You can check the events calendar on the website for upcoming events. (A big part of our mission is offering age-appropriate nutrition classes to children. You can learn more about the children's programs on our website.)
+ Through facilitator training programs: We have a certification training program on DVD that prepares individuals to become Certified Processed-Free™ Facilitators.
+ By gathering signatures: We're collecting signatures to petition the FDA to ban some of the most egregious food additives—the ones scientific studies show are harmful, and especially the ones that have already been banned in other countries but

are still being used in the United States. Please visit the website to sign our petition!

PRODUCE CONVERTER:

www.howmuchisin.com (a smartphone app is also available)

Produce Converter will help you convert the "juice of 1 lemon" and other similar recipe instructions into tablespoons, cups, and other concrete measurements. Produce Converter can also be used to figure out how many vegetables to buy when you need, for instance, "a cup of diced onion." The site has an easy conversion tool to figure out exactly how many onions you need to buy at the store in order to end up with the amount you need for your cooking. This is a must-have in the kitchen and will make planning your meals a snap.

TROPICAL TRADITIONS:

www.tropicaltraditions.com

Not only is Tropical Traditions the best online source for high-quality organic coconut products at competitive bulk discount prices, the website also houses a wealth of health and nutrition information, as well as an extensive collection of recipes. The best things about Tropical Traditions are their frequent offers for free shipping and two-for-the-price-of-one specials on a wide variety of items.

ENVIRONMENTAL WORKING GROUP (EWG):

www.ewg.org

EWG is the nonprofit organization that produces the annual "Dirty Dozen" and "Clean 15 Shopper's Guide to Pesticides in Produce" that is available for download from www.foodnews .org (a smartphone app is also available). EWG provides practical information that will assist your efforts to protect the health and well-being of your family and community.

THE CORNUCOPIA INSTITUTE:

www.cornucopia.org

The Cornucopia Institute is a nonprofit organization that conducts research and investigations on food issues and provides reports to consumers and the media. Notable works by the institute are their "scorecards," which rate how well companies adhere to organic practices. Check out their scorecards on eggs, dairy, and soy and their "Shopping Guide to Avoiding Carrageenan in Organic Foods."

THE WESTON A. PRICE FOUNDATION:

www.westonaprice.org

A fascinating and informative website devoted to teaching people about the healthfulness of traditional foods. See the Soy Alert Page and Sally Fallon's "The Dirty Secrets of the Food Processing Industry."

PRICE-POTTENGER NUTRITION FOUNDATION:

www.ppnf.org

The Price-Pottenger Nutrition Foundation has been teaching people how to attain optimal health for over sixteen years. The website is a storehouse of cutting-edge articles, research, and videos on whole-foods nutrition. The foundation offers classes, lectures, and information on healthful foods and lifestyle practices that enable people to take steps to lead a healthier life.

Notes

CHAPTER 1: The Science: Foods That Steal and Foods That Heal

1. Robert H. Lustig, Laura A. Schmidt, Claire D. Brindis, "Public Health: The Toxic Truth About Sugar," *Nature* 482 (February 2, 2012):27.

CHAPTER 2: The Skinny: Processed-Free Superfoods and Ingredients

1. Dr. Michael Saska and Dr. Chung Chi Chou, "Antioxidant Properties of Sugarcane Extracts" (paper presented at Proceedings of First Biannual World Conference on Recent Developments in Sugar Technologies, Delray Beach, Florida, May 16–17, 2002), http://www.esugartech.com/documents/Properties%20Sugarcane%20Extracts.pdf.

2. S. Klenow, et al., "Does an Extract of Carob (Ceratonia siliqua L.) Have Chemopreventive Potential Related to Oxidative Stress and Drug Metabolism in Human Colon Cells?" *Journal of Agriculture, Food and Chemistry* 57, no. 7 (April 8, 2009).

CHAPTER 6: Power Juices and Green Smoothies

1. E. Hedrén, V. Diaz, U. Svanberg, "Estimation of Carotenoid Accessibility from Carrots Determined by an In Vitro Digestion Method," *European Journal of Clinical Nutrition* 56, no. 5 (May 2002):425–430.

2. University of Kentucky, "Watermelon Reduces Atherosclerosis, Animal Study Finds," *ScienceDaily*, November 1, 2011, http://www.sciencedaily.com/releases/2011/10/111027125153.htm (October 23, 2013); M. P. Tarazona-Díaz, et al., "Watermelon Juice: Potential Functional Drink for Sore Muscle Relief in Athletes," *Journal of Agricultural Food Chemistry* 61, no. 31 (2013):7522–7528.

3. Orie Yoshinari, Hideyo Sato, Kiharu Igarashi, "Anti-Diabetic Effects of Pumpkin

and Its Components, Trigonelline and Nicotinic Acid, on Goto-Kakizaki Rats," *Bioscience Biotechnology and Biochemistry* 73, no. 5 (June 2009):1033–1041.

CHAPTER 7: Outside-the-Cereal-Box Breakfasts

1. S. Nongtaodum, et al., "Oil Coating Affects Internal Quality and Sensory Acceptance of Selected Attributes of Raw Eggs During Storage," *Journal of Food Science* 78, no. 2 (February 2013):S328–335.

CHAPTER 11: Sensational Salads and Versatile Veggies

1. Linda Stradley, "Balsamic Vinegar—Aceto Balsamico Tradizionale Vinegar," What's Cooking America, http://whatscookingamerica.net/balsamic.htm.

2. Elisa Zied, "Potatoes May Help Lower Blood Pressure. Purple Ones, That Is," Diet and Nutrition on NBC News.com, September 1, 2011, http://www.nbcnews.com/id/44345789/ns/health-diet_and_nutrition/t/potatoes-may-help-lower-blood-pressure-purple-ones/#.UZoIkLUceHg.

Index

Milk. *See also* Almond Milk; Coconut Milk
    cow's, healthy swaps for, 45
    substituting types of, in recipes, 52, 133
Millet
    Ancient Grains Tabbouleh, 228
    Pilaf with Braised Carrots and Fennel,
        226–27
Mint
    Apple Vitamin Water, 82
    Chocolate Bliss Smoothie, 109
    Cool and Collected Cucumber Juice, 94
    Cucumber Vitamin Water, 82
    Dandelion Greens Salad with Sweet Citrus
        Dressing, 198
    Fresh, Ice Cream, 258
    Ginger Asian Slaw, 203–4
    Lassi, Fresh, 84
    Tea, Fresh, 79
Miso
    heating, note about, 218
    Tahini Dressing with Orange and Ginger,
        152–53
    Vegetable Soup, Hearty, 219
    Wakame Soup, Easy, 218
Molasses
    blackstrap, about, 47
    blackstrap, health benefits, 24
    Blackstrap, Vinegar Tonic, 78
    Mocha, Iced, 84–85
    Whole Grain Gingerbread Cookies,
        255–56
Monosodium glutamate (MSG), 10
Moroccan Carrot Salad, 192–93
Mousse, Choco-cado, 259
Muesli, Coconut Currant Breakfast, 117
Muffins
    Banana Blueberry Flourless Oat Bran
        (variations), 132–33
    substituting milk types in, 133

Nut Butter(s)
    Banana, and Hemp Seed Bites, 170–71
    Cacao–Stuffed Dates, 172–73
    Homemade (variations), 72–74
    storing, 74
Nut-milk strainer bags, 62, 282
Nutritional yeast, about, 26
Nut(s). *See also* Nut Butter(s); *specific nuts*
    Better-Than-Boxed Almond/Nut Milk
        (variations), 62–63
    Coconut Currant Breakfast Muesli, 117
    on pantry list, 30
    soaked, drying, 37
    soaking, notes on, 39
    soaking and sprouting, 34–39
    Sweet 'n' Spicy Mixed, 186

Oat(s)
    Baked Oatmeal with Sweet Potato and
        Apples, 119
    Bran, Creamy Pumpkin (variations), 120
    bran, health benefits, 22, 27
    bran, soaking overnight, 133
    Bran Muffins, Blueberry Banana Flourless
        (variations), 132–33
    Coconut Currant Breakfast Muesli, 117
    groats, about, 26
    health benefits, 26–27
    High-Protein Granola Bars, 177–78
    Pumpkin-Spiced Quinoa Granola, 121
    rolled, about, 27
    Scottish oatmeal, about, 27
    soaking, to use for baking, 41
    steel cut, about, 26–27
Obesogens, 9–10
Oils
    cooking with, 33–34
    olive, extra-virgin, 21
    on pantry list, 30